GOSSYPOL
A Potential Contraceptive for Men

REPRODUCTIVE BIOLOGY

Series Editor: Sheldon J. Segal
The Rockefeller Foundation
New York, New York

GOSSYPOL: A Potential Contraceptive for Men

Edited by Sheldon J. Segal

A Continuation Order Plan is available for this series. A continuation order will bring delivery of each new volume immediately upon publication. Volumes are billed only upon actual shipment. For further information please contact the publisher.

GOSSYPOL
A Potential Contraceptive for Men

Edited by

Sheldon J. Segal
The Rockefeller Foundation
New York, New York

PLENUM PRESS • NEW YORK AND LONDON

Library of Congress Cataloging in Publication Data

Main entry under title:

GOSSYPOL, a potential contraceptive for men.

  (Reproductive biology)
  Bibliography: p.
  Includes index.
    1. Infertility, Male. 2. Gossypol—Physiological effect. 3. Gossypol—Testing. 4. Oral con-
traceptives, Male. I. Segal, Sheldon Jerome, 1926–   . II. Series. |DNLM: 1. Gossypol—
pharmacodynamics. 2. Gossypol—toxicity. 3. Contraceptive Agents, Male. QV 177
G681|

RC889.G67 1984   613.9′432   84-18230
ISBN-13: 978-1-4612-9729-1   e-ISBN-13: 978-1-4613-2809-4
DOI: 10.1007/978-1-4613-2809-4

This volume is dedicated to the researchers of China, who persevered for many years in studying gossypol, and who in so doing have made a substantial contribution to the field of male fertility regulation.

PREFACE

The search for a reversible male contraceptive has centered upon the suppression of sperm production or sperm motility. Gossypol, a natural substance extracted from the cotton plant, appears to cause both of these effects. Its ability to reduce spermatogenesis in men is undeniable and has been demonstrated in both large studies in China and a smaller confirmatory study in Brazil. These investigations have revealed the remarkable fact that with gossypol, it is possible to separate an effect on the testis' gamete-producing function from an effect on its hormone-producing function. Thus, it is possible to maintain normal testosterone levels and libido while sperm counts (and motility) fall.

Because of this unique and important action, gossypol warrants the fullest possible evaluation as a potential male contraceptive.

Sheldon J. Segal

ACKNOWLEDGMENT

Lynn C. Landman played a major role in
this publication by skillfully editing the
manuscripts which were submitted for inclusion
in this volume. Janet O'Connell added her efforts
in editing, assembling texts and figures and
handling final details required for publication.
I thank these talented colleagues for their
invaluable contributions.

                              Sheldon J. Segal

CONTENTS

INTRODUCTION AND HISTORY OF GOSSYPOL

Whether one's perspective is directed toward the effects of high fertility on individual couples or to its impact on nations and the world community, reduced fertility levels are a desirable, even urgent, objective. Some degree of decline in the birth rate can be expected as a consequence of social progress. In many nations and subgroups within nations, however, high fertility itself retards social progress. If fertility could be reduced while other social developments are pursued, a multiplier effect would occur, thus accelerating the overall process. Many nations, particularly in the Third World, have instituted national programs to educate individuals about the personal benefits of fertility regulation and to provide greater access to existing contraceptive methods. Because existing technology has limitations, however, many countries also are encouraging research directed at new and improved techniques for fertility regulation.

These are complementary and, indeed, necessary components of a successful national program. A decline in the birth rate would be expected from a vigorous family planning program that effectively distributes currently available contraceptive technology. In addition, new methods would contribute to program success, particularly if they are better adapted to the circumstances of nations lacking sufficient health resources. More effective methods, which can be distributed simply and inexpensively, would increase the acceptability of family planning at any level of personal motivation toward fertility control.

Since the development of oral contraceptives for women, there have been efforts to identify suitable drugs for inhibition of male fertility. A variety of antimetabolic agents and steroid hormones are known to suppress the production of sperm by the testis. However, the antimetabolic agents cannot be seriously considered as potential contraceptives because of their general systemic toxicity. At appropriate dose levels, the various hormones, including estrogens, progestins, androgens, and antiandrogens, block the production of sperm, through interference with endocrinological mechanisms.

1

Estrogens are among the most potent agents for this purpose; but long-term administration of estrogens to men can cause breast enlargement, loss of libido, and an increase in thromboembolic disease. Nevertheless, limited clinical investigations are still being conducted in the hope that these problems can be minimized by using very low doses of estrogens combined with testosterone. The preliminary results of these clinical studies confirm the observation first made by researchers in the mid-1970s that suppression of sperm production can be achieved in the short-term without evident side effects [1, 2]. Any extensive development of this approach, however, is not likely because of the toxicity of estrogens in long-term administration.

Although progestins are less potent than estrogen in inhibiting spermatogenesis, they have been much more widely tested in men because there is no firm evidence linking them to an increased incidence of cardiovascular disease in men. Sperm production can indeed be suppressed using progestins supplemented with androgens. Normal plasma testosterone levels are maintained, and sperm production can be restored when treatment stops. Current research, continuing the efforts begun a decade ago [3, 4, 5], still seeks to identify effective hormonal combinations without unacceptable side effects in dosages to be administered as either monthly injections or daily pills. Success is still elusive.

Testosterone itself inhibits sperm production if given in sufficiently high doses. Frequent intramuscular injections are necessary, however, and there is concern about long-term health hazards, vascular problems in particular, because of the high doses required. In an attempt to reduce toxicity, researchers have done some work with orally active steroids less androgenic than testosterone [6, 7, 8, 9, 10, 11]. However, relatively high doses of the anabolic agents studied have been only partially effective [12].

It is precisely because all avenues to the development of a reversible male contraceptive seem blocked that interest in gossypol, a polyphenolic compound isolated from the seeds, stems, and roots of the cotton plant Gossypium sp., is so great. For more than 10 years, researchers in the Peoples Republic of China have been working on developing the substance into a male contraceptive. They have clinical experience with the agent [13], which has thus far been used by more than 10,000 men. There are now data on its efficacy as a contraceptive and on its toxicity - but much remains to be done to elucidate its mechanism of action, its safety, its reversibility, and the dose levels at which it achieves its effects. The research reported in this book aims to answer some of these questions. Meanwhile, a look at its recent history is of interest.

The Discovery of Gossypol's Antifertility Property

In the late 1960's, people in many rural areas of China, including in Hubei and Hebei provinces, complained of fatigue and of
burning of the face, extremities, and other exposed parts of the
bodies. The farms in the areas raised cotton. The afflicted people
could not work in the fields, but hid in the shade, lying on rocks
to get cool. Local doctors were puzzled. The disease had reached
epidemic proportions, but the cause remained unknown. The peasants
called their disease "the burning fever" [14, 15].

Burning fever was especially prevalent in Xingtai, a county in
Hebei province. A local doctor discovered that these affected
peasants consumed raw, homemade, cotton seed oil. Commercially
manufactured cotton seed oil had been used in cooking for many years,
but only in the 1960's, did the peasants begin to make oil from un-
cooked seeds, using their own pressing machines. Raw cotton seeds
contain gossypol which is destroyed by heat. Unlike the commercial
process, preparation of homemade oil does not include heating. Consequently, gossypol remains dissolved in homemade oil. This substance was discovered to be the cause of the burning fever.

Gossypol was first discovered by J. J. Longmore in 1886 [16],
and was purified in crystalline form by the Russian chemist, L.
Marchlewski, in 1889 [17]. Researchers have often tried to make
use of all parts of the cotton plant. The seeds contain protein
and oil, and attempts have been made to adapt cotton meal as an animal feed and as infant food. However, the plant was found to be
toxic and such attempts were not successful.

As soon as crude cotton seed oil was identified as the source
of burning fever, Xingtai doctors advised their patients to stop
pressing their own raw oil. The burning and fatigue stopped. Several years later however, many couples were found to be experiencing
fertility problems. A large number of women had amenorrhea, and many
men were impotent. These cases of infertility were regarded as a
sequel of burning fever. When women remained on gossypol-free
diets, many eventually recovered from amenorrhea. Very few men,
despite the elimination of gossypol from their diets, recovered from
their infertility and impotency. Further examination of these men
revealed azoospermia or oligospermia. In addition, some men noted
a decrease in testicular size. Medical and scientific research
workers from universities and hospitals were sent to the area to investigate these problems. They confirmed the findings of the local
doctors. Infertility was prevalent, and women seemed to recover at
a much higher rate than men. Men who did recover were found to have
consumed a lower total amount of cotton seed oil for shorter periods
of time. This information led investigators to hypothesize whether
controlled doses of purified gossypol could be used effectively as
a male fertility-control agent. Observational studies in the

countryside had shown that burning fever, fatigue, and infertility were the most serious effects of gossypol ingestion. Mortality was not observed as a result of burning fever. Because the rate of recovery from male infertility was dependent on the amount of cotton oil a man had consumed, scientists conjectured that infertility would most likely be reversible if the gossypol dosage could be limited. Cessation of intake would probably lead to restoration of fertility.

Animal Studies Testing Gossypol for its Effectiveness and Toxicity

Researchers began animal experiments in the late 1960s and studies using male rats, mice, rabbits, hamsters, dogs, and monkeys yielded almost identical infertility results [18]. In addition, the absorption, distribution, and excretion of gossypol were also found to be similar in these animals [19].

The biological half-life of gossypol in the gastrointestinal tract of the rat is about 10 hours. Elimination of gossypol takes place mainly through the bile-fecal pathway, while excretion through the kidney is minimal [20]. Its elimination from the body is slow, taking a rat 19 days to eliminate 97% of the dose from its body [21]. Continued administration, therefore could lead to accumulation.

The half-life of gossypol in mice and dogs is longer than in rats [22]. This might explain the more obvious toxic reactions in the former two species. Dogs are more sensitive to the toxic action of gossypol. They are more likely to die as a result of anorexia and of pulmonary and myocardial disturbances. Monkeys, however, exhibit few adverse reactions at the antifertility dosage [23, 24].

The order of gossypol distribution throughout the body in all animals studied is liver, gastrointestinal tract, spleen, lymph nodes, kidneys, heart, lungs, pancreas, salivary glands, muscle, adipose tissue, testes, blood, urinary bladder, brain and spinal cord [25]. Although the testes do not retain much gossypol, sperm cells are vulnerable to the substance. Because gossypol concentration is high in the liver and kidneys, there should be special concern about toxic effects on these organs.

Research carried on during the 1970s helped elucidate many aspects of the mechanism of action of gossypol, its effects on endocrine function, on the various reproductive structures, on its toxicity and on its antifertility effects in a wide variety of animals including mice, rats, hamsters, rabbits, bulls, and monkeys. Its effects on human males was also studied closely by Chinese investigators and was reported at numerous conferences and in scientific journals.

Research continues today in laboratories around the world. This book presents an up-to-date report on many facets of gossypol research. The findings, considered with earlier results, suggest that while much remains to be learned, gossypol is still a promising male antifertility lead. Its antifertility properties have been confirmed. It is now fairly certain that it acts locally, at the level of the reproductive organs themselves, and does not interfere with testicular hormone production. During the first few weeks of treatment, gossypol attaches to maturing sperm stored in the epididymis and renders them immotile. In the course of longer treatment, the drug also acts in the testes to check sperm production. These characteristics, the direct action on the motility of mature spermatozoa and on the growth of immature sperm cells is what sets gossypol apart from other potential chemical fertility-regulating agents. Gossypol acts without interfering with the Leydig cells or with the pituitary-gonadal system. Therefore, it should not affect a man's sex drive and should not disturb the general hormonal regulatory system. Research reported here is also reassuring on the issue of the drug's possible teratogenic effects.

All of this is not to say that gossypol is without disadvantages. Optimism must be tempered. The risks of sterility and hypokalemia, as well as possible toxic effects on the heart and liver, cannot be ignored. Nor should they be exaggerated, however. One should remain aware of the results of animal experiments using dogs and other sensitive species, keeping in mind that still other animal species, especially primates, exhibit a much lower toxic reaction and require a lower antifertility dose. Nonetheless, toxicity remains an issue of concern.

Clearly, much more study is required. Nontheless it is important to recognize that gossypol is a major and promising lead in the search for a safe, effective, reversible, and inexpensive fertility-regulating agent.

Guo-zhen Liu and Sheldon J. Segal

REFERENCES

1. M. Briggs and M. Briggs, Oral contraception for men, Nature, 252:585 (1974).
2. L. L. Ewig, Effects of testosterone and estradiol, silastic implants, on spermatogenesis in rats and rhesus monkeys, in: "Proceedings Hormonal Control of Male Fertility," DHEW Publication No. (NIH) 78-1097, p. 173 (1978).
3. E. M. Coutinho and J. F. Melo, Successful inhibition of spermatogenesis in man without loss of libido: A potential new approach to male contraception, Contraception, 8:207 (1973).
4. J. Frick, Control of spermatogenesis in men by combined administration of progestin and androgen, Contraception, 8:191 (1973).

5. J. Frick and G. Bartsch, Inhibition of spermatogenesis, in: "Physiology and genetics of reproduction, Part A" (E. M. Coutinho and M. Fuchs, eds.), Plenum Press, New York, p. 230 (1974).

6. G. R. Cunningham, V. E. Silverman, and P. O. Kohler, Clinical Evaluation of testosterone enanthate for induction and maintenance of reversible azoospermia in man, in: "Proceedings Hormonal Control of Male Fertility," DHEW Publication No. (NIH) 78-1097, p. 71 (1978a).

7. C. G. Heller, W. O. Nelson, J. C. Hill, E. Henderson, W. O. Maddock, and E. C. Jung, The effect of testosterone administration upon the human testis, J. Clin. Endocrinol. Metab., 10: 816 (1950b).

8. R. S. Hotchkiss, Effects of massive doses of testosterone propionate upon spermatogenesis, J. Clin. Endocrinol., 4:117 (1944).

9. J. Mauss, G. Börsch, E. Richter, and K. Bormacher, Investigations on the use of testosterone enanthate as a male contraceptive agent: a preliminary report, Contraception, 10:281 (1974).

10. P. R. K. Reddy and J. M. Rao, Reversible antifertility action of testosterone propionate in human males, Contraception, 5: 295 (1972).

11. E. Steinberger and K. D. Smith, Testosterone enanthate: a possible reversible male contraceptive, Contraception, 16:261 (1977a).

12. J. M. Leonard and C. A. Paulsen, Contraceptive development studies for males: Oral and parenteral steroid hormone administration, in: Proceedings Hormonal Control of Male Fertility, DHEW Publication No. (NIH) 78-1097, p. 223 (1978).

13. National Coordinating Group on Male Antifertility Agents: Gossypol - a new antifertility agent for males, Chinese Med. J., 4:417 (1978).

14. Ibid.

15. X. R. Wu, Study of antifertility action of cottonseeds and their effective component - gossypol, papers presented at the National Conference on Recent Advances of Family Planning Research, Beijing, March, 1972 and at the First National Conference on Male Antifertility Agents, Wuhan, September, 1972.

16. J. J. Longmore, Cottonseed oil: Its coloring matter mucilage, and description of a new method of recovering the loss occurring in the refining process, J. Soc. Chem. Ind., 5:200 (1886).

17. L. Marchlewski, Gossypol, ein Bestandteil der Baumwollsamen, J. Prakt. Chem., 60:84 (1899).

18. National Coordinating Group on Male Antifertility Agents, 1978, op. cit. (see Ref. 13).

19. N. G. Wang and H. P. Lei, Antifertility effect of gossypol acetic acid on male rats, Natl. Med. J. Clin., 59:402 (1979).

20. S. P. Xue, Studies on the antifertility effect of gossypol, a
     new contraceptive for males, in: "Recent Advances in Fertility
     Regulation, Proc. Symp. Beijing, September, 1980" (C. F. Chang,
     D. Griffin, and A. Wollman, eds.), Atar, Geneva (1983).
21. Ibid.
22. X. C. Tang, M. Zhu, and Q. X. Shi, Comparative studies on the
     absorption, distribution and excretion ^{14}C-gossypol in four
     species of animals, Acta Pharmacol. Sin., 15:212 (1980).
23. National Coordinating Group on Male Infertility Agents, 1978,
     op. cit. (see Ref. 13).
24. S. P. Xue, in press, op. cit. (see Ref. 20).
25. X. C. Tang, et al., 1980, op. cit. (see REf. 22).

TRIAL OF GOSSYPOL AS A MALE CONTRACEPTIVE

Guo-zhen Liu,* Katherine C. Lyle,†
and Jian Cao*

*Capital Hospital
 The Chinese Academy of Medical Sciences
 Beijing, The People's Republic of China

†The Rockefeller Foundation
 New York, U.S.A.

INTRODUCTION

In the 1950's gossypol was identified as the cause of male infertility in many rural communes in China where ingestion of raw cotton seed oil was common. Since, then efforts have been made by the China National Coordinating Group on Male Anti-fertility Agents to develop this compound as a pill for men. If successful, gossypol could be a valuable addition to the existing methods of contraception. In the late 1960's and early 1970's, studies were undertaken to determine the toxic effects of gossypol in animals and in human beings. In 1972, a multicenter study, in-volving 14 centers and 8806 volunteers, was carried out to gather data on the efficacy, side-effects and clinical pharmacology of gossypol when used as a male contraceptive.

The efficacy study showed that there is an optimal dose as well as a preferred route of administration. The oral administration of 20 mg of gossypol per day for 75 days is highly effective in sup-pressing spermatogenesis to below 4 million spermatozoa per cc as can be seen in Table 1. Table 2 demonstrated that a maintenance dose of 50 mg per week is necessary to maintain suppression at that level.

Although data relating to subjective symptoms, such as fatigue, changes in libido, loss of appetite, and headache, among others, were elicited from the volunteers, no valid inferences could be drawn both because of a lack of uniformity in the protocol in the 14 cen-ters and of a control group.

9

TABLE 1.   Efficacy of Gossypol Taken Orally, 20 mg/day,
           for Varying Intervals

Interval (No. of days)	No. of subjects	Sperm count <4 m/cc No. of subjects	Efficacy rate	χ^2
50	87	26	28.89	
60	110	66	60.00	
75	2437	2400	98.48	10.63 (P < 0.01)
Total	2634	2492		

Source: China National Coordinating Group on Male Antifertility
         Agents Report, 1980.

TABLE 2.   Weekly Dosage Required to Maintain Suppres-
           sion of Spermatozoa to <4 Million per cc,
           by Regimen

Dosage regimen	No. of subjects	No. of subjects with sperm count <4 mm/cc	Efficacy rate	χ^2
30 mg/wk	353	326	92.3	
40 mg/wk	1492	1430	95.8	
50 mg/wk	429	425	99.1	10.43 (P < 0.01)
60 mg/10th day	95	85	89.5	
100 mg/15th day	156	144	92.3	
20 mg/daily days	172	155	90.1	
Total	2697	2565		

Source: See Table 1.

     With respect to safety, blood chemistry and other pharmacologi-
cal studies have been carried out on many of the 8806 men. A reduction of serum potassium levels to below normal was observed in 66
out of the 8806 subjects. Serum potassium levels returned to normal
after oral administration of potassium salts. However, concerns
about toxicity caused a division of opinion among both Chinese and
western scientists about the usefulness of gossypol for suppression
of human sperm production. Work done outside China since 1978 has
essentially confirmed the Chinese observation of gossypol efficacy,

TABLE 3. Demographic and Medical Characteristics of the
Men in the Gossypol Group and in the Placebo
Group, by Characteristic

Characteristics	Gossypol Mean SD (N = 75)		Placebo Mean SD (N = 77)	
Age (yrs)	31.7	4.2	31.0	4.2
Education (yrs)				
1-6	11		9	
7-9	57		57	
10-12	3		9	
13+	4	2		
Occupation				
Worker	70		71	
Clerical (office)	5		5	
Med./Prof.	0		1	
Sexual Intercourse				
(per wk.)	1.5	0.5	1.6	0.5
Blood pressure				
Systolic (mm Hg)	116.1	11.2	114.4	11.8
Diastolic (mm Hg)	82.1	8.4	80.5	9.1
Hemoglobin				
(gm/100 ml)	15.1	1.2	15.5	1.2
Serum potassium				
(MEQ/L)	4.25	0.43	4.32	0.48
Sperm count				
(m/cc)	79.9	46.6	87.9	50.4

both in animal and in human studies. In early 1980, a group within
the China National Coordinating Group on Male Antifertility Agents
recommended to the Chinese Ministry of Health that a gossypol pill
be introduced for general use. However, another group recommended
further research because certain efficacy and safety issues remained unresolved.

In June 1980, The Rockefeller Foundation made a grant to the
Chinese Academy of Medical Sciences to conduct a study evaluating
gossypol as a male contraceptive agent. The study was to be conducted by staff of the Capital Hospital in Beijing. A clinical
trial was started in December 1981. We report here some of the preliminary results.

SUBJECTS AND METHODS

One hundred and fifty-two men recruited from various factories
in the Beijing metropolitan area who met entry criteria participated
in this trial. The participants were randomly allocated into 2
groups. Seventy-five received 20 mg of gossypol per day for 75
days, while 77 participants received placebos for the same period.

TABLE 4. Reasons for Withdrawal from the Study, by Group to which Assigned (P = Placebo Group, G = Gossypol Group)

No.	Participant code	No. of pills taken	Reasons for withdrawals	Inclusion in analysis safety data	subject data
1	007 (P)	0	Unwillingness	No	No
2	017 (G)	15	Increased libido	No	Yes
3	018 (G)	0	Unwillingness	No	No
4	027 (G)	8	Decreased libido	No	Yes
5	047 (G)	0	Unwillingness	No	No
6	048 (P)	0	Vomiting	No	No
7	051 (G)	19	Vomiting	No	Yes
8	059 (G)	10	Hepatic disease*	No	No
9	062 (G)	0	Moved	No	No
10	064 (P)	0	Unwillingness	No	No
11	074 (G)	0	Moved	No	No
12	082 (G)	0	Unwillingness	No	No
13	094 (G)	45	Irregulary pill taking	No	Yes
14	116 (G)	36	Hospitalized due to accident	No	Yes

*This subject should not have been permitted to enter the study.

TABLE 5.   Sperm Count after 75 Days of Gossypol
           Treatment (N = 64)

Sperm count (m/cc)	Participants No. %
0	20 (31%)
1-4	39 (61%)
5-9	2 (3%)
10-125	3 (5%)

The demographic and physiologic characteristics of the two treatment groups are shown in Table 3. As can be seen, the two groups were similar in all respects. A double-blind technique was employed to control for subjective symptoms of fatigue, decreased libido and appetite changes. Two follow-ups were scheduled, one on the 37th day and the other on the 75th day after the start of the study.

The follow-ups provided data on participants' subjective symptoms and on safety as derived from laboratory measurement of body weight, blood pressure, hemoglobin, serum potassium, sperm count and electrocardiograms.

A total of 14 participants withdrew before the end of the study, 11 from the gossypol treatment group and three from the placebo group. Table 4 provides details on the reasons for withdrawal. None were included in the analyses of safety; five were included in the subjective analyses. Comparison of variables of withdrawals with the original groups to which they were assigned showed no statistical difference. The final analysis of the double-blind study is based on the findings of 64 gossypol and 74 placebo participants for the safety data analysis. For the subjective data, the sample size was 69 for the gossypol and 74 for the placebo group.

RESULTS

Table 5 shows that among the 64 gossypol-treated participants, 31% achieved azoospermia and 61% had a sperm count of less than 4 million per cc; 3% (two participants) had a sperm count between 5-9 million per cc, and the remaining 5% (three participants), sperm counts above 10 million per cc. In sum, a 92% efficacy rate was achieved. Sperm counts for the placebo group remained unchanged.

A comparison of the incidence of fatigue, decreased libido and gastro-intestinal disturbance of the two groups showed no statistically significant differences (Table 6). Similarly, as Table 6 shows, no differences were observed in hemoglobin, serum K, body weight or blood pressure between the gossypol- and placebo-treated groups. In

TABLE 6. Number and Percent of Participants in Each
          Group (Gossypol and Placebo) Who Experienced
          Side Effects, by Specific Side Effect

Side effect	Gossypol (N = 69)		Placebo (N = 74)	z
	No.	%	%	
Fatigue	9	13	4 5	1.3 (P < .05)
GI disturbance	5	7	5 7	-0.2 (P < .05)
Libido decrease	6	9	4 3	1.2 (P < .05)

view of the particular interest in the serum K levels specifically,
the distributions for the two treatment groups at admission and at
the end of the study phase are given in Table 8. No statistically
significant difference was found at either time, but a slight lowering of the mean values for the placebo group in a self-paired comparison was evident.

DISCUSSION

     The present study confirms the previous Chinese observation of
gossypol efficacy. Of the three participants who had sperm counts
over 10 million per cc at the end of the loading phase, 2 had failed
to take the pills for about 2 weeks. Only one participant was a
bonafide failure. This man had a starting sperm count of 214 m/cc
which was reduced to 34 m/cc after 75 days of gossypol treatment.

     The Chinese studies in the 70's indicated a 12.61% rate of
fatigue. The present study indicates 13%, but it remained statistically insignificant when compared with a control group incidence of 5%.

     In the previous Chinese studies, high rates of altered libido
was found among Beijing participants while none or very low rates
were found among Nanjing participants. The reason for this discrepancy may be that the doctors in the Beijing area were very interested in the libido problem and repeatedly queried their patients
on this score; Nanjing doctors on the other hand, were apparently
less interested and did not try adequately to elicit responses from
their patients. Thus, the difference in libido may be entirely
artifactual. This assumption is supported by our present study
which found no statistically significant difference between the
gossypol- and placebo-treated groups.

     The most serious side-effect of gossypol contraception in
earlier reports was the presumed lowering of serum K levels. As

TABLE 7. Comparison of Mean and Standard Deviation of the 2 Treatment Groups at the End of Double-Blind Study

Characteristic	Gossypol (N = 64)	Placebo (N = 74)	t
Hemoglobin (g/100 ml)	15.8 ± 1.02	15.6 ± 1.03	1.3 (P > .05)
Serum K (MEQ/L)	4.16 ± 0.42	4.18 ± 0.41	-0.3 (P > .05)
Weight (kgs)	64.3 ± 8.7	61.5 ± 8.4	1.9 (P > .05)
Blood Pressure			
Systolic (mm Hg)	115.8 ± 9.3	113.9 ± 9.5	1.9 (P > .05)
Diastolic (mm Hg)	81.4 ± 7.9	79.2 ± 7.6	1.6 (P > .05)

TABLE 8. Mean and Standard Deviation of Serum K Levels (MEQ/L) of the 2 Treatment Groups at Admission and at the End of the Double-Blind Study

Level	Gossypol (N = 64)	Placebo (N = 74)	t (independent sample)
At admission	4.25 ± 0.43	4.32 ± 0.48	.9 (P > .05)
End of study	4.16 ± 0.42	4.18 ± 0.41	-.3 (P > 0.5)
t (paired sample)	1.6 (P > .05)	2.0 (P > .05)	

TABLE 9.   Serum Potassium Levels Found in a Base-Line
           Study Conducted in Nanjing, Where Rice is a
           Staple of the Diet, and Tai-an Where Wheat
           is a Main Element of the Diet

Location	No. of cases	Mean + S.D.	P value
Nanjing	40	3.92 ± 0.1	$t_{75} = 4.29$
Tai-an	37	4.11 ± 0.26	(P < 0.001)

noted earlier, there were 66 hypokalemic (with serum K levels 2.00–
2.73 mEq/L) cases among the 8806 volunteers in the previous Chinese
studies. It is noteworthy that the incidence of hypokalemia unrelated to gossypol treatment has a regional variation in China. A
base-line study on serum K levels was carried out in 2 geographically
varied locations, Nanjing, south of the Yangtze River, where rice is
the main staple food and Tai-an, in Shandong Province, north of the
Yangtze, where wheat is consumed in large quantity. The findings
are presented in Table 9. In addition, the dietary intake of potassium in these 2 places was analyzed. The mean intake in Nanjing
was 26.9 mEq/L compared with 53.2 mEq/L in Tai-an. The higher serum
K level in Tai-an, attributable to the higher dietary intake of potassium, may protect the people there from developing hypokalemia.
Consequently, there were no known cases of hypokalemia in the Tai-an
area following gossypol treatment. The much higher incidence of
hypokalemia found in the areas of Nanjing (and Shanghai) may be due
to the lower dietary potassium. In our present study in Beijing,
the serum K level at admission (4.25 ± 0.43) was comparable to that
in the Tai-an area (4.11 ± 0.26). However, the mechanism of gossypol-
induced hypokalemia is not yet well understood. Some speculate that
fatigue may be a prodromal symptom of impending hypokalemic paralysis.
Nine of the study participants in the gossypol group and four in the
placebo group complained of fatigue. It may be important to compare
the serum K levels of these two groups with non-fatigue groups to
detect any difference in serum K distributions.

The double-blind study reported here covers only the 75th-day
loading phase. While the findings on efficacy and safety are encouraging the long-term effects of gossypol contraception require
further study.

EFFECT OF GOSSYPOL ON HUMAN TESTICULAR FUNCTION:

EVALUATION OF SEMINAL AND HORMONAL PARAMETERS

Julian Frick and C. Danner

Urological Department
General Hospital
Salzburg, Austria

INTRODUCTION

There have been a number of reports from the National Research Group for Male Fertility Control of the People's Republic of China concerning the use of gossypol as a safe antifertility agent for men. The efficacy has been said to be 99.9%. The men usually recovered fertility three or more months after termination of treatment, and several apparently healthy babies were born to wives of men who stopped using gossypol [2, 3, 4, 5]. The study presented here was performed in 1981. The aim was to study gossypol's effect on the tubular compartment in human males and on the hormonal and electrolyte status.

MATERIAL AND METHODS

Five subjects, aged 47-65, were enrolled in this study and treated for 3 months with an oral dosage of 20 mg gossypol daily. The parameters examined before and during treatment are shown in Table 1. In two subjects, 47 and 48 years old, the function of the tubular compartment was examined by sperm analyses. In the remaining three cases, aged 62-65, the effect on testicular function was determined by pre-treatment and post-treatment testicle biopsies. In the two younger men regular sperm analyses were also undertaken during the recovery phase.

The sperm analyses were done according to the recommendations of Eliasson [6]. The plasma hormone values were determined by radioimmunological techniques [7, 8].

TABLE 1.   Parameters Examined in Five Men Before and
During Treatment with 20 mg of Gossypol
Given Orally Per Day for 12 Weeks

Testicle biopsy	x			x
Prostate biopsy	x			x
Sperm analysis	x	x	x	x
T, LH, FSH, E_2, prolactin	x	x	x	x
Blood counts	x	x	x	x
SMA 12 with potassium	x	x	x	x
Cortisol	x	x	x	x
Urine analysis	x	x	x	x
	0	4	8	12 weeks

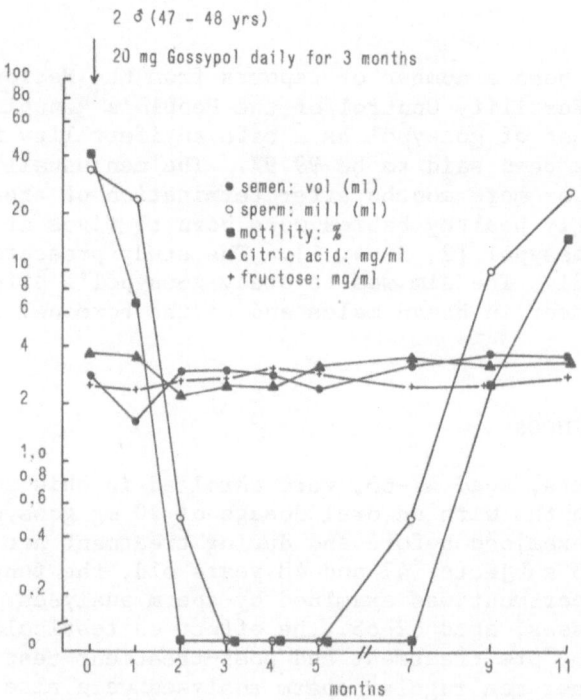

Fig. 1.   Sperm analysis data in 2 men, aged 47 and 48, before, during and after treatment with 20 mg gossypol orally/day for
3 months. Each point represents the mean of two values.

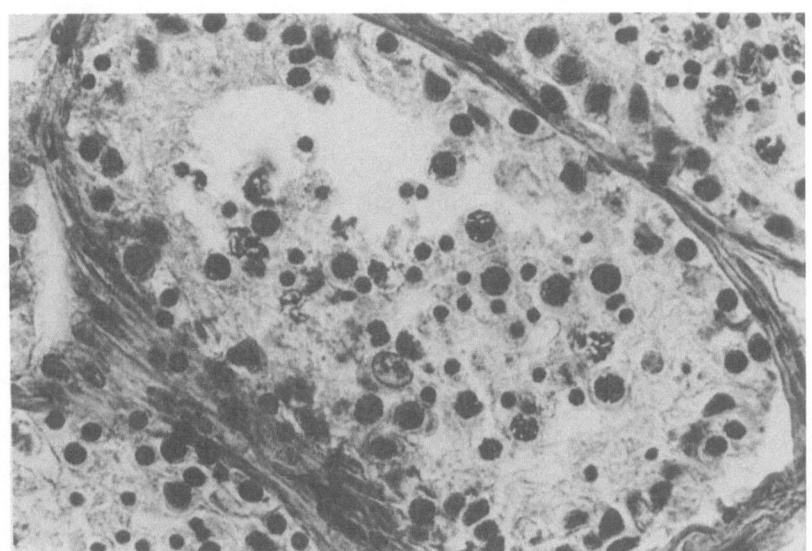

Fig. 2. Pretreatment testicle biopsy of a 63 year old man. The
         histology shows almost all steps of spermatogenesis (hema-
         toxilin-eosin, magnification: 672:1).

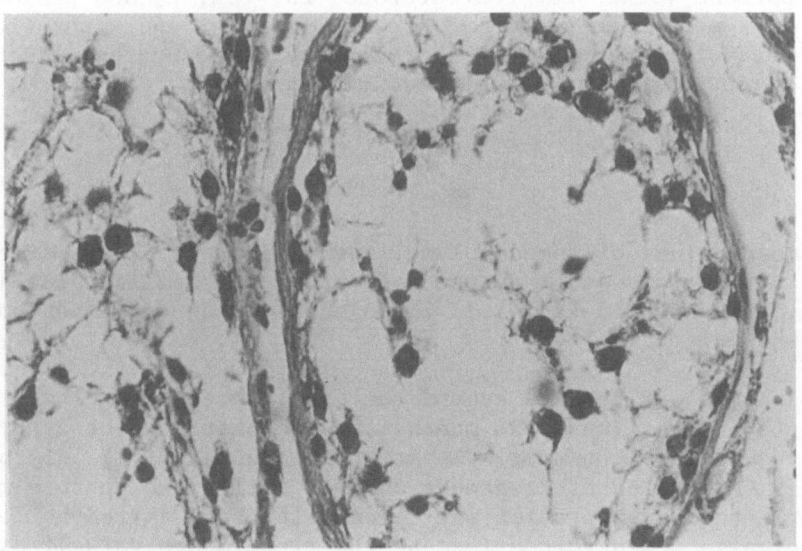

Fig. 3. Testicle biopsy of the same man as in Fig. 2 taken 11 weeks
         after initiation of gossypol treatment (20 mg gossypol
         orally/day for 3 months). The histology reveals a
         complete arrest of spermatogenesis (hematoxilin-eosin,
         magnification: 672:1).

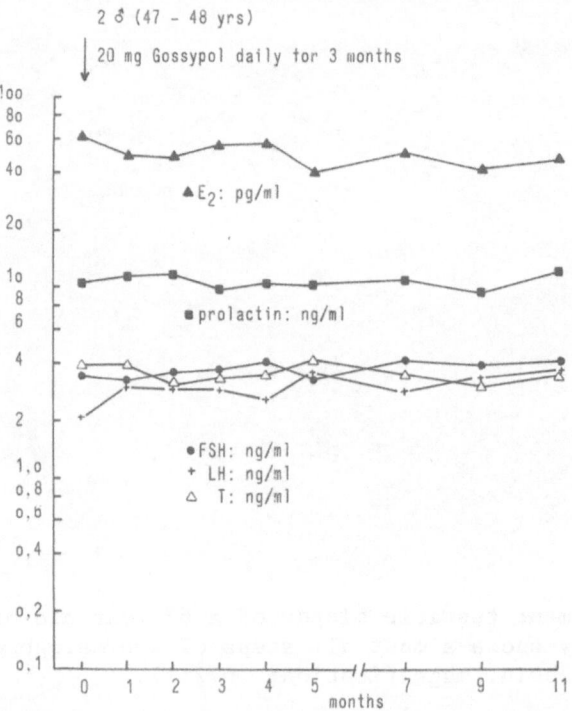

Fig. 4.   Hormone values for testosterone, LH, FSH, E₂ and prolactin
          in 2 men, aged 47 and 48, before, during, and after treat-
          ment with 20 mg gossypol orally/day for 3 months. Each
          point represents the mean of two values.

RESULTS

     The mean values of semen volume, sperm density, progressive
motility, citric acid and fructose content of the seminal plasma at
zero time, are shown in Fig. 1 in 2 subjects during treatment and
recovery phases.

     Azoospermia was reached around the eighth week of treatment and
was present until at least two months after cessation of therapy.
Progressive motility, however, was markedly lowered (<8%) only one
month after initiation of treatment and was still zero up to 4 months
after the last gossypol tablet was taken. It then started to return to normal: semen volume (except the first month value), citric
acid and fructose content of the seminal plasma underwent no marked
changes during the treatment and recovery phases.

     The pretreatment testicle biopsies in the remaining three cases,
aged 62-64, showed a fairly normal distribution of germinal elements

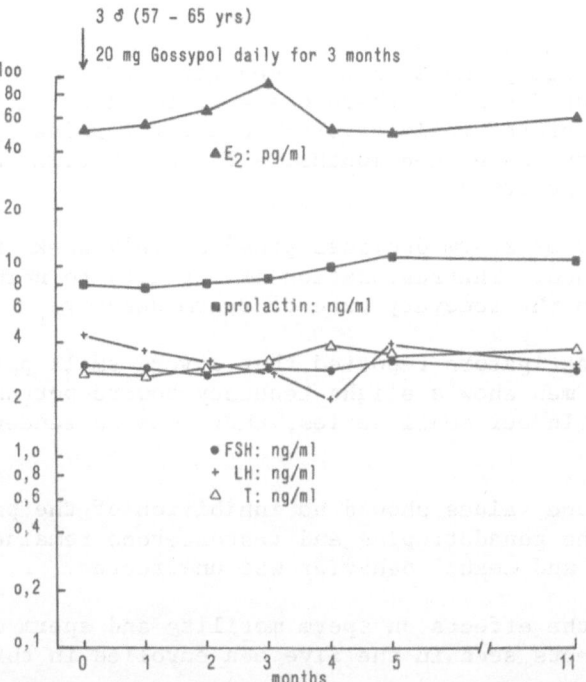

Fig. 5.   Hormone values for testosterone, LH, FSH, E_2 and prolactin
          in 3 men, aged 57-65, before, during, and after treatment
          with 20 mg gossypol orally/day for 3 months. Each point
          represents the mean of three values.

for that age group (Fig. 2). The biopsy taken between 10 and 12
weeks of treatment revealed empty tubules with an almost complete
arrest of spermatogenesis (Fig. 3).

Plasma Hormone Levels during Treatment and Recovery

    The hormone levels showed similar patterns in all subjects
(Figs. 4 and 5). LH, FSH, testosterone (T), E_2 and prolactin fluc-
tuated within normal range during the treatment and recovery phases.
A suppression of the pituitary gonadal axis could not be found.

Pharmacology, Clinical Findings, and Side Effects

    Measurements of various urine and serum components (SMA 12,
cortisol) showed no marked changes during the treatment period. We
found no case of hypokalemia. The electrocardiograms were also normal during the treatment period, and none of the subjects enrolled
in this study complained of decrease of libido or changes in sexual
behavior.

DISCUSSION

The present study shows that in men given 20 mg of gossypol orally per day for 3 months, there was a profound effect on spermatogenesis. This proved fully reversible after termination of treatment. Infertility lasted 4-6 months, after which time full recovery of fertility was achieved.

The motility of sperm declines progressively weeks before azoospermia is reached. The restoration of motility to normal is delayed compared to the recovery rate of sperm density.

Chinese investigators reported that a very small percentage of gossypol-treated men show a slight tendency toward potassium decrease [9, 10]. In our small series, there was no tendency toward hypokalemia.

Plasma hormone values showed no inhibition of the pituitary-gonadal axis. The gonadotropins and testosterone remained unchanged during treatment and sexual behavior was unaffected.

Other than the effects on sperm motility and sperm count, there were no side effects seen in the five men enrolled in this study.

REFERENCES

1.   National Coordinating Group on Male Antifertility Agents, Gossypol. A New Antifertility Agent for Males, Chin. Med. J., 4:417 (1978).
2.   E. J. Coutinho, J. F. Melo, S. J. Segal, and I. Barbosa, Suppression of spermatogeneis in men by gossypol, Israel Med. Sci. J., 31:20 (1981).
3.   G. Z. Liu, Clinical study of gossypol as a male contraceptive, in: "Proc. Tenth World Congress on Fertil. Steril.," p. 96, Madrid (1980).
4.   Z. Q. Liu, G. Z. Liu, L. S. Hei, R. A. Zhang, and C. Z. Yu, Clinical trial of gossypol as a male antifertility agent, in: "Recent Advances in Fertility Regulation (C. F. Chang and D. Griffin, eds.), p. 160, Atar, S. A. (1981).
5.   National Coordinating Group on Male Antifertility Agents, 1978, op. cit. (see Ref. 1).
6.   R. Eliasson, Standards for investigation of human semen, Andrologia, 3:49 (1971).
7.   A. Bartke, R. E. Steels, N. Musto, and B. V. Caldwell, Fluctuations in plasma testosterone levels in adult male rats and mice, Endocr., 92:1223 (1973).
8.   P. G. Crosignani, R. M. Nakamura, D. N. Hovland, and D. R. Mishell, Jr., A method of solid phase radioimmunoassay utilizing polypropylene disc, J. Clin. Endocrinol. Metab., 30:153 (1970).

9. National Coordinating Group on Male Infertility Aents, 1978, op. cit. (see Ref. 1).
10. M. R. N. Prasad and E. Diczfalusy, Gossypol, Int. J. Androl., 5:53 (1982).

BIPHASIC ACTION OF GOSSYPOL IN MEN

Elsimar M. Coutinho, Sheldon J. Segal,
Jose F. Melo and Ione Barbosa

Maternidade Climerio de Oliveira
Federal University of Bahia
School of Medicine
Salvador, Bahia, Brazil

and

Population Sciences
The Rockefeller Foundation
New York, New York, U.S.A.

INTRODUCTION

Gossypol appears to have several advantages over other potential systemic contraceptives for use by men. Its action is independent of the hormonal events of the hypothalamo-hypophysial
gonadal axis, so that a suppression of the testis' gamete-producing
function can be achieved without suppressing the gonad's hormone-
producing function [1]. The range of reported side effects in men
is far more limited than reported when hormonal steroids have been
used experimentally for male contraception. The use of androgens,
progestins, or combinations of the two by men has been associated
with breast tenderness, gynecomastia, weight gain, loss of libido,
changes in blood chemistry indicative of altered liver function and
hemoconcentration [2]. None of these problems have been associated
with the use of gossypol.

When used experimentally in China, gossypol clearly elicited
an anti-spermatogenic effect in over 90% of men who used the drug
for six months to four-and-one-half years. Two important issues
which require further attention evolved from these pioneering
clinical studies: (a) delay or failure in restoration of spermatogenesis after cessation of treatment and (b) drug-induced reduction in
serum potassium associated with muscle weakness and/or paralysis in

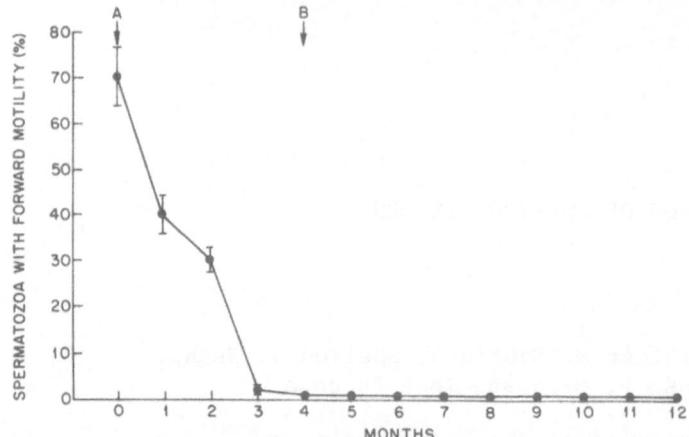

Fig. 1.   Effect of gossypol on sperm motility.   A) Start of daily
dosage of 20 mg; B) start of weekly dosage of 60 mg.   Note
significant decrease in motility at the end of the first
month of treatment.   Values are mean ± standard error
(S.E.M.) n = 10.

some cases [3].   The quantification of these phenomena is difficult
because of the design of the initial clinical studies.   Hypokalemia,
a condition which occurs idiopathically in some sub-groups of the
Chinese, was observed in some of the gossypol study centers, but
not in others.   Reported cases of fatigue were not always evaluated
for serum potassium values.   With regard to reversibility, little
information is available on pretreatment fertility or testicular
status of gossypol-treated men, so that the influence of co-variants
associated with secondary infertility is not known.

The need for a confirmatory study of the effectiveness and important side effects of gossypol in a non-Chinese population prompted
us to evaluate this compound's activity in a group of Brazilian men
desiring to cease their fertility through elective vasectomy, thus
giving the volunteers the option of achieving their contraceptive
objectives while retaining the potential for reversibility.

METHOD

Twelve men were selected out of a group of volunteers who
sought sterilization in our Family Planning Unit.   Selection was
based on recently proved fertility between ages 25 and 40, and free-
dom from uro-genital disease and endocrinopathies.   Patients having
clinically detectable varicocele were not accepted.   Blood chemistry,
which included C.B.C. cholesterol, glucose, tri-glycerides, acid

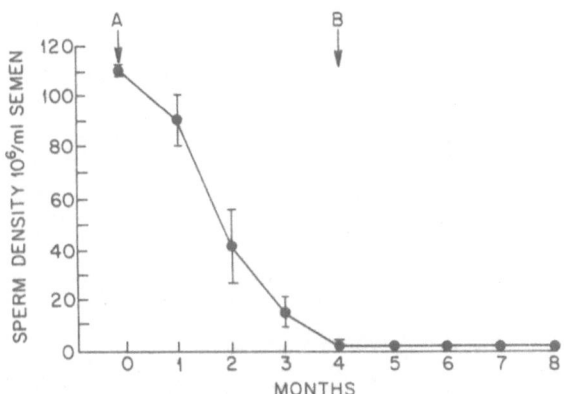

Fig. 2. Effect of gossypol on sperm count. A) Start of daily dosage of 20 mg; B) start of weekly dosage of 60 mg. Significant reduction is noted at 2 months; azoospermia occurs at the end of the fourth month of treatment. Values are mean ± S.E.M., n = 10.

phosphatase, urea, transaminases, sodium and potassium, was carried out before and monthly during treatment. Sperm counts were performed twice before treatment and every month during gossypol administration. Following discontinuation, sperm counts were performed monthly until reversal was documented.

Luteinizing hormone releasing hormone (LHRH) response was investigated in eight subjects before and during treatment. Two basal blood samples were collected at 5 min intervals and then 100 μ. of LHRH was injected subcutaneously. Blood samples were collected every $^1/_4$ hour for an additional two hours in order to quantitate the LH response. Leydig cell function was evaluated by measuring basal blood testosterone before and monthly during treatment with gossypol. Stimulating tests with hCG were carried out before and three to six months after initiation of treatment in 5 men. Test procedure was as follows; basal blood testosterone on day 0 before the intramuscular injection of 2000 I.U. of hCG. Testosterone levels were measured at 24-h intervals for four days following the hCG injection.

Gossypol

Each patient received a monthly supply of gossypol monoacetic acid coated tablets containing 20 mg of the drug. The drug was manufactured at the Institute of Materia Medica, Nanjing, China. One 20 mg tablet was given daily for four months. The dose was then reduced to 60 mg weekly (20 mg three times a week). This dose was maintained for 4-6 months, extending the total treatment duration to 10-12 months. Two of the 12 cases had a slightly altered regimen, as described below.

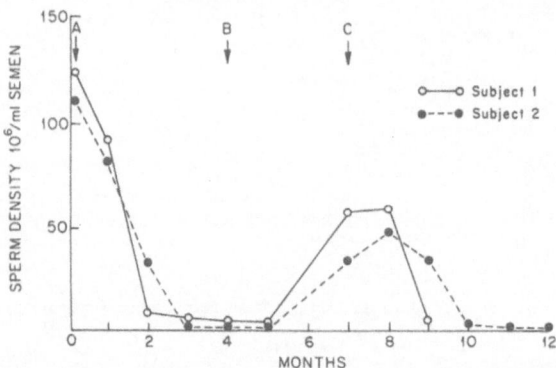

Fig. 3.   Effect of gossypol on sperm count in two subjects: A)
start of daily dosage of 20 mg; B) reduction of dosage to
20 mg weekly; C) resumption of daily dosage of 20 mg.

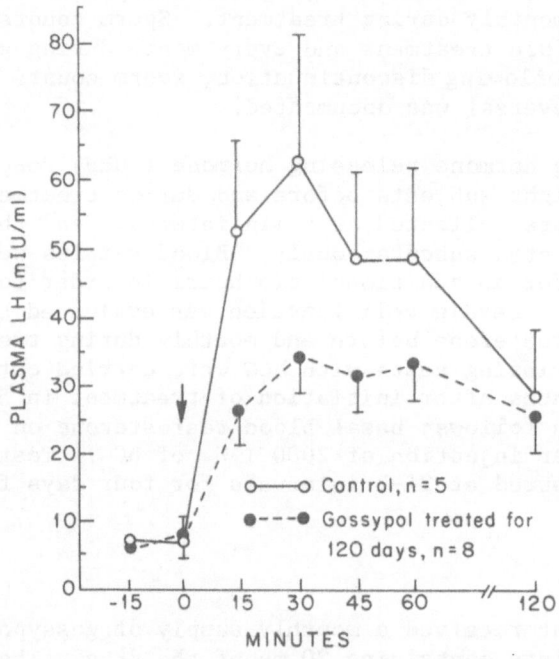

Fig. 4.   LH levels following injection of LHRH (100 μg) at time 0
in gossypol treated and control men. No significant difference between the two groups.

TABLE 1

Sub- ject No.	Before gossypol	Sperm count in millions/ml		One year after dis- continua- tion
		Third month	Fourth month	
1	129	27	Azoo	42
2	108	11*	Azoo	Azoo
3	115	0	Azoo	106
4	118	25	Azoo	122
5	86	24	Azoo	Azoo
6	88	10	0.2*	48
7	123	28	Azoo	111
8	95	26	0.5*	104
9	91	22	Azoo	98
10	108	0.2*	Azoo	Azoo
11	87	0.8*	Azoo	77
12	96	6.0	Azoo	Azoo

*Necrospermia

RESULTS

Only a small reduction (less than 20%) in sperm count occurred after the first month of treatment. However, a significant (p < 0.005) reduction in sperm motility was detected in all the subjects (Fig. 1). An increase in the number of immature cells forms in the ejaculate was also observed in all cases. By the end of the second month, sperm count was significantly reduced in most but not all subjects. Severe oligospermia with few immotile spermatozoa or azoospermia developed only after four months of daily gossypol administration. Reduction to the 60 mg weekly regimen following the loading phase allowed continued inhibition of spermatogenesis, as illustrated in Fig. 2. By the end of the fifth month all men were azoospermic or had few immotile spermatozoa in the ejaculate. Thus, the effect of gossypol was biphasic. The initial effect was the motility of stored spermatozoa; subsequently, there was a reduction in sperm production. No significant change in semen volume was detected throughout the study period. In two subjects in whom the dose was reduced further to 20 mg weekly there was a rebound in the sperm count. Sixty days after reducing the dose to 20 mg weekly, there was a rebound in the sperm count; this rebound amounted to 50% of the pretreatment level. By returning to the initial daily schedule of 20 mg, azoospermia was re-established in both men (Fig. 3).

Following discontinuation of gossypol, sperm count returned to original pretreatment levels in six men. In two other men, sperm

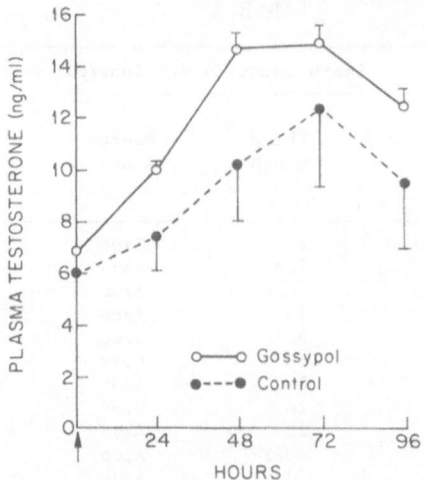

Fig. 5. Testosterone levels in gossypol treated men (n = 5) fol-
         lowing injection of 5000 I.U. of hCG. Note normal rise
         reaching maximum at 72 h. No significant difference be-
         tween the two groups.

count rose to 50% of pretreatment levels and remained at this reduced levels as long as two years after discontinuation. Motility
was fully restored by the end of the second year. In four men, as
long as one year following discontinuation of gossypol treatment,
the sperm count remained zero (Table 1). Follow-up of these subjects is reported elsewhere [6].

     Despite some individual variation, no significant changes oc-
curred in the response to LHRH during gossypol treatment. Prompt
rise in LH could be detected in all men following the LHRH injection (Fig. 4). No significant changes in basal testosterone levels
occurred. The response to an hCG stimulation test was likewise unchanged during treatment as compared to controls (Fig. 5).

     Blood levels of glucose, cholesterol, acid phosphatase, trans-
aminases, triglycerides, urea, sodium and potassium remained within
the normal range throughout the treatment period.

     None of the 12 subjects reported changes in libido or in the
frequency of intercourse. There were no significant changes in body
weight or in blood pressure. Transient fatigue was reported by one
subject.

COMMENTS

    The first observed effect of gossypol in men is a rapid loss
of sperm motility. Initially, therefore, gossypol appears to affect
the function of stored, epididymal sperm. This effect is noted one
month after initiation of treatment, and possibly sooner. Whether
this effect, by itself, would reduce male fertility is not known.
Subsequently, production of sperm within the seminiferous tubules
is reduced with continued exposure to gossypol. The second phase
may, in fact, be initiated earlier than semen analysis would suggest, considering the length of the seminiferous cycle in man.
Nevertheless, as far as the semen analysis is concerned, gossypol
first reduces sperm motility and then reduces sperm count.

    The present study confirms Chinese reports that gossypol in-
hibits spermatogenesis in men at a dose level which in short-term
treatment (up to 12 months) appears to be free of side effects. In
order to induce azoospermia in this selected group of Brazilian men,
a daily dose of 20 mg of gossypol had to be maintained for four
months. Although this duration is slightly longer than that reported by Chinese investigators, it should be noted that in the
Chinese clinical trials, subjects were unselected and included older
men in whom the response to gossypol may have been more rapid [4].
The failure of four subjects to restore spermatogenesis for one year
after cessation of gossypol treatment has not escaped our attention
and has been investigated further. The results of these investigations, which suggest an association of this secondary infertility with
varicocele, will be published elsewhere [5].

REFERENCES

1.   National Coordinating Group on Male Infertility Agents, A new
      antifertility agent for males, Chin. Med. J., 9 (new series
      No. 4):417 (1978).
2.   J. Frick, Effect of Steroids on Spermatogenesis, "Control of
      Male Fertility" (J. H. Sciarra, C. Markland, and J. J. Speidel,
      eds.), Harper and Row, New York.
3.   Qian Shaozhen, Jing Guangwei, Wu Xiaoyng, Xu Ye, Li Yaoging, and
      Zhao Zhihong, Gossypol related to hypokalemia. Clinicopharma-
      cological studies, Chin. Med. J., 93:477 (1980).
      Male Fertility" (J. H. Sciarra, C. Markland, and J. J. Speidel,
      eds.), Harper and Row, New York.
4.   National Coordinating Group on Male Infertility Agents, 1978,
      op. cit. (see Ref. 1).
5.   E. Coutinho, et al., Fertility and Sterility, in press (1984).

EFFECT OF GOSSYPOL ON THE FERTILITY

OF THE MALE BONNET MONKEY

Natwar R. Kalla,* J. Foo,*
T. W. Kalpana,† S. Hurkadli,†
and A. R. Sheth†

*Department of Biophysics
Panjab University
Chandigarh, India

†Institute for Research in Reproduction
Bombay, India

INTRODUCTION

The discovery of gossypol as a male antifertility agent by
Chinese investigators has aroused considerable interest among
students of reproductive biology [1]. The antifertility activity
has been verified in laboratory animals by a number of researchers
[2, 3, 4, 5]. In none of the reported studies was gossypol found
to have any deleterious effect on the health of the animals. En-
couraged by these observations, the present investigations were
designed to establish the antifertility potential of gossypol in a
sub-human primate model, the bonnet monkey, Macaca radiata, in the
hope that these observations would provide baseline data for the
development of gossypol as a suitable male contraceptive pill.

MATERIAL AND METHODS

Animals, Dose, and Treatment Schedule

Six male adult bonnet monkeys (Macaca radiata) were used in
the present investigations. The animals were fed monkey food
(Hindustan Lever) supplemented with fresh fruits and vegetable.
Gossypol acetic acid suspended in Tonoferon tonic(R) (East India
Pharmaceutical Ltd., Bombay; composition per 5 ml: Colloidal iron
hydroxide 500 mg (250 mg elemental iron), folic acid IP 1.75 mg,

33

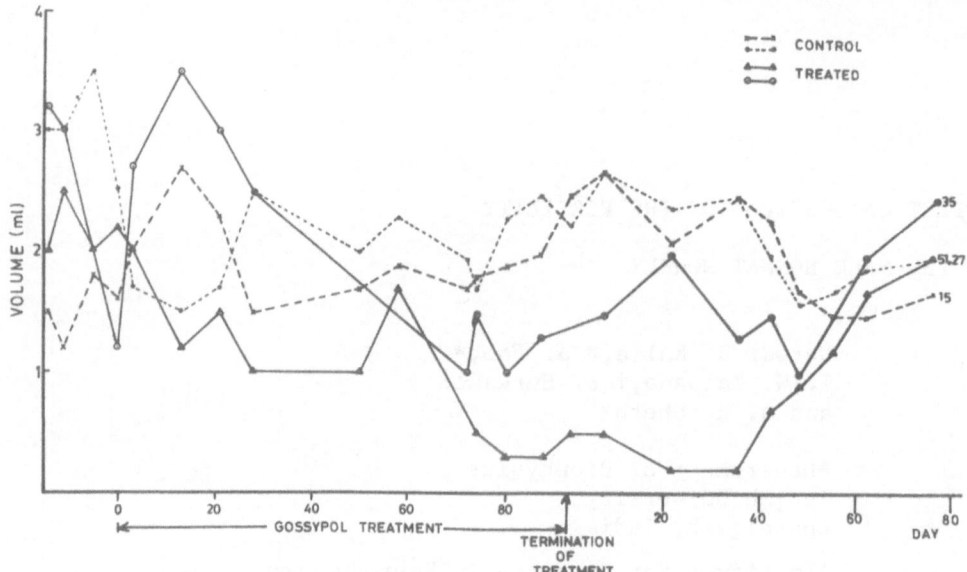

Fig. 1.   Effect of gossypol acetic acid on the semen volume in
          bonnet monkey.

vitamin B_{12} IP 7.5 mg, ethyl alcohol 9.5% by volume, syrup and
falvour) was fed to monkeys, 4 mg/animal/day (0.5 mg/kg body weight)
five days a week (Monday-Friday) for three months. The same tonic
was given to control monkeys. Two monkeys (Nos. 27 and 35) were exposed to gossypol from July-September and the other two monkeys
(Nos. 3 and 4) were exposed to gossypol from December-March. Control monkeys (Nos. 15 and 51) were the same in both the experiments.
In both cases gossypol treatment was discontinued after 3 months for
recovery studies.

Semen Analysis

     Using the penile stimulation method of Settlage for electro-
ejaculation [6], semen samples were collected from the monkeys at
intervals of 6-8 days for 3 months during the gossypol-treatment
period. The sperm motility was calculated by the method of Settlage.
The total number of spermatozoa in the semen samples were counted
by the method of Hukeri [7]. The estimation of citric acid and
fructose from the seminal plasma was made by the methods of Beulter
and Yeh [8] and Sheth and Rao [9].

Hematological Studies

     The general health of the animals was evaluated during the
gossypol-treatment phase and the recovery phase. During the course

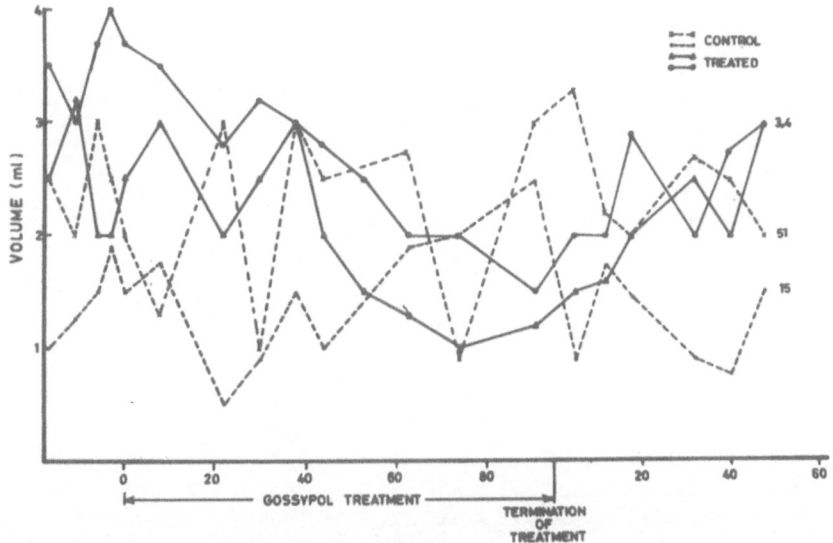

Fig. 2.   Effect of gossypol acetic acid on the semen volume in
          bonnet monkey.

of drug treatment blood was drawn after every 6-8 days for the following investigations: a) total erythrocyte count; b) total leucocyte count; c) differential leucocyte count; d) hematocrit; e) total
hemoglobin; and f) mean corpuscular volume (MCV), mean corpuscular
hemoglobin (MCH) and mean corpuscular hemoglobin concentration
(MCMC).   These observations were made by the standard hematological
procedures.   Gossypol acetic acid (GA-19-3-98.55%) was obtained from
Dr. Angelo V. Graci, U.S.D.A., New Orleans, U.S.A.   All the data
were analyzed using Student's test.

RESULTS

Semen Analysis

     Figures 1 and 2 summarize the changes in the semen volume in
both treated and control monkeys.   The percentage of motile spermatozoa in the ejaculate decreased markedly in the course of the 90
days of gossypol treatment.   However, 50 days after terminating
treatment, the normal level of motile sperm in the ejaculate returned (Figs. 3 and 4).   The sperm density/ejaculate was significantly lowered in the gossypol-treated monkeys after 75 days of
treatment.   It returned to the normal level 60 days after termination of gossypol treatment (Figs. 5 and 6).

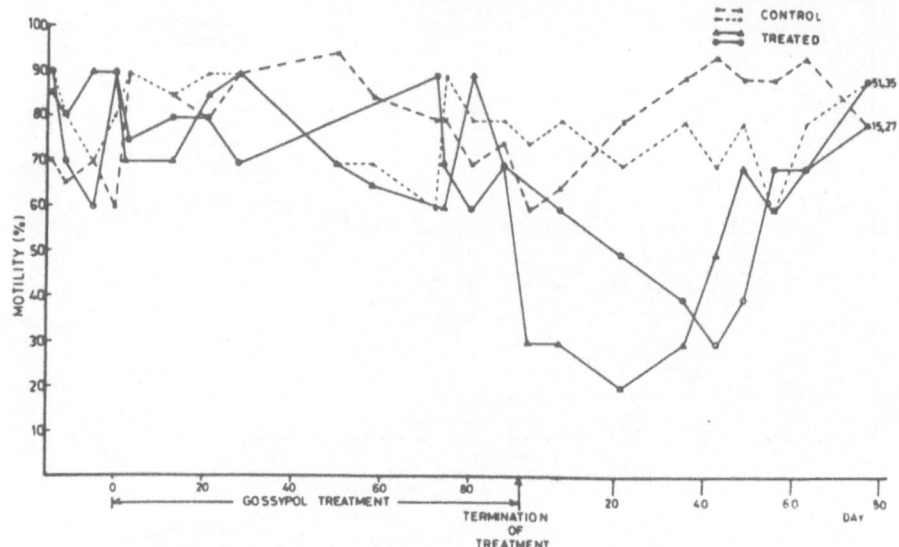

Fig. 3.   Effect of gossypol acetic acid on the sperm motility in
          bonnet monkey.

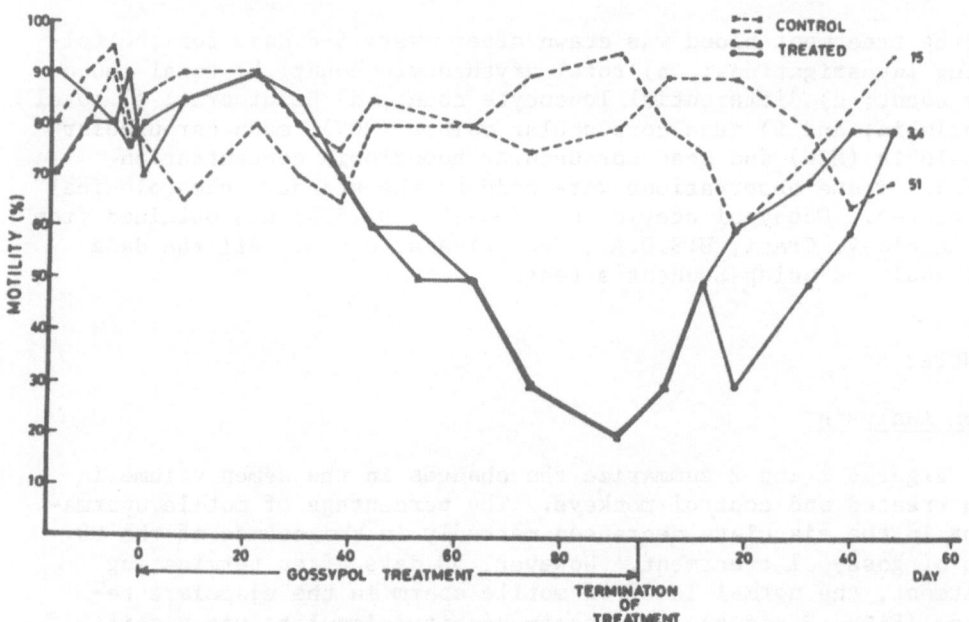

Fig. 4.   Effect of gossypol acetic acid on the sperm motility in
          bonnet monkey.

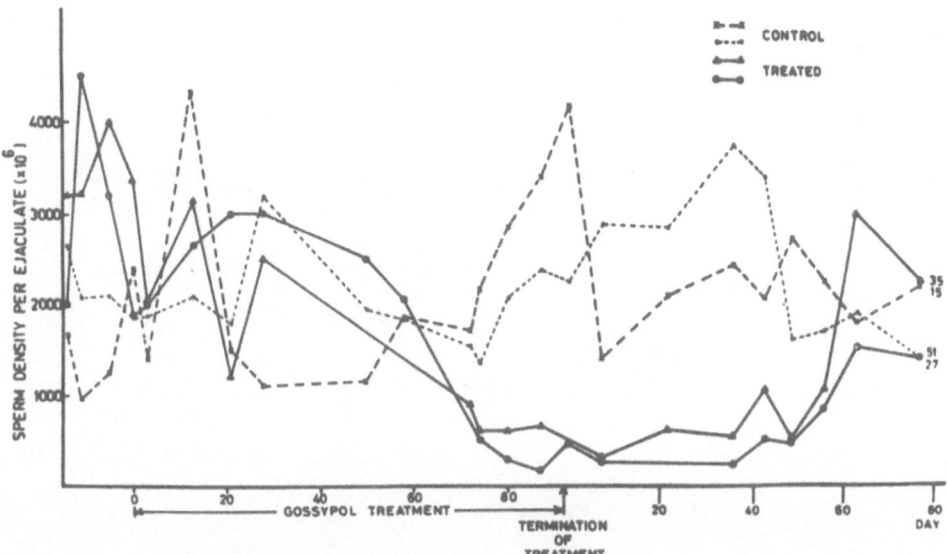

Fig. 5. Effect of gossypol acetic acid on the sperm density per ejaculate in bonnet monkey.

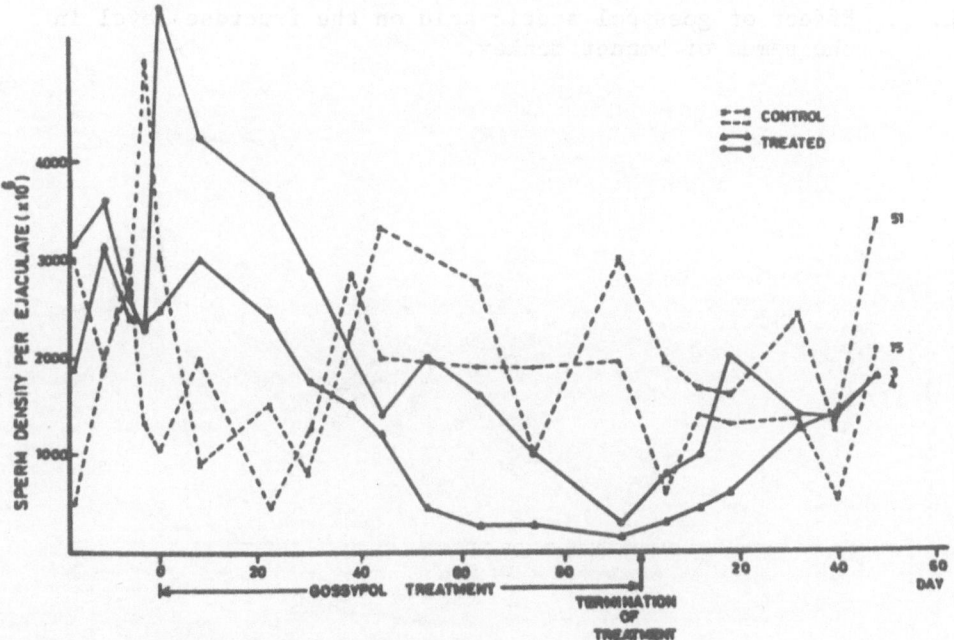

Fig. 6. Effect of gossypol acetic acid on the sperm density per ejaculate in bonnet monkey.

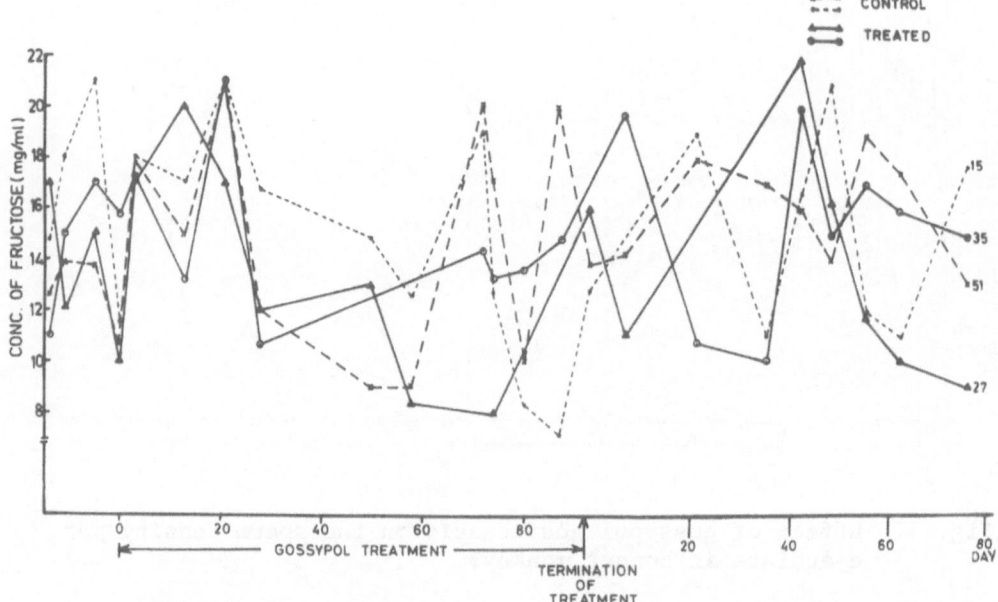

Fig. 7.   Effect of gossypol acetic acid on the fructose level in
          the semen of bonnet monkey.

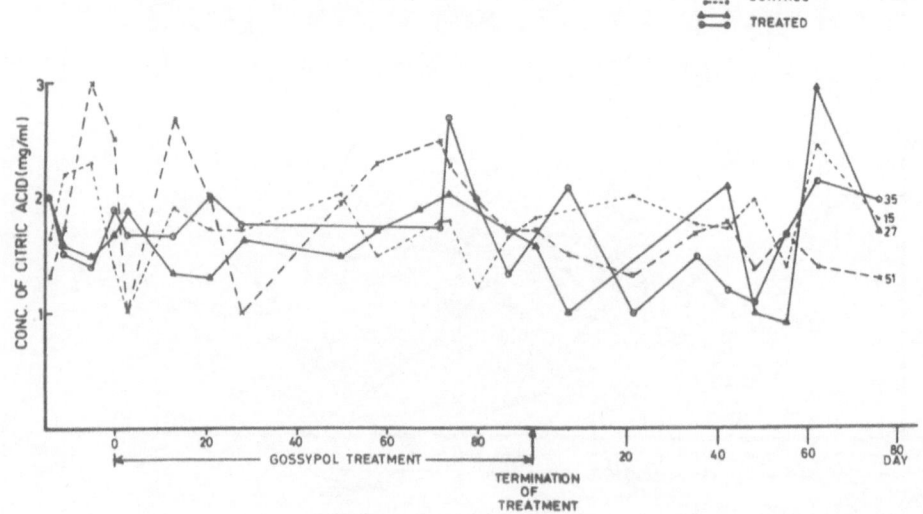

Fig. 8.   Effect of gossypol acetic acid on the citric acid level
          in the semen of bonnet monkey.

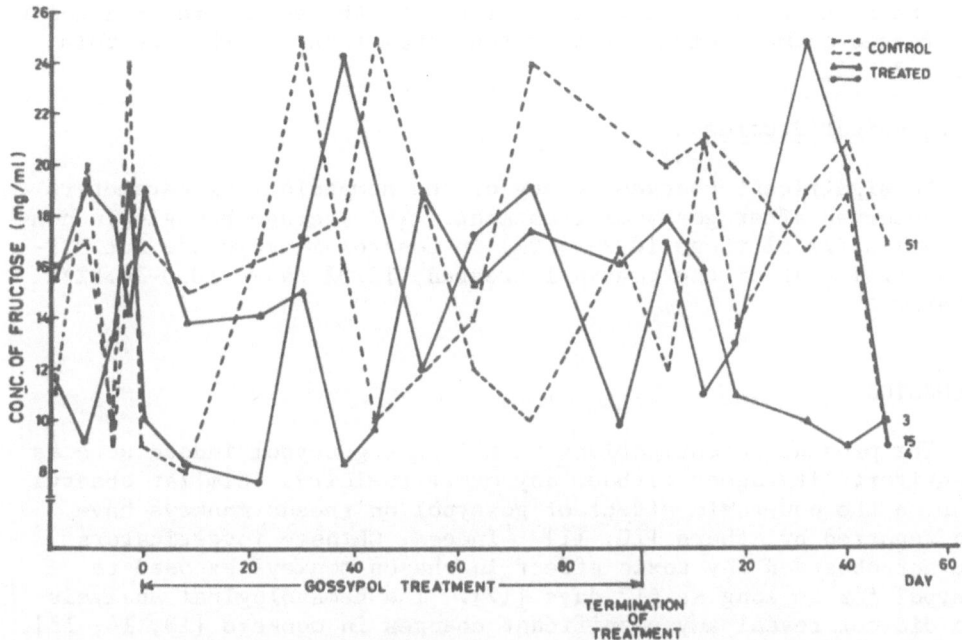

Fig. 9.   Effect of gossypol acetic acid on the fructose level in
the semen of bonnet monkey.

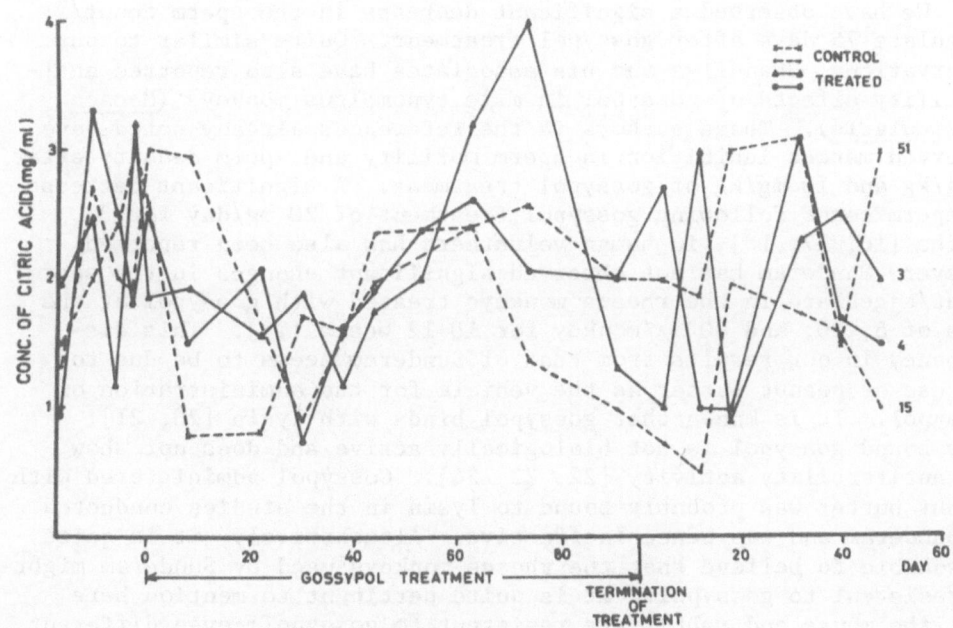

Fig. 10. Effect of gossypol acetic acid on the citric acid level
in the semen of bonnet monkey.

The fructose and citric acid levels in the semen from the gossypol-treated animals were not different from those of the controls (Figs. 7-10).

Hematological Studies

No significant changes in any of the hematological parameters were observed after gossypol treatment. The average hemoglobin concentration (12.5% range 10.2-14.0%) in control monkeys was not different from that of the gossypol-treated (13.0% range 10.0-14.5%) monkeys.

DISCUSSION

The present investigations reveal that gossypol indeed acts as an antifertility agent without any overt toxicity. Similar observations on the non-toxic effect of gossypol on rhesus monkeys have been reported by others [10, 11]. Indeed, Chinese investigators have not observed any toxic effect in rhesus monkeys exposed to gossypol for as long as 617 days [12]. The hematological analysis also did not reveal any significant changes in monkeys [13, 14, 15], nor did the gossypol treatment (4 mg/day for 2 years) have any deleterious effects on the histoarchitecture of the liver, heart, kidneys, and adrenals.

We have observed a significant decrease in the sperm count/ejaculate 75 days after gossypol treatment. Quite similar to our observations, Shandilya and his associates have also reported antifertility effects of gossypol in male cynomolgus monkeys (Macaca fuscicularis). These authors in the references already noted have observed marked inhibition in sperm motility and sperm density after 5 mg/kg and 10 mg/kg of gossypol treatment. A significant decrease in sperm count following gossypol treatment of 20 mg/day for 3 months [16, 17, 18], in human volunteers has also been reported. However, Sunderam has not observed significant changes in the sperm count/ejaculate in the rhesus monkeys treated with gossypol at the dose of 5, 20, and 80 mg/monkey for 10-12 weeks [19]. This discrepancy in our results from that of Sunderam seems to be due to his use of peanut butter as the vehicle for the administration of gossypol. It is known that gossypol binds with lysin [20, 21]; this bound gossypol is not biologically active and does not show any antifertility activity [22, 23, 24]. Gossypol administered with peanut butter was probably bound to lysin in the studies conducted by Sunderam and was hence ineffective. Alternatively, it is quite reasonable to believe that the rhesus-monkeys used by Sunderam might be resistent to gossypol. It is quite pertinent to mention here that the mouse and rabbit are resistent to gossypol; even different strains of rats exhibit varied degrees of resistence to gossypol [25, 26, 27]. However, Sunderam has not observed any toxic effect even at the dose of 80 mg/monkey (the antifertility dose for human is 20 mg/day for 3 months).

Insignificant changes in the fructose and citric acid levels in the semen after gossypol treatment suggest that gossypol treatment to monkeys does not interfere in androgen synthesis. Frick and his associates have also not observed any changes in the citric acid and fructose levels in the semen of human volunteers exposed to gossypol, 20 mg/day, for 12 weeks [28]. Our observations that gossypol does not interfere in androgen synthesis are further supported by the fact that the plasma level of testosterone remains unchanged after gossypol treatment [29, 30, 31, 32]. Similarly, the plasma level of LH is also not affected by gossypol treatment [33, 34, 35, 36, 37, 38].

During the course of the present investigations, using light microscopy, we have not observed any changes in the morphology of the spermatozoa after gossypol treatment. We have, however, observed marked changes in the morphology of the spermatozoa at the ultrastructure level (disorganization of mitochondrial cristae in the mid-piece, detachment of the plasma membrane in the mid-piece and head region, complete or partial detachment of the head from the tail) after 90 days of gossypol treatment (unpublished). Similar ultrastructure changes have been reported in rat [39, 40], monkey [41], and human spermatozoa [42] after gossypol treatment. These observations suggest that gossypol may be interfering with spermatogenesis and/or acting directly on the spermatozoa by the mechanisms/s that affects both sperm production and sperm motility.

In conclusion, our preliminary studies by the findings of other investigators, provide evidence that gossypol is indeed a potential male antifertility agent without any overt toxicity in primates.

REFERENCES

1. National Coordinating Group on Male Antifertility Agents, Gossypol - A new antifertility agent for males, Chinese Med. J., 8:417 (1978).
2. M. J. Nadakavukaren, H. R. Sorensen, and J. N. Tone, Effect of gossypol on the ultrastructure of rat spermatozoa, Cell Tissue Res., 204:293 (1979).
3. M. C. Chang, Z. Gu, and S. K. Saksena, Effect of gossypol on the fertility of male rats, hamsters, and rabbits, Contraception, 21:461 (1980).
4. N. R. Kalla, M. Vasudev, and G. Arora, Studies on the male antifertility agent - Gossypol acetic acid. III. Effect of gossypol acetic acid on rat testis, Andrologia, 13:242 (1981).
5. M. K. Hadley, Y. C. Lin, and M. Dym, Effect of gossypol on the reproductive system of male rats, J. Andrology, 2:190 (1981).

6. D. S. F. Settlage, Establishment of normal parameters in semen analysis of Rhesus monkey (Macaca mulatta), M.S. Thesis, University of California (1972).

7. V. B. Hukari, Influence of the various dilutors on the motility, livability, and morphology of bovine spermatozoa and their significance during preservation, Ph.D. Thesis, Nagpur University, India, p. 37 (1969).

8. E. Beulter and N. K. Y. Yeh, A simplified method for the determination of citric acid J. Lab. Clin. Med., 54:125 (1959).

9. A. R. Sheth and S. S. Rao, Fructose and fructolysis in human semen determined chromatographically, Experientia, 15:314 (1959).

10. Y. E. Wang, Y. D. Luo, and X. C. Tang, Studies on the antifertility actions of cotton seed meal and gossypol, Acta Pharmacol. Sinica, 14:662 (1979).

11. K. Sunderam, Effect of gossypol on rhesus monkeys, Proc. Workshop on Gossypol, Chicago, Abstract No. 14 (1980).

12. Y. E. Wang, et al., 1979, op. cit. (see Ref. 10).

13. K. Sunderam, 1980, op. cit. (see Ref. 11).

14. L. N. Sandilya and T. B. Clarkson, a. Hypolipidemic effects of gossypol in Cynomolgus monkeys (Macaca fascicularis), Lipids, 17:285 (1982).

15. L. N. Shandilya, T. B. Clarkson, M. R. Admas, and J. C. Lewis, Effect of gossypol on reproductive and endocrine functions of male Cynomolgus monkeys (Macaca fascicularis), Biol. Reprod., 27:241 (1982).

16. National Coordinating Group on Male Antifertility Agents, 1978, op. cit. (see Ref. 1).

17. E. Coutinho, J. F. Melo, S. J. Segal, and I. Barbosa, Suppression of spermatogenesis in men by gossypol, Israel J. Med. Sci., 17:741 (1981).

18. J. Frick, Ch. Danner, R. Kohle, and G. Kunit, Male fertility regulation, in: "Research on Fertility and Sterility" (J. Cortes Prieto, Campos da Paz, and M. Neves-e-Castro, eds.), p. 291, MTP Press Ltd., Lancaster (1981).

19. K. Sunderam, 1980, op. cit. (see Ref. 11).

20. B. P. Baliga and C. M. Lyman, Preliminary report on the nutritional significance of bound gossypol in cotton seed meal, J. Am. Oil. Chem. Soc., 34:21 (1957).

21. A. J. Clawson, F. H. Smith, J. C. Osborne, and E. R. Barrick, Effect of protein source, autoclaying and lysin supplementation of gossypol toxicity, J. Anim. Sci., 20:547 (1961).

22. F. Hale and C. M. Lyman, Lysine supplementation of sorghum grain cotton seed meal rations for growing pigs, J. Anim. Sic., 20:734 (1961).

23. Qian S. Z., Jing G. W., Wu X. Y., Li Y. Q., Zhou Z.H., Gossypol Related Hypokalemia Clinicopharmacologie studies. Chineese Medical Jrnl., 93:477, (1980).

24. G. S. Lu, Purification of gossypol and preparation of the derivatives, Proc. Workshop on Gossypol, Chicago, Abst. No. 21 (1980).

25. M. C. Chang, et al., 1980, op. cit. (see Ref. 3).
26. D. W. Hahn, C. Rusticus, A. Probst, R. Hahn, and A. N. Johnson, Antifertility and endocrine activities of gossypol in rodents, Contraception, 24:97 (1981).
27. G. I. Zatuchni and C. K. Osborn, Gossypol: A possible male antifertility agent, Report of a Workshop, Research Frontiers in Fertility Regulation 1.
28. J. Frick, et al., 1981, op. cit. (see Ref. 18).
29. A. R. Sheth and S. S. Rao, 1959, op. cit. (see Ref. 9).
30. L. N. Shandilya, et al., 1982, op. cit. (see Ref. 15).
31. E. Coutinho, et al., 1981, op. cit. (see Ref. 7).
32. H. Y. Wang, Y. S. Xu, L. C. Jiang, S. L. Dei, Y. A. Shi, and Z. M. Zhou, The effects of sex steroid hormones and gossypol on LH secretion of rat pituitary by radioimmunoassy, Acta Physiol. Sinica, 31:337 (1979).
33. National Coordinating Group on Male Antifertility Agents, 1978, op. cit. (see Ref. 1).
34. A. R. Sheth and S. S. Rao, 1959, op. cit. (see Ref. 9).
35. E. Coutinho, et al., 1981, op. cit. (see Ref. 17).
36. J. Frick, et al., 1981, op. cit. (see Ref. 18).
37. H. Y. Wang, 1979, op. cit (see Ref. 32).
38. N. R. Kalla, J. Foo, T. W. and A. R. Sheath, Studies on the male antifertility agent - Gossypol acetic acid. V. Effect of gossypol acetic acid on the fertility of male rats, Andrologia, 14:492 (1982).
39. M. J. Nadakavukaren, et al., 1979, op. cit. (see Ref. 2).
40. M. K. Hadley, et al., 1981, op. cit. (see Ref. 5).
41. Shandilya, L. N., et al., 1982, op. cit. (see Ref. 15).
42. National Coordinating Group on Male Antifertility Agents, 1978, op. cit. (see Ref. 1).

ASSESSMENT OF TOXICITY AND ANTIFERTILITY EFFICACY

OF GOSSYPOL IN MALE RATS

Chin-Chuan Chang and Sheldon J. Segal

Center for Biomedical Research
The Population Council
New York, New York, U.S.A.

and

Population Sciences
The Rockefeller Foundation
New York, New York, U.S.A.

INTRODUCTION

The discovery by Chinese scientists of gossypol as an anti-fertility agent for men aroused a great deal of interest around the world in assessing its fertility regulating action in a variety of laboratory animals. In addition to its widely reported toxic effects in animals, it had been reported that when given at high doses, gossypol also caused death in some animal species characterized by generalized edema, hemorrhages, and necrosis of the liver [1, 2]. Tolerance levels for gossypol differed by species. For example, dogs were more sensitive to gossypol, while other animals, including the rabbit, appeared to be less sensitive to it [3, 4, 5, 6].

Studies on the antifertility effects of gossypol in rats demonstrated that: 1) epididymal sperm exhibited a distinct ultrastructural degeneration of the midpiece mitochondria [7, 8, 9, 10]. Sperm became totally immotile and many were decapitated or had sharply bent tails [11, 12]. The cell types within the cycle of the seminiferous epithelium were damaged sequentially beginning with the most advanced stages; spermatids were damaged early, followed by pachytene spermatocytes, leptotene/zygotene spermatocytes, and finally type B and intermediate spermatogonia [13, 14]. Leydig cells showed no detectable changes [15, 16]. The time to onset of infertility and the time to recovery of fertility after discontinua-

45

tion of treatment were dose related [17, 18, 19, 20, 21, 22, 23].
Mating behavior of gossypol-treated rats was not affected at the
time that gossypol inhibited fertility. Reduction of serum levels
of testosterone and luteinizing hormone were observed, was related
to dose and duration of treatment [24, 25, 26].

In view of the diversified results in many laboratories in
toxicity testing and fertility in rats, our objectives in the present
study in male rats was (1) to examine the toxicity of gossypol acetic
acid in different strains; (2) to determine dosing and food consumption in relation to toxicity and fertility; and (3) to evaluate
the toxicity of "pure" and "impure" gossypol and their effects on
antifertility efficacy.

MATERIALS AND METHODS

General Conditions

Adult male rats of Sprague-Dawley strain (Charles River Breeding
Laboratories, Waltham, MA), each weighing between 290-320 gm were
used, except for the experiment that was designed to examine gossypol
toxicity in different strains of rats as described below. Animals
were housed in a temperature (24.5-26.5°C) and illumination (14 hr
light and 10 h dark) controlled room and maintained on Purina Laboratory Chow and tap water ad libitum.

Gossypol acetic acid powder (Beijing Institute of Zoology,
Beijing, China; 99.2% pure by HPLC at 254 nm) was kept in a brown
glass bottle covered with black paper and stored at -20°C. Gossypol
acetic acid suspension was prepared for oral administration by suspending it in sesame oil (Sigma) with the aid of 0.5% tragacanth gum
(Simga). Doses of 7.5, 15.0, and 40.0 mg/kg/day of gossypol in 0.4-
0.5 ml of the suspending vehicle were given 6 times a week by means
of a gavage needle inserted into the stomach of the animal. Control
animals were administered an equal volume of the vehicle.

The body weight and food intake were recorded 3 times a week and
the growth rate and weekly food consumption were calculated. The
weights of testes, epididymides, seminal vesicles, prostate, liver,
spleen, kidneys, thymus, adrenals, thyroid, and pituitary were determined at autopsy.

Gossypol Toxicity in Different Strains

In addition to the Sprague-Dawley strain obtained from Charles
River (MA), the same strain from Camm (NJ), the Wistar strain from
Toconic (Penn), the Fisher strain, F 344, and the Long Evans strain
from Charles River (MA) were evaluated. The animals were treated
with a daily dose of 40 mg/kg of gossypol acetic acid for 2 weeks.
The body weight and mortality were recorded.

Dosing in Relation to Food Consumption

In this experiment one group of animals were treated with 15 mg/kg/day of gossypol acetic acid by gavage 6 times a week for 6 weeks. Another group of animals were administered 15 mg/kg/day of gossypol acetic acid for the first 3 weeks and were then dosed at 7.5 mg/kg/day for the 4th, 5th, and 6th weeks. Control animals received an equal volume of the vehicle. The body weight and food consumption of the animals were calculated weekly.

Impurities of Gossypol in Relation to Toxicity and Antifertility Efficacy

Two lots of gossypol acetic acid labelled CDB-1371-A and CDB-1371-B were supplied by National Institute of Child Health and Human Development. Lot CDB-1371-A (92% pure) was made by Calbiochem (CA). Lot CDB-1371-B (99% pure) was assayed by analytical high pressure liquid chromatography (HPLC) using reverse phase C_{18u}-Bondapak column (acetonitrile:water, 70:30 with 1% acetic acid; 4 ml/min, 0.5 cm/min, UV detector at 254 nm). The sample was dissolved in acetone before injection. The HPLC traces were xeroxed and the peaks of gossypol acetic acid and accompanying impurities were cut and weighed. The weight thus obtained was divided by the total weight of both peaks and multiplied by 100 to give the percentage of gossypol acetic acid and impurities in each sample.

Animals were administrered 15 mg/kg/day of either CDB-1371-A or CDB-1371-B by gavage 6 days a week for 8 weeks. The control group received the vehicle. Eight animals were assigned to each group. Body weight was taken twice a week. At autopsy, one cauda epididymis from each animal was minced to release the sperm into 2 ml of medium 199 (Grand Island Biological Co.). The suspension was thoroughly mixed and serially diluted in two steps by transferring 50 µl into 2 ml of the medium at each step. The morphology, motility, and the number of spermatozoa in each cauda were examined in 4 hemocytometer chambers and the total and differential sperm counts in the cauda computed. The weights of testes, epididymis, seminal vesicles, prostate, adrenals, thyroid, pituitary, spleed, kidneys, and liver were recorded.

Fertility tests were carried out at 5, 6, 7, and 8 weeks of treatment by cohabitating each male overnight with 2 females in proestrus. Positive mating were verified by the presence of either copulation plugs or sperm in the vagina. The mating behavior was determined and the mated females were autopsied on day 9 after mating and the number of implantation sites were counted.

The results were expressed as mean plus/minus standard error of the mean. The data were analyzed for statistical significance by Student's t-test.

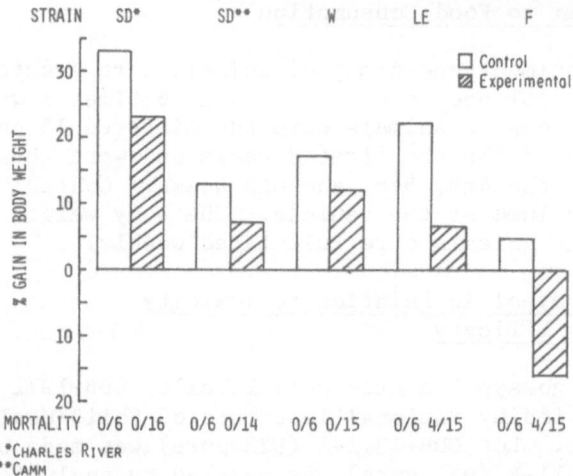

Fig. 1.   Growth rate of male rats of different strains administered
          gossypol acetic acid at 40 mg/kg/day for 2 weeks. SD =
          Sprague-Dawley; W = Wistar; LE = Long Evans; F = Fisher.

RESULTS

Growth Rate and Mortality in Different Strains

     The growth rate of the rats treated for 6 consecutive days/wk
for 2 weeks with 40 mg/kg of gossypol acetic acid is shown in Fig.
1. At this high dose level, the animals of Sprague-Dawley strain
from Charles River, Sprague-Dawley strain from Camm, Wistar strain
from Long Evans strain gained in weight in a differential way; the
Sprague-Dawley strain from Charles River showed less toxic affects
than the other strains tested. The weight gain in all these three
strains was significantly depressed as compared with that of the
controls. The animals of Fisher strain even lost 15% in weight by
the end of treatment. During the treatment period, there was no
mortality in Sprague-Dawley and Wistar strains. However, 4 out of
15 animals of Long Evans strain and 3 out of 15 animals of Fisher
strain died within the first 3 days of treatment.

Dosing in Relation to Food Consumption

     The growth rate of the animals administered 15 mg/kg/day of
gossypol acetic acid for 6 consecutive weeks and the growth rate of
the animals treated with 15 mg/kg/day for the first 3 weeks and then
dosed at 7.5 mg/kg/day for the 4th, 5th, and 6th weeks are presented
in Fig. 2.   There were no significant differences in the body weight
gain of the animals treated with 15 mg/kg during the first 3 weeks
of treatment as compared to that of the controls. However, treat-

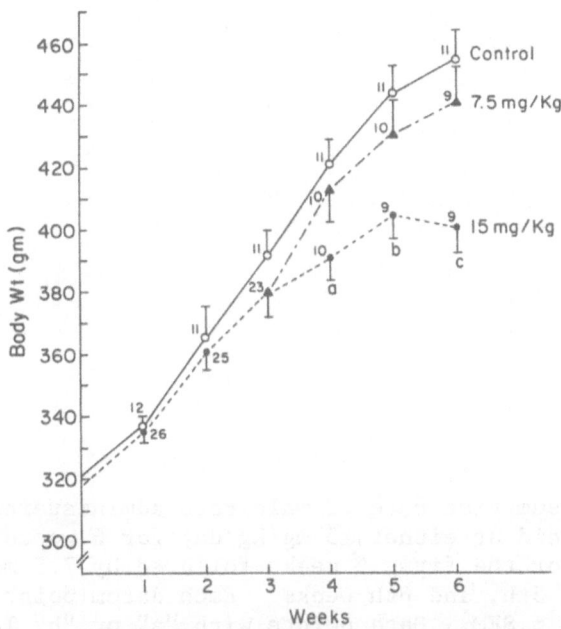

Fig. 2. Growth rate of male rats administered gossypol acetic acid at either 15 mg/kg/day for 6 weeks or 15 mg/kg/day for the first 3 weeks followed by 7.5 mg/kg/day for the 4th, 5th, and 6th weeks. Each datum point represents the mean ± SEM of the number of animals indicated in parentheses. Data points with "a," "b," or "c," letters are significantly different ([a]p < 0.02; [b]p < 0.01; [c]p < 0.001) by Student's t-test.

ment of gossypol acetic acid continued with 15 mg/kg dose level significantly depressed body weight gain (p < 0.02, p < 0.01, and p < 0.001 in the 4th, 5th, and 6th weeks, respectively), whereas there were no significantly effects on the growth rate when gossypol acetic acid was dosed at 7.5 mg/kg after the third week of treatment.

Food consumption of the animals receiving either 15 mg/kg/day of gossypol acetic acid for 6 consecutive weeks or 15 mg/kg/day for the first 3 weeks and then 7.5 mg/kg/day for the 4th, 5th, and 6th weeks of treatment is illustrated in Fig. 3. There were no significant differences in food intake between the treated animals and controls during the first 3 weeks of treatment. Food consumption of the animals receiving 15 mg/kg for the 4th, 5th, and 6th weeks was significantly reduced as compared with the controls (p < 0.001 in each of the 3 weeks of treatment). However, there were no significant effects on food intake when dosed at 7.5 mg/kg/day for the 4th, 5th, and 6th weeks.

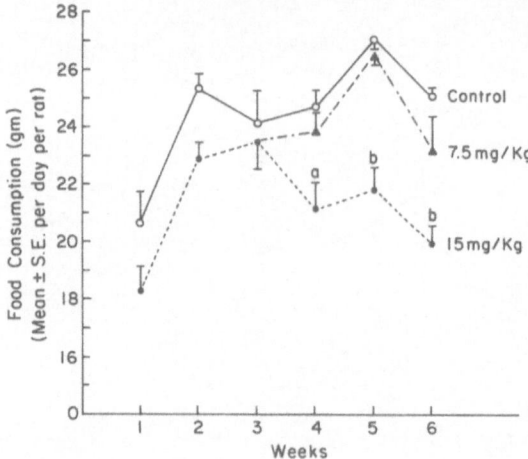

Fig. 3.   Food consumption rate of male rats administered gossypol
          acetic acid at either 15 mg/kg/day for 6 weeks or 15 mg/
          kg/day for the first 3 weeks followed by 7.5 mg/kg/day for
          the 4th, 5th, and 6th weeks. Each datum point represents
          the mean ± SEM. Data points with "a" or "b" letters are
          signifiantly different ([a]p < 0.01; [b]p < 0.001) by Student's
          t-test.

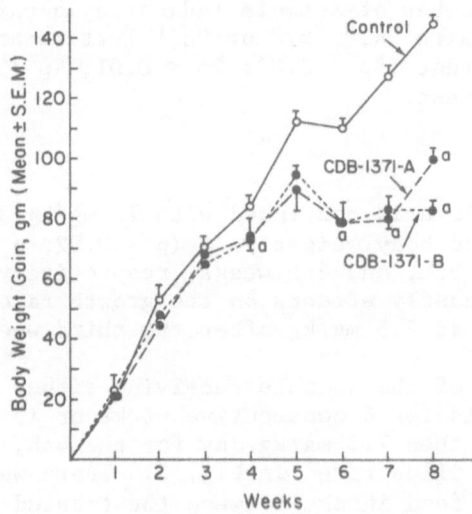

Fig. 4.   Growth rate of male rats treated with impure and pure
          gossypol acetic acid at 15 mg/kg/day for 8 weeks. Each
          datum point represents the mean ± SEM. Data points with
          "a" or "b" letters are significantly less than vehicle-
          treated control ([a]p < 0.001; [b]p < 0.02) by Student's t-test.

TABLE 1. Effect of Gossypol Dosing on Epididymal Sperm in Male Rats

| Treatment | | Number of sperm/cauda (mean + SEM × 10^6) | | | Non-motile | |
Dose mg/kg/day (No of rats)	Time period (weeks)	total	motile	normal appearance	head only	bent tail
Control (5)	1-6	182.4 ± 90.4	104.0 ± 75.8	76.8 ± 13.0	1.6 ± 1.6	0
15.0 (5)	1-6	115.6 ± 24.5	0	28.0 ± 7.4	46.4 ± 6.9	41.6 ± 10.2
15.0/7.5 (5)	1-3/4-6	131.8 ± 29.5	0.6 ± 0.6	44.8 ± 13.3	51.3 ± 7.4	35.2 ± 8.2

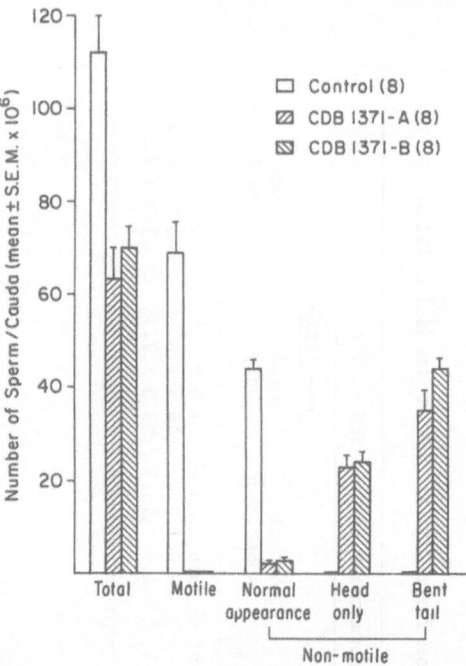

Fig. 5. Sperm concentration and differential sperm counts in male
         rats treated with impure and pure gossypol acetic acid at
         15 mg/kg/day for 8 weeks. CDB-1371-A = impure gossypol
         (92% pure); CDB-1371-B = pure gossypol (99% pure). The
         number of animals is indicated in <u>parentheses</u>.

     The effects of gossypol acetic acid treatment on epididymal
sperm are shown in Table 1. The spermatozoa recovered from the cauda
epididymis at the time of sacrifice showed abnormal morphology and
motility. Morphological abnormalities included sharply bent tails
and complete separation of the tail from the head. The total numbers
of sperm were significantly reduced in both treated groups. No motile sperm were found in animals receiving 15 mg/kg for 6 consecutive weeks. There were about 0.5% motile sperm found in animals receiving 7.5 mg/kg for the 4th, 5th, and 6th weeks.

Impurities of Gossypol in Relation to Toxicity and Antiferility Efficacy

     The growth rate of the animals receiving 15 mg/kg/day of impure
(CDB-1371-A) and pure (CDB-1371-B) gossypol acetic acid for 8 weeks
is shown in Fig. 4. There were no significant differences in body
weight gain between the two treated groups after 7 weeks' dosing.
The weight gain of the pure gossypol acetic acid treatment group was
significantly depressed by 4 weeks (p < 0.001) as compared with that

TABLE 2. Effect of Pure and Impure Gossypol on Fertility in Male Rats

Lot	Treatment* duration (weeks)	No. of positive matings / No. of animals used	No. of mated ♀s with implantation sites (%)	No. of implantation sites, mean ± SEM
Control	5	8/8	8 (100)	11.5 ± 1.5
CDB-1371-A†	5	7/7	3 (43)	1.6 ± 1.0
CDB-1371-B‡	5	6/8	0 (0)	0
Control	6	8/8	8 (100)	9.3 ± 1.4
CDB-1371-A	6	6/7	0 (0)	0
CDB-1371-B	6	8/8	0 (0)	0
Control	7	7/8	7 (100)	14.4 ± 0.6
CDB-1371-A	7	5/6	0 (0)	0
CDB-1371-B	7	5/6	0 (0)	0
Control	8	6/6	6 (100)	10.3 ± 1.2
CDB-1371-A	8	6/6	0 (0)	0
CDB-1371-B	8	4/6	0 (0)	0

*Animals received 15 mg/kg daily 6 times daily a week.
†Impure gossypol (impurity: 8%).
‡Pure gossypol (impurity: 0.999%).

of the controls. The growth rate of the animals receiving impure gossypol acetic acid was markedly reduced by 5 weeks of treatment.

Figure 5 shows the differential sperm counts of the animals treated with the impure and pure gossypol acetic acid. The sperm concentration was reduced by about 40% but none of the sperm were motile in both treatment groups. The numbers of non-motile sperm between the two treatment groups did not differ.

A summary of the results of fertility tests on animals receiving 15 mg/kg/day of impure and pure gossypol acetic acid after 5, 6, 7, and 8 weeks of treatment is presented in Table 2. There were no effects on the incidence of successful matings in both treatment groups during the 8-week treatment. None of the females mated with the males receiving pure gossypol acetic acid had implantation sites after 5 weeks of treatment. Three of 7 females mated with the males receiving impure gossypol acetic acid had implantation sites. However, the average number of implantation sites was significantly reduced.

There were no significant differences in organ weights of both treated groups.

DISCUSSION

Loss of body weight is one of the common symptoms of gossypol toxicity in laboratory animals. A variety of studies demonstrated that tolerance levels for gossypol were associated with the species. We first presented our preliminary data (at the PARFR Workshop on Gossypol) that gossypol toxicity was even related to the strain of rats [27]. In our previous study, there was no mortality at 15-30 mg/kg dose levels for 6-12 weeks when given to Sprague-Dawley strain of rats [28]. A dose of 40 mg/kg/day was chosen to insure that a response of strain differences would be seen in the present study. The data presented here demonstrate that the sensitivity to gossypol of the four strains of rats was markedly different. The same strain from different sources, such as Sprague-Dawley strain from Charles River and from Camm, responded differently. There are no apparent explanations for these differences. It is evident that Fisher strain was more sensitive to gossypol in regard to toxicity; Sprague-Dawley strain in the present study appeared to be more resistant to gossypol. There was no mortality in Sprague-Dawley and Wistar strains. Necropsies of animals of Long Evans strain and Fisher strain showed hemorrhages in the lung, liver, and spleen. The stomach and intestines were empty and ballooned. The loss of body weight and the symptoms of gossypol intoxication observed in our laboratory are similar to those found in the rats by others [29, 30, 31, 32].

We have demonstrated that administration of gossypol to rats of the Sprague-Dawley strain at a dose of 15 mg/kg/day caused significant reduction in growth rate. However, there is little or no depression of weight gain by a daily dose of 7.5 mg/kg, although this dose did not totally induce sterility after 12 weeks of treatment [33]. These findings prompted us to examine whether or not proper dosing would overcome the toxic effects of gossypol. In addition, it is relevant to examine whether or not food intake would be associated with dosing. The finding presented here demonstrated that body weight gain and food intake were not affected within the first three weeks of treatment at high dose (15 mg/kg). The body weight and food intake depressing effects became evident by the 4th week (Figs. 2 and 3). There were, however, no depression of body weight gain and food intake by reducing to one-half dose (7.5 mg/kg) given from the 4th week. Furthermore, under this 15/7.5 mg/kg dosing regimen, the animals were considered to be infertile on the basis of sperm count, and there were virtually no motile sperm in the cauda epididymis. In clinical trials in China, a loading dose was usually 20 mg/day for 60-75 days followed by a maintenance dose of 50-60 mg/week. Antifertility effects, as judged by sperm counts (below 4 million/ml), were manifested by the end of the loading phase [34, 35]. The common side effects noticed in the Chinese clinical trials were fatigue, intestinal symptoms, decreased libido, dizziness, and dryness of the mouth. It is unknown whether the side effects could be ascribed to the prolonged, high loading dose. Based on the present findings in the rat, clinical testing of a new protocol of the loading phase would be worthwhile.

Some investigators have speculated that part or all of the antifertility effect and toxicity of gossypol were caused by impurities in gossypol. The data presented in this study clearly show that the body weight gain (Fig. 4) and fertility rate of the impure gossypol-treated animals did not significantly differ from that of the pure gossypol-treated animals. In fact, the results indicated that the fertility rate of the impure gossypol-treated group was not reduced to zero until the 6th week of treatment, whereas the pure gossypol-treated group were totally sterile by the 5th week of treatment (Table 2). The results of the present experiment in the rats are in agreement with that of others, who reported that male rats became infertile when treated with 20 mg/kg/day for 6 weeks [36]. One team of researchers reported that in the hamster, pure gossypol (36 mg/kg) reduced fertility rate to zero and depressed weight gain after 6 weeks of dosing [37]. However, animals treated with impure gossypol (40 mg/kg, 90% pure) maintained constant fertility rates throughout the duration of the experiment. The investigators postulated that the impurities may inhibit the antifertility action of gossypol. In contrast, the data obtained in this experiment indicate that impure gossypol acetic acid (92% pure) given to the rat on a dose of 15 mg/kg induced immotile sperm in the cauda epididymis and, in fact, infertility occurred after 6 weeks of treatment. In the rat, we did not observe any differences between pure and impure gossypol in toxicity as well as in antifertility action. The differences in these two studies may be due to the different species and the different gossypol forms used. Since there are variances on the efficacy of gossypol as an antifertility agent in laboratory animals and as a potential method of human male fertility regulation, standardization of procedures for purification of gossypol or gossypol acetic acid and defining criteria for evaluation of its purity will be necessary.

REFERENCES

1. M. B. Abou-Donia, Physiological effects and metabolism of gossypol, Residue, Rev., 61:125 (1976).
2. L. C. Berardi and L. H. Goldblatt, Gossypol, in: "Toxic Constituents of Plant Foodstuffs" (I. E. Liener, ed.), p. 183, Academic Press, New York (1980).
3. M. B. Abou-Donia, 1976, op. cit. (see Ref. 1).
4. M. C. Chang, Z. P. Gu, and S. K. Saksena, Effects of gossypol on the fertility of male rats, hamsters, and rabbits, Contraception, 21:461 (1980).
5. S. K. Saksena, R. Salmonsen, I. F. Lau, and M. C. Chang, Gossypol: Its Toxicological and Endocrinological Effects in Male Rabbits, Contraception, 24:203 (1981).
6. M. R. N. Prasad and E. Diczfalusy, Gossypol, in: "Physiological and Medical Aspects of Andrology," International J. Andrology, Supplementum 5, pp. 53-70, Scriptor, Copenhagen (1982).
7. National Coordinating Group on Male Antifertility Agents, Gossypol - A new antifertility agent for males, Chinese Med. J., 4:417 (1978).
8. M. J. Nadakavukaren, R. H. Sorensen, and J. N. Tone, Effect of gossypol on the ultrastructure of rat spermatozoa, Cell Tissue Res., 204:293 (1979).
9. M. A. Hadley, Y. C. Lin, and M. Dym, Effects of gossypol on the reproductive system of male rats, J. Androl., 2:190 (1981).
10. A. P. Hoffer, Ultrastructural studies of spematozoa and the epithelial lining of the epididymis and vas deferens in rats treated with gossypol, Archives Androl., 8:233 (1982).
11. L. F. Zhou, C. C. Chen, N. G. Wang, and H. P. Lei, Observations on long-term administration of gossypol acetic acid to rats, Nat. Med. J., 60:343 (1980).
12. C. C. Chang, Z. P. Gu, and Y. Y. Tsong, Studies on gossypol. I. Toxicity, antifertility, and endocrine analyses in male rats, Int. J. Fertil., 27:213 (1982).
13. National Coordinating Group on Male Infertility Agents, 1978, op. cit. (see Ref. 7).
14. S. P. Xue, Studies on the antifertility effect of gossypol, a new contraceptive for males, in: "Recent Advances in Fertility

Regulation" (C. F. Chang, D. Griffin, and A. Woolman, eds.),
pp. 122-146, Atar, Geneva (1982).

15. M. A. Hadley, et al., 1981, op. cit. (see Ref. 9).
16. S. P. Xue, 1982, op. cit. (see Ref. 14).
17. R. X. Dai, S. N. Pang, X. K. Lin, Y. B. Ke, Z. L. Liu, and
    R. H. Dong, A study of antifertility effect of cottonseed,
    Acta Biol. Exp. Sinica, 11:1 (1978).
18. R. X. Dai, S. N. Pang, and Z. L. Liu, Studies on the anti-
    fertility effect of gossypol. 2. A morphological analysis of
    the antifertility effect of gossypol, Acta Biol. Exp. Sinica,
    11:27 (1978).
19. N. G. Wang and H. P. Lei, Antifertility effect of gossypol
    acetic acid on male rats, Chinese Med. J., 59:402 (1979).
20. M. A. Hadley, et al., 1981, op. cit. (see Ref. 9).
21. D. W. Hahn, C. Rusticus, A. Probst, R. Homm, and A. N. Johnson,
    Antifertility and endocrine activities of gossypol in rodents,
    Contraception, 24:97 (1981).
22. C. C. Chang, et al., 1982, op. cit. (see Ref. 12).
23. L. F. Zhou and H. P. Lei, Recovery of fertility in rats after
    gossypol treatment, in: "Recent Advances in Fertility Regula-
    tion" (C. F. Chang, D. Griffin, and A. Woolman, eds.), pp.
    147-151, Atar, Geneva (1982).
24. M. A. Hadley, et al., 1981, op. cit. (see Ref. 9).
25. C. C. Chang, et al., 1982, op. cit. (see Ref. 12).
26. S. P. Xue, 1982, op. cit. (see Ref. 14).
27. G. I. Zatuchni and C. K. Osborn, Gossypol: a possible male
    antifertility agent. Report of a workshop, Res. Frontiers in
    Fert. Reg., 1:1 (1981).
28. C. C. Chang, et al., 1982, op. cit. (see Ref. 12).
29. E. Eagle and H. F. Bialek, Toxicity and body weight-depressing
    effects in the rat of water-soluble combination products of
    gossypol, gossypol and cottonseed pigment glands, Food Res.,
    17:543 (1952).
30. F. H. Smith and A. J. Clawson, Effect of dietary gossypol on
    animals, J. Amer. Oil Chemist's Soc., 47:443 (1970).
31. M. C. Chang, et al., 1980, op. cit. (see Ref. 4).
32. D. W. Hahn, et al., 1981, op. cit. (see Ref. 21).
33. C. C. Chang, et al., 1982, op. cit. (see Ref. 12).
34. National Coordinating Group on Male Antifertility Agents, 1978,
    op. cit. (see Ref. 7).
35. G.-Z. Liu, et al., Trial of Gossypol as a Male Contraceptive,
    this volumer, pg. 9.
36. D. W. Hahn, et al., 1981, op. cit. (see Ref. 21).
37. D. P. Waller, H. H. S. Fong, G. A. Cordell, and D. D. Soejarto,
    Antifertility effects of gossypol and its impurities on male
    hamsters, Contraception, 23:653 (1981).

THE ARRHYTHOMOGENIC EFFECT OF GOSSYPOL

IN THE RAT HEART

Wei-min Huang,* Charles R. Katholi,†
and W. T. Woods‡

*Cardiovascular Research and Training Center
†Biostatistics and Biomathematics
‡Department of Physiology and Biophysics
 The University of Alabama
 School of Medicine
 Birmingham, Alabama

INTRODUCTION

Gossypol has been used as a male contraceptive for more than 10 years in China [1, 2]. It is considered to be highly effective, reversible, and inexpensive, but it has some reported side effects, one of which is cardiac arrhythmias. Gossypol has been at least circumstantially associated with sinus bradycardia, bundle branch block, premature beats, and ventricular fibrillation in some patients and experimental animals [3, 4, 5, 6, 7, 8]. However, the direct cardiac electrophysiologic effects of gossypol are virtually unknown. We report here on our investigation of the effects of gossypol on the transmembrane action potentials and impulse conduction velocities in atrial and ventricular muscle cells of isolated rat hearts.

MATERIALS AND METHODS

Hearts were rapidly removed from 24 ether-anesthetized rats and submerged in a physiologic solution at room temperature. The solution contained (in millimoles (mmol) per liter) Na^+, 145; K^+, 4.20; Ca^{2+}, 1.27; Mg^{2+}, 0.85; Cl^-, 124; SO_4^{2-}, 0.85; $H_2PO_4^-$, 2.40; HCO_3^-, 25; dextrose, 5.6. The solution was bubbled with 95% O_2 and 5% CO_2 so that in this and all test solutions PO_2 exceeded 500 mm Hg and pH was 7.4; temperature was maintained at 36 ± 1°C. Glass microelectrodes filled with 2.5 molar KCl and suspended on 30 gauge silver

wires were used to record action potentials and to display them on
an oscilloscope screen as previously described [9, 10]. Stimulation
of the cells was performed by a Grass S4 stimulator with SIU5 isolation unit and CCU IA constant current unit. Pulses were delivered
to the tissue via two silver wires spaced 2 mm apart. Stimulus
pulses (2 ms duration) were adjusted to be as close to threshold as
possible.

The cardiac apices were pinned to a wax-bottomed perfusion
bath (40 ml volume) at $36 \pm 1°C$. The aortae were perfused at 3 ml
per min through an 18 gauge stainless steel cannula within 5 min
after the heart was excised. A vent was cut in the apex of each
ventricle to allow perfusion fluid to drain into the bath. The
perfusate accumulated in the chamber to submerge the entire heart.

Action potentials were recorded continually in different atrial
and ventricular cells during exposure to gossypol for 60 min. Action
potential contours and relative conduction velocities (relative because they were measured between 2 points only) recorded at different
elapsed times (2 or more for each of the 24 atria and ventricles)
were plotted against time for each gossypol perfusion experiment.

From plots of the data versus time it was determined that a
straight line was a satisfactory model to describe the time trend
in each of the variables measured. A general linear model [11] of
the form

$$\text{variable} = \beta_0 + \sum_{i=1}^{p} \beta_i X_i + \alpha \text{ time} \tag{1}$$

$$X_i = \begin{cases} 1, & i^{th} \text{ sample} \\ -1, & (p+1)^{st} \text{ sample} \\ 0, & \text{otherwise} \end{cases}$$

$$p = (\text{number of tissue samples}) - 1$$

which assumes a common slope for the observations from all tissue
samples and allows different intercepts for each sample, was used as
the basis for the statistical analysis of the data. For any variable,
only the tissue samples which had data at two or more distinct points
in time were included in the analysis. The null hypothesis tested
was that of no time trend; that is $\alpha = 0$. A conservative approach
to testing this hypothesis was adopted in that a significant overall
regression was required as well as a rejection of the null hypothesis before concluding that a significant time trend was present.
The requirement of significant overall regression was included to
insure that the model [12] was adequate and appropriate to describe
the variation in the data. All tests were carried out at the 0.05
level of significance. All calculations were performed on an IBM
4341-2 using the Statistical Analysis System [13].

TABLE 1. Action Potentials Recorded in Rat Heart 3 ± 1 h After Excision

Rate (beats/min)	MDP (mv.)	V_{max} (v./s.)	Osht (mv.)	Ampl (mv.)	APD_{20} (ms.)	APD_{50} (ms.)	APD_{80} (ms.)	CV_{rel} (mm./sec)
Atrial Working Cells								
158	-77	240	14	90	7	19	37	637
±57	± 6	±50	± 5	± 6	± 4	± 9	±16	±426
(30)	(30)	(31)	(30)	(31)	(31)	(30)	(29)	(19)
Ventricular Working Cells								
	-80	230	9	89	6	13	28	853
	± 6	±50	± 6	± 6	± 3	± 6	±11	±365
	(23)	(24)	(23)	(24)	(24)	(24)	(23)	(18

MDP = maximum diastolic potential; V_{max} = maximum upstroke velocity; Osht = overshoot; Ampl = amplitude; APD_{20}, APD_{50}, APD_{80} = action potential durations at 20%, 50%, and 80% repolarization; CV_{rel} = relative conduction velocity (measured between 2 points only).

TABLE 2. Effects of Gossypol on Rat Heart Action Potentials

Measure-ment	Change	Prediction equation*	(P value)†	Correlation coefficient	N
		Atrial Working Cells			
Sinus rate	Decrease	= 193.1-1.9t (beats/min.)	<0.002	0.82	58
MDP	Decrease	= -75-0.2t (mv.)	<0.002	0.64	96
V_{max}	Decrease	= 204-1.6t (v./sec.)	<0.001	0.66	99
Osht	Decrease	= 11-0.1t (mv.)	<0.007	0.61	96
Ampl	Decrease	= 85-0.5t (mv.)	<0.002	0.66	100
APD_{20}	N. S.	--	--	--	54
APD_{50}	N. S.	--	--	--	94
APD_{80}	N. S.	--	--	--	91
CV_{rel}	N. S.	--	--	--	72
		Ventricular Working Cells			
MDP	N. S.	--	--	--	48
V_{max}	Decrease	= 227-3.3t (v./sec.)	<0.001	0.76	55
Osht	N. S.	(Decreased in more than half)	--	--	54
Ampl	Decrease	= 88-0.9t (mv.)	<0.006	0.73	55
APD_{20}	N. S.	--	--	--	94
APD_{50}	N. S.	--	--	--	54
APD_{80}	Decrease	= 32-0.6t (ms.)	<0.007	0.74	52
CV_{rel}	Decrease	= 861-11t (mm./sec.)	<0.016	0.82	31

*In these prediction equations, t = time of exposure to gossypol in minutes; N = number of data points used in fitting the regression model. Other abbreviations are the same as those used in Table 1.

†H_0: $\alpha = 0$ versus H_a: $\alpha = 0$.

RESULTS

Action Potentials of Rat Atrial and Ventricular Fibers

Only those action potentials recorded in the first 4 h after excision of hearts were analyzed (see Table 1). The gossypol vehicle (0.2% acetone or 0.1% ethanol in normal perfusate) was perfused into 3 hearts for one hour without gossypol. No significant (P = n.s.) changes in action potential morphologies or conduction velocities were observed. Therefore, the changes in cardiac action potentials in hearts that underwent gossypol perfusion were attributed to the presence of the drug.

Effects of Gossypol

The concentration of gossypol (1.0 mg/liter) tested in this study is less than the maximum possible blood concentration of gossypol (3.0 mg/liter) that could be theoretically achieved in humans taking the drug by mouth. Within 45 ± 15 min gossypol elicited the statistically significant changes in rat heart action potentials described in Table 2. After 60 ± 15 min all impaled cells in atria and ventricles were quiescent. Impulses delivered to the hearts directly by stimulating electrodes were unable to elicit action potentials.

Since these effects were time-dependent, all data were plotted with respect to the time elapsed since gossypol perfusion began. The significance (P < 0.05) of the resultant slope (effect/time) was tested, but this slope was considered significant only if the overall regression was also significant (P < 0.05). The prediction equation for the behavior of an arbitrary (as yet unmeasured) tissue sample is

$$\text{variable} = \hat{\beta}_0 + \hat{\alpha} \text{ time} \tag{2}$$

where $\hat{\beta}_0$ and $\hat{\alpha}$ are the least squares estimators of β_0 and α in Eq. (1). For each measurement, this prediction equation and the multiple correlation coefficient, R, from fitting the model (Eq. (1)) are given in Table 2. Actual P-values for the tests of the null hypothesis are given as well.

DISCUSSION

The tabulated results of this study show that gossypol elicited electrophysiologic changes in the rat heart that are potentially arrhythmogenic. Conduction velocity was reduced in ventricular cells, and this may be related to the fact that action potential maximum upstroke velocity in ventricular cells was markedly reduced by gossypol. Action potential duration was decreased in ventricular cells only, but any functional significance is questionable since this effect was

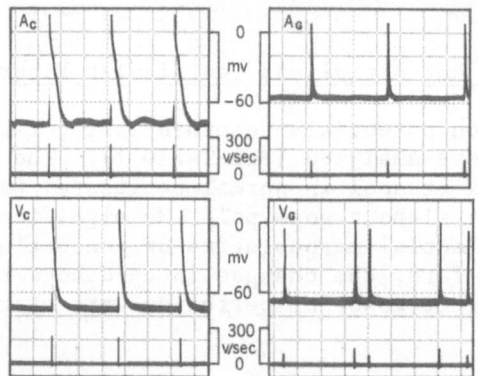

Fig. 1.   Action potentials were recorded in atrial cells (A_c) and
          ventricular cells (V_c) before gossypol was perfused. A_g
          and V_g show the effects of gossypol perfusion on an atrial
          cell after 33 min and on a ventricular cell after 31 min;
          all of these action potentials were recorded in the same
          heart.   Sinus rate slowing is illustrated in A_g and a typi-
          cal arrhythmia is illustrated in V_g.   Action potential up-
          strokes were electronically differentiated and displayed
          below the action potentials.   Calibrations are identical in
          each panel.   Each major horizontal division is 0.1 sec.
          Records were retouched to enhance clarity.

relatively small (only 18 ms decrease after 30 min).   Maximum diastolic potentials remained constant in ventricular cells and fell
very slowly in atrial cells.   Therefore, changes in resting potential
cannot be responsible for the other electrophysiologic effects.   The
predominant and consistent effects of gossypol were decreases in
heart rate, maximum upstroke velocity, overshoot, and amplitude.

     This combination of factors can promote arrhythmias.   Lowering
the firing rate normally causes lengthening of the ventricular action
potential and, therefore, longer refractory period.   But this pro-
tective event was counteracted by gossypol which shortened ventricular action potential duration.   This makes the ventricles more vulnerable to rapid repetitive stimulation (ventricular tachycardia).
Conduction velocity was substantially reduced in the rat ventricles
by gossypol.   Slow conduction of the ventricular impulse can lead to
re-entrant ventricular tachycardia [14].   Accordingly, ventricular
tachyarrhythmias were observed in over 80% of the hearts exposed to
gossypol for 30 min or more (example in Fig. 1).   Conduction velocity
was not decreased in atrial cells, but the maximum diastolic potential
fell progressively.   Depolarization of the diastolic potential continuing over a long period of time can eventually lead to slower impulse conduction and emergence of ectopic atrial pacemakers [14].

Some of gossypol's effects on action potentials could be mediated by cardiac nerves. However, it appears unlikely that acetylcholine (possibly released from parasympathetic nerves) accounts for the changes, since in the isolated canine right atrium it increases maximum diastolic potential and shortens action potential duration when its concentration is adequate to reduce sinus rate to the extent we observed [15]. We cannot rule out a possible attenuation of norepinephrine effects (from sympathetic nerves) as a minor part of the mechanism for the negative chronotropic action of gossypol.

Gossypol has a potent effect on action potentials in the rat heart. Whether the potency of this drug is similar in other mammals, including humans, remains to be demonstrated. The minimal effect on resting transmembrane potential suggests that future studies should also explore effects of gossypol on transmembrane ion flux during cardiac action potentials.

ACKNOWLEDGMENTS

The authors thank Dr. Stephen M. Cain and Dr. Keith V. Kuhlemeier for providing the experimental subjects. This research was supported by grants from The Rockefeller Foundation, the National Heart, Lung, and Blood Vessel Institute, and the U.S. Army Medical Research and Development Command.

REFERENCES

1. National Coordinating Group on Male Fertility, A new male contraceptive drug - cotton phenol (Gossypol), Chinese Medical Journal, 4:417 (1978).
2. G. I. Zatuchni and C. K. Osborn, Gossypol: A possible male antifertility agent. Report of a Workshop, in: "Research Frontiers in Fertility Regulation," Vol. 1, No. 4, pp. 1 (1981).
3. Pei-de Chang, et al., Study of toxicity of gossypol in the dog. Symposium on gossypol research at Shandong Institute of Chinese Traditional Medicine, p. 163 (1980).
4. Ru-huan Gao, et al., The effects of high doses of gossypol on phrenic nerve, diaphragm, and myocardial electrical activity, presented at the Chinese National Meeting on Gossypol at Qin Huang Dao (1980).
5. Shaanxi Clinical Coordinating Group on Male Fertility, Clinical observations concerning gossypol acetate in 508 cases, presented at the Chinese National Meeting on Gossypol at Quin Huang Dao (1980).
6. Shanghai Clinical Study Group on Gossypol, Male contraceptive - gossypol: Clinical results in 330 trial cases, presented at the Chinese National Meeting on Gossypol at Qin Huang Dao (1980).

7.   National Coordinating Group on Gossypol, Gossypol as oral con-
     traceptive for males; 880 cases clinical trial report, pre-
     sented at the Chinese National Meeting on Gosypol at Qin Huang
     Dao (1980).
8.   Beijing Coordinating Group on Gossypol, Results of Clinical
     trials of gossypol in the Beijing area, presented at the
     Chinese National Meeting on Gossypol at Quin Huang Dao (1980).
9.   W. T. Woods, F. Urthaler, and T. N. James, Spontaneous action
     potentials of cells in the canine sinus node, Circulation Re-
     search, 39:76 (1976).
10. W. T. Woods, L. Sherf, and T. N. James, Structure and function
     of specific regions in the canine atrioventricular node, Am.
     J. Physiol., 243:H41 (1982).
11. N. R. Draper and H. Smith, Applied Regression Analysis, 2nd
     Edition, John Wiley and Sons, Inc., New York (1981).
12. SAS User's Guide, SAS Institute, Inc., Cary, North Carolina
     (1982).
13. P. F. Cranefield, The Conduction of the Cardiac Impulse,
     Futura Press, Mt. Kisco, New York (1975).
14. Ibid.
15. W. T. Woods, F. Urthaler, and T. N. James, Electrical activity
     in canine sinus node cells during arrest produced by acetyl-
     choline, J. Molec. Cell. Cardiol., 13:349 (1981).

GOSSYPOL STUDIES IN MALE RATS

Chin-Chuan Chang, Zhiping Gu,
and Yun-Yen Tsong

Center for Biomedical Research
The Population Council
New York, New York

INTRODUCTION

Gossypol, a yellow phenolic pigment of the cotton plant [1], has occupied the attention of agricultural research groups for many years because of its toxicity to monogastric animals. The usual manifestations of toxicity are depressed appetite, loss of body weight and inefficient protein utilization [2, 3, 4]. New interest in gossypol emerged from the finding that it inhibits the fertility of males of several species [5]. Although the initial observations were made in man, studies have also been made in laboratory animals. For example, male rats became infertile when gossypol acetic acid was administered orally for several weeks [6, 7]. The time to onset of infertility and the appearance of toxic signs were dose related. Decapitated spermatozoa, spermatozoa with bent tails, spermatids and spermatocytes were observed in the cauda epididymidis and vas deferens of gossypol-treated rats. Normal mating behavior was maintained in spite of infertility. The time until recovery of fertility after discontinuation of treatment was dependent on the dose and duration of treatment.

Although gossypol has been tested clinically in China as a male contraceptive with encouraging results, details of its physiological effects, mode of action and reversibility are imperfectly understood. Several studies suggest that the laboratory rat is a satisfactory model for such studies [8, 9, 10, 11, 12]. Although it is less sensitive than man to the antifertility effects of gossypol, it is more sensitive than several other species such as the mouse and rabbit. We have therefore used the rat in the present study to examine the relation between effective and toxic doses; the effects

on spermatogenesis, mating behavior, and fertility; and the effects
on hormones known to play a role in spermatogenesis.

MATERIALS AND METHODS

    Adult male rats of Sprague-Dawley strain weighing 280-300 gm
obtained from the Charles River Breeding Laboratories (Waltam, MA)
were used. Animals were housed in a temperature (76-80°F) and illumination (14 h light and 10 h dark) controlled room and maintained
on Purine laboratory chow and tap water ad libitum. Twelve animals
were assigned to each treatment group and 12 to control groups. The
body weight was recorded weekly and the weights of the following
organs were determined at autopsy: testes, epididymides, seminal
vesicles, prostate, liver, spleen, kidney, thymus, adrenals, thyroid,
and pituitary. The primary and accessory sex organs were fixed in
Bouin's solution. Histological sections were stained with hema-
toxylin and eosin. Animals treated with the highest dose (30 mg/
kg/day) were killed after 6 weeks of treatment and animals with the
lower doses (15 and 7.5 mg/kg/day) were killed after 12 weeks, except for a cohort of 6 animals treated at the 15 mg/kg level which
were permitted a 6-week recovery period before sacrifice.

    Blood was collected at the termination of treatment by decapi-
tation. The blood was allowed to clot at room temperature for several hours and then at 4°C overnight and subsequently centrifuged
at 3000 rpm for 20 min. Serum was separated and stored at -24°C
until assayed.

    Fertility tests were carried out after various durations of
treatment by mating each male with a 30-day old female rat treated
with 10 IU of pregnant mare serum gonadotropin (Sigma) in accord-
ance with the procedure described elsewhere [13]. Positive matings
were verified by the presence of either copulation plugs or by a
finding of sperm in the vaginal smear taken the following morning.
The mated females were autopsied on Day 9 after mating and the implantation sites counted.

Gossypol Acetic Acid Treatment

    Three batches of gossypol acetic acid were used in the experi-
ment. Two were obtained from the Beijing Institute of Zoology,
Beijing, China, and one from the Shanghai Institute of Materia Medica.
The purity of the three batches of gossypol acetic acid was assayed
(by Dr. H. K. Kim of the Center for Population Research, National
Institute of Child Health and Human Development, Bethesda, Md.) by
analytical high pressure liquid chromatography (HPLC) using reverse
phase $C_{18\mu}$-Bondapak column (acetonitrile:water, 70:30 with 1% acetic
acid; 4 ml/min, 0.5 cm/min, UV detector at 254 nm). The sample was
dissolved in acetone before injection. The HPLC traces were xeroxed

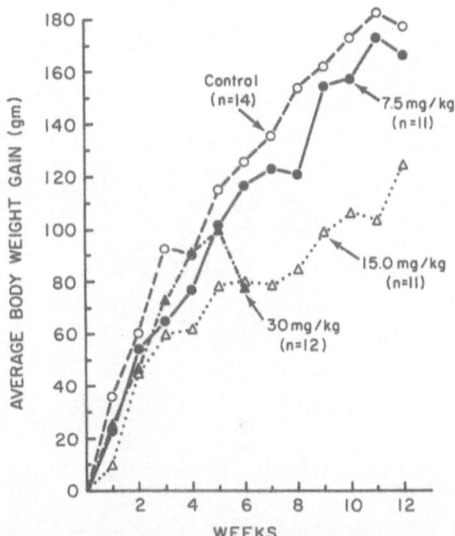

Fig. 1. Growth rates of male rats administered gossypol by gavage
         at 7.5 and 15 mg/kg daily for 12 weeks, and 30 mg/kg daily
         for 6 weeks.

and the peaks of gossypol acetic acid and impurities were cut and
weighed. The weight thus obtained was divided by the total weight
of both peaks and multiplied by 100 to give the percentage of gossypol acetic acid and impurities in each sample. Not more than 1.5%
impurity was found in any of the batches.

       Gossypol acetic acid powder was placed in a brown bottle covered
with black paper and stored at -20°C. Gossypol acetic acid suspension was prepared twice a week for oral administration by suspending
it in sesame oil (Sigma) with the aid of 0.5% trigancanth gum (Sigma).
Doses of 7.5, 15.0, and 30.0 mg/kg of body weight/day of gossypol in
0.4-0.5 ml of the suspending vehicle were given 6 times a week for
either 6 or 12 weeks by means of a gavage needle inserted into the
stomach of the animal. Control animals were administered an equal
volume of the vehicle.

Epididymal Spermatozoal Count

       At autopsy, one cauda epididymis from each animals was minced
to release the sperm into 2 ml of Medium 199 (Grand Island Biological
Co.) containing 1% deactivated fetal calf serum. The suspension was
thoroughly mixed and serially diluted in two steps by transferring
50 µl into 2 ml of the Medium at each step. The morphology, motility, and the number of spermatozoa in each cauda were examined in
4 hemacytometer chambers and the total sperm in the cauda computed.

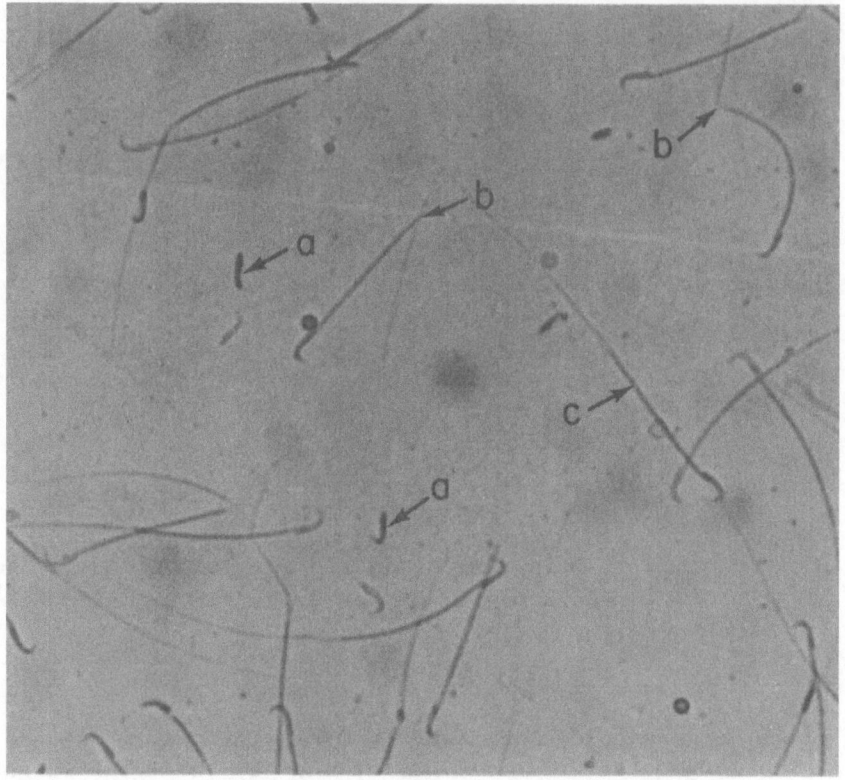

Fig. 2.   Photomicrograph of epididymal spermatozoa of a rat treated
          with 7.5 mg/kg of gossypol. a) Decapitated sperm; b) bent
          tail sperm; c) motile sperm (original magnification,
          ×200).

Radioimmunoassays

The double antibody RIA technique was used to determine serum
LH and FSH levels [14].   Results were expressed in nanograms per
milliliter of serum.   Standards were NIH-LH-RP1 (biological potency,
0.03 × NIH-LH-S1) and NIH-FSH-RP1 (biological potency, 2.1 × NIH-
FSH-S1) for LH and FSH, respectively.   Serum testosterone levels
were estimated by RIA as described by Midgley [15]. $[1,2-^3H]$ testosterone (43.5 Ci/mmol, SA) and the antiserum against testosterone-
3-oxime-BSA were purchased from New England Nuclear.   All assays
were performed in duplicate.

Statistical Evaluation

The results were expressed as mean plus or minus standard error
of the mean.   The data were analyzed for statistical significance
by Student's t-test.

TABLE 1.   Effect of Gossypol on Fertility in the Male Rat

Duration (wk)	Dose (mg/kg)	No. of positive matings / No. of animals used	No. of mated females with implantation sites (%)	No. of implantation sites per animal mean ± SEM
Treatment				
-	Control	7/8	7 (100)	12.0 ± 0.3
	7.5	8/10	8 (100)	9.8 ± 1.0
	15.0	7/10	2 (28.6)	2.5 ± 0.5
8	Control	6/8	5 (83.3)	10.2 ± 1.4
	7.5	6/10	3 (50)	9.6 ± 2.0
	15.0	7/10	1 (14.3)	3.0
12	Control	7/8	6 (85.7)	10.3 ± 1.8
	7.5	8/10	1 (16.7)	2.0
	15.0	6/10	0 (0)	0
Posttreatment[b]				
6	Control	5/5	4 (80)	12.0 ± 0.7
	15.0	5/5	5 (100)	12.4 ± 0.4

[a] Each Sprague-Dawley male was exposed to a 30-day old female which had been ovulated with 10 IU pregnant mare serum gonadotropin. A positive mating was verified by observing a vaginal plug or sperm in the vagina. Implantation sites were counted 9 days after mating.

[b] Fertility of the rats treated at 7.5 mg/kg dose of gossypol was not tested.

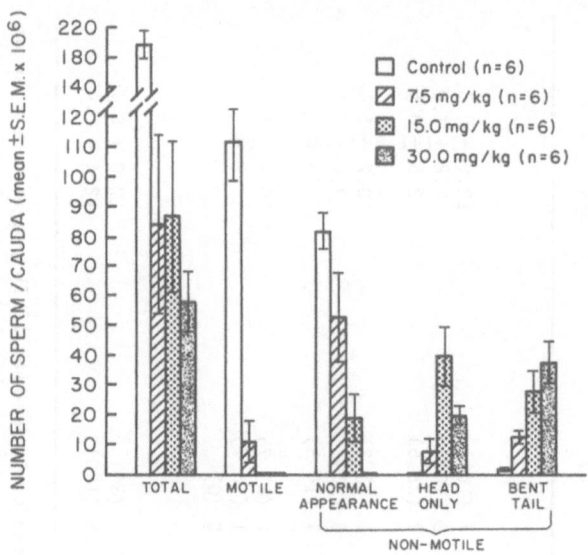

Fig. 3.   Sperm concentrations and differential sperm counts after
dosing rats at 7.5 or 15 mg/kg/day for 12 weeks or 30 mg/
kg/day for 6 weeks.

RESULTS

Growth Rate

     The growth of rats treated 6 days with 7.5, 15.0, or 30.0 mg/kg
of gossypol are shown in Fig. 1.   Animals receiving the 7.5 mg/kg
dose gained weight nearly as rapidly as the controls.   A dose of
15.0 mg/kg markedly slowed the growth and at the end of the 12-week
treatment period, animals in this group had gained only 70% as much
as control animals.   When they were terminated at 6 weeks, animals
receiving 30 mg/kg had gained 61% as much as control animals.

Fertility Test

     A summary of the results of fertility tests on animals receiv-
ing 7.5 or 15 mg/kg after 4, 8, and 12 weeks' treatment is presented
in Table 1.   There were no significant effects on the incidence of
unsuccessful matings at the 7.5 and 15 mg/kg dose levels during the
12 weeks' treatment.   There was, however, a marked reduction in fertility after 4 weeks' treatment at the 15 mg/kg dose level and after
12 weeks at the 7.5 mg/kg dose level.   To examine recovery of fertility after discontinuation of treatment, a mating test was carried
out on 5 rats treated for 12 weeks at the 15 mg/kg dose level and
then allowed a six-week recovery period.   Their fertility matched

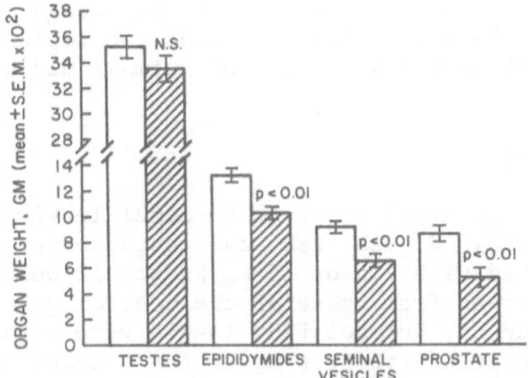

Fig. 4. Effect of gossypol at 30 mg/kg dose level for 6 weeks on
         the weights of accessory sex organs of rats compared with
         control animals sacrificed at the same time. The average
         body weight of treated animals was 61% as much as that of
         controls. Open bars represent controls and hatched bars
         gossypol treated animals.

that of the untreated controls and thus indicated that recovery had
occurred (Table 1).

Sperm Motility, Morphology, and Concentration

     The spermatozoa recovered from the cauda epididymidis showed
abnormal motility and morphology at the time of sacrifice - 6 weeks
for animals receiving 30 mg/kg/day and 12 weeks for animals receiving 7.5 or 15 mg/kg/day. Morphological abnormalities included
sharply bent tails and complete separation of the tail from the head
(Fig. 2). The effects of gossypol treatment on epididymal sperm are
shown graphically in Fig. 3. All dose levels reduced the total number of sperm to less than 50% of those in control animals and most
of the sperm from treated animals were immotile. In fact, at the
two highest dose levels, no motile sperm were found. The number of
spermatozoa with normal appearance decreased progressively with increasing dose, the numbers with bent tails and separated heads increased.

Organ Weights

     There were no significant differences in the weights of testes,
epididymides, seminal vesicles, prostate, liver, spleen, kidney,
thymus, adrenals, thyroid or pituitary of the animals treated with
either 7.5 or 15.0 mg/kg of gossypol for 12 weeks as compared to
those of the control animals. However, gossypol at 30.0 mg/kg significantly reduced the weights of epididymides, seminal vesicles and

prostate by 6 weeks (p < 0.01); the testicular weight was not affected (Fig. 4). Histological examinations of the testes, epididymides,
prostate and seminal vesicles of treated animals did not show deviation from normal.

Serum Hormonal Levels

The effects of gossypol on serum hormonal levels of male rats
are summarized in Table 2. LH, FSH, and testosterone serum levels
among animals treated with 7.5 or 15 mg/kg for 12 weeks were not
significantly different from those of the control group. However,
the testosterone and LH, but not FSH, levels were significantly
lower in animals treated with 30.0 mg/kg for 6 weeks (p < 0.01).

DISCUSSION

It has been previously reported that administration of gossypol
to rats at doses of 20 to 40 mg/kg per day causes retarded weight
gain [16, 17, 18]. In the present experiments, there was little or
no depression by doses 7.5 mg/kg/day. However, body weight gain of
male rats was significantly depressed by 15 mg/kg per day. The animals receiving 30 mg/kg per day grew almost as rapidly as controls
for 5 weeks but then lost weight rapidly; they were sacrificed at
6 weeks because of their poor health.

Although the pattern of toxicity observed in the present study
matched those of several subsequent experiments in our laboratory
in which gossypol was administered for different purposes, we observed much greater toxicity in two earlier trials of gossypol (results not shown). In these earlier trials, 41 of 54 rats dies within
10 days on a dose of 20 mg/kg/day, and 18 of 54 and 3 of 16 died
within 6 weeks at 10 mg/kg/day. Animals characteristically showed
loss of body weight, sluggish behavior and a yellow hair color.
Necropsies showed hemorrhages in the lung, liver, and spleen. The
stomach and intestines were empty and ballooned. The body weight-
depressing effect and the symptoms of gossypol toxicity observed in
our laboratory are similar to those found in the rat by Eagle and
Bialek [19] and Smith and Clawson [20]. No explanation for these
differences in dose levels required for gross toxicity are apparent.
The rats were of the Sprague-Dawley strain (Camm, N.J.) and were
administered gossypol in the same vehicle and in the same volume as

TABLE 2. Effect of Gossypol on Serum Hormonal Levels of Male Rats

Treatment			Serum hormonal levels, ng/ml $\pm$ SEM		
Dose (mg/kg)	Duration (wk)	No. of animals	Testosterone	LH	FSH
Control	1?	5	8.3 $\pm$ 1.6	64.0 $\pm$ 4.6	471.2 $\pm$ 42.1
7.5	12	6	7.1 $\pm$ 2.5	71.9 $\pm$ 5.6	396.6 $\pm$ 55.5
15.0	12	6	7.7 $\pm$ 2.4	84.0 $\pm$ 10.6	387.5 $\pm$ 28.1
30.0	6	5	3.7 $\pm$ 0.7[a]	46.3 $\pm$ 2.1[a]	553.5 $\pm$ 66.9

[a] Significantly different from controls (P<0.01).

in the present experiments. HPL chromatography of the gossypol showed less than 2% impurity, an amount not greater than in the gossypol used in later experiments. Technical errors would seem to be ruled out since there was no mortality at 5.0 and 7.5 mg/kg/day given in the same volume in the earlier experiments (16 weeks) or with the 15 mg or 30 mg/kg/day doses in the present study (12 and 6 weeks, respectively).

The findings in the present study are in rough agreement with others who reported that male rats became infertile but maintained nomral mating behavior when treated with 15 to 40 mg/kg by gavage 5 times a week [21]. The time required to attain infertility was, however, greater in the present study (12 vs. 2 to 4 weeks). Our findings are also in agreement with the studies showing that the onset of antifertility effect is dose-related and is characterized by a reduction in sperm concentration [22]. The data obtained in the present study clearly demonstrate that as the number of sperm in the epididymides decreases, the number of motile sperm decreases and the proportion of non-motile sperm increases. Immotile sperm include decapitated and bent-tail sperm as well as sperm of normal appearance.

Our observations on the reduction in serum levels of testosterone and LH, but not FSH, in animals treated with 30 mg/kg for 6 weeks

are in accord with other data [23]. The decrease in LH and testosterone could be a function of weight loss since similar decreases
are found in starvation and diabetes [24, 25].

The weights of testes, epididymides, seminal vesicles, prostate,
liver, kidney, spleen, adrenals, thyroid, and pituitary of the animals treated with 7.5 and 15 mg/kg of gossypol for 12 weeks were not
significantly different from those of the control groups. In contrast, one team of investigators have observed that the weight of
the adrenals after 8 weeks' treatment was significantly increased
with a 5 mg/kg dose and significantly decreased with a 10 mg/kg dose
[26]. In the present study, the weights of the accessory sex organs,
but not the weight of testes, were significantly reduced at the 30
mg/kg dose level for 6 weeks. These changes probably resulted from
the reduction in the sperm levels of testosterone and LH with this
regimen. Since in the present study there was no significant change
in serum levels of testosterone, LH, or FSH in animals receiving 7.5
and 15 mg/kg doses of gossypol, it appears that the mechanism of contraceptive action of gossypol at these levels is independent of any
change in the endocrine system. At the highest dose level, however,
depressed testosterone and LH levels may play a role in infertility.
The decreased levels may reflect effects on the Leydig cells.
Whether the observed effects on growth and reproduction are related
to the effects of gossypol on iron metabolism and protein utilization [13] is unknown.

REFERENCES

1.   R. Adams, T. A. Geissman, and J. D. Edwards, Gossypol, a pig-
     ment of cottonseed, Chem. Rev., 60:555 (1960).
2.   L. C. Berardi and L. H. Goldblatt, Gossypol, in: "Toxic Con-
     stituents of Plant Foodstuffs" (I. E. Liener, ed.), Academic
     Press, New York (1969).
3.   L. A. Jones and F. H. Smith, Effect of bound gossypol and amino
     acid supplementation of glandless cottonseed meal on the growth
     of weanling rats, J. Animal Sci., 44:401 (1977).
4.   L. A. Jones and F. H. Smith, Effect of gossypol on the removal
     of nitrogen and amino acids from feed in digestion of the rat,
     J. Animal Sci., 44:410 (1977).
5.   National Coordinating Group on Male Antifertility Agents:
     Gossypol - A New Antifertility Agent for Males, Chinese Med. J.,
     5:517 (1978).
6.   Ibid.
7.   R. X. Dai, S. N. Pang, X. K. Lin, Y. B. Ke, Z. L. Liu, and
     R. H. Dong, A study of antifertility of cottonseed, Acta Biol.
     Exp. Sinica, 11:1 (1978).
8.   National Coordinating Group on Male Antifertility Agents, 1978,
     op. cit. (see Ref. 5).

9. R. X. Dai, et al., 1978, op. cit. (see Ref. 7).
10. R. X. Dai and R. H. Dong, Studies on antifertility effect of gossypol. 1. An experimental analysis of epididymal ligature, Acta Biol. Exp. Sinica, 11:15 (1978).
11. S. P. Hsueh, S. T. Tsong, S. Y. Su, Y. W. Wu, Y. Liu, T. H. Chou, and H. H. Ma, Cytological, radioautograph and ultrastructural observations on the antispermatogenesis action of gossypol in the rat, Scientia Sinica, 9:915 (1979).
12. R. X. Dai, S. N. Pang, and Z. L. Liu, Studies on the antifertility effect of gossypol. 2. A morphological analysis of the antifertility effect of gossypol, Acta Biol. Exp. Sinica, 11:27 (1978).
13. J. T. Wu and R. K. Meyer, Delayed implantation in gonadotropin-treated immature rats, Proc. Soc. Exp. Biol. Med., 123:88 (1966).
14. G. D. Niswander, A. R. Midgley, S. E. Monroe, and L. E. Reichert, Radioimmunoassay for rat luteinzing hormone with anti-ovine LH serum and ovine LH-^{131}I, Proc. Soc. Exp. Biol. Med., 128:807 (1968).
15. A. R. Midgley and G. D. Niswender, Radioimmunoassay of steroids, Acta Endocrinol. (Kbh) 147:320 (1970).
16. L. A. Jones and F. H. Smith, 1977, op. cit. (see Ref. 4).
17. J. E. Braham and R. Brensani, Effect of different levels of gossypol on transaminase activity, on non-essential to essential amino acids ratio, and on iron and nitrogen retention in rats, J. Nutrition, 105:348 (1975).
18. E. Eagle and H. F. Biacek, Toxicity and body weight-depressing effects in the rat of water-soluble combination products of gossypol, gossypol and cottonseed pigment glands, Food Res., 17:543 (1952).
19. Ibid.
20. F. H. Smith and A. J. Clawson, Effect of dietary gossypol on animals, J. Am. Oil Chemist's Soc., 47:443 (1970).
21. R. X. Dai, et al., 1978, op. cit. (see Ref. 7).
22. National Coordinating Group on Male Antifertility Agents, 1978, op. cit. (see Ref. 5).
23. Y. C. Lin, N. A. Hadley, D. Klingener, and M. Dym, Effects of gossypol on the reproductive system of male rats, Biol. Reprod., 22 (Suppl. No. 1) abstract p, 95a (1980).
24. W. O. Maddock and C. G. Heller, Dichotomy between hypophyseal content and amount of circulating gonadotropins during starvation, Proc. Soc. Biol. Med., 66:595 (1947).
25. P. Horstmann, Excretion of androgens in human diabetes mellitus, Acta Endocrinol., 5:261 (1950).
26. M. C. Chang, Z. P. Gu, and S. K. Saksena, Effects of gossypol on the fertility of male rats, hamsters, and rabbits, Contraception, 21:461 (1980).

EMBRYONIC AND REPRODUCTIVE TOXICITY

EVALUATION OF GOSSYPOL

Gerhard F. Weinbauer,* Natwar R. Kalla,†
and Julian Frick‡

*Zoological Institute
 University of Salzburg
 Salzburg, Austria

†Department of Biophysics
 Panjab University
 Chandigarh, India

‡Urological Department
 General Hospital
 Salzburg, Austria

INTRODUCTION

Increased attention is now being given to gossypol, and researchers are studying its ability to act as a male fertility-regulating agent. The non-mutagenicity of gossypol has been documented
by several investigators [1, 2, 3], and we present evidence for the
embryonic and reproductive non-toxicity of gossypol acetic acid in
rats.

MATERIALS AND METHODS

Adult male and female Wistar rats were purchased from Chemie
Linz AG. Animals were kept under controlled environmental conditions with a commercial diet and tap water ad libitum. Gossypol
acetic acid (GAA) solutions were prepared according to the method
of Reiser and Fu [4]; GAA was dissolved in ethanol, glycerol was
added and the alcohol was evaporated under reduced pressure. The
mixture was then diluted with water for appropriate concentrations
of GAA.

GAA was administered daily by oral intubation (0.2 ml) without
anesthesia at concentrations of 5 mg/kg (N = 7), 10 mg/kg (N = 9),
and 25 mg/kg (N = 7) on days 5-15 of pregnancy. Control animals received the vehicle (glycerol, N = 6) or were left untreated (N = 7).
Females were cohabited with 2 or 3 males overnight, and the presence
of the copulatory plug was evaluated as day 1 of gestation.

Body weight was recorded daily until parturition. Animals who
did not give birth were killed, and the uteri were checked for implants. Litter sizes and weights were recorded on days 1 and 21
after birth. No sex distinction was made. Some of the young males
(5 per group) were sacrificed 50-55 days after birth. Main organs
and viscera were examined macroscopically for alterations. The
testes were excised and weighed. Other male and female pups were
raised to adulthood (F_1-generation). Males from GAA-treated mothers
were mated with females from control mothers and vice versa.

Parts of the litters (F_2-generation) were weighed on day of
birth, and were raised and mated as described for the F_1-generation.

Statistical Evaluation

Data from litters were analyzed by ANOVA, Kruskal-Wallis-test
and χ^2-test as recommended for this type of study [5]. For the
analysis of variance procedures, the mean fetal characteristics
(equivalent to number of mothers per group) rather than the individual ones (numbers of litters per group) were used as sample
units [6].

For group body weight analysis throughout the time period, the
Spearman correlation coefficient (r_s) was tested for significance
[7]. The relative body weight gain was estimated by the body weight
ratios between days 15:5 and 21:15. Values are expressed as mean ±
S.E.M.

RESULTS

Maternal Effects

Of the females exhibiting the copulatory plug after mating,
66% (25 out of 38) were impregnated. Birth occurred in 57% (8 out
of 14) of the control and in 71% (17 out of 24) of the GAA-treated
animals (p > 0.10). In the 5 mg/kg GAA-group one animal which did
not deliver was found to have 3 normally developed fetuses in the
uterus.

As Table 1 shows, non-pregnant control animals maintained their
body weight throughout the experimental period. Animals given 10
mg/kg and 25 mg/kg of GAA showed significantly negative body weight

TABLE 1. Body Weight Responses of Non-Pregnant Rats during Gossypol Acetic Acid (GAA) Treatment (mg/kg/d)

Treatment	No. of animals	Mean body weight (±S.E.M.)				Correl. Coeff. significance
		A	B	C	D	
Control	2	264 ±13	277 ±14	275 ±25	272 ±14	0.153 >0.10
Placebo	3	250 ± 6.1	277 ± 8.3	271 ±10	273 ±10	0.273 >0.10
10 mg GAA	3	240 ± 5.8	239 ±13	246 ±24	236 ±35	-0.412 <0.05
25 mg GAA	4	237 ± 7.5	238 ± 5.2	225 ±11	216 ±13	-0.640 <0.01

Note: A = start of experiment; B = start of treatment (for 10 days consecutively); C = termination of treatment; and D = one week after termination.

TABLE 2. Body Weight Responses of Pregnant Rats during Gossypol Acetic Acid (GAA) Treatment (mg/kd/d) on Days 5-15 of Pregnancy

Treat-ment	No. of animals	Mean body weight (±S.E.M.)				Correl. coeff. signifi-cance	Body weight ratio	
		A	B	C	D		C/B	D/C
Control	5	247 ± 8.2	261 ± 8.4	288 ±11	366 ±16	0.927 <0.01	1.100	1.26
Placebo	3	253 ± 3.3	263 ± 7.2	289 ± 6.1	360 ±22	0.886 <0.01	1.100	1.28
5 mg GAA	6	246 ± 4.4	258 ± 5.3	277 ± 6.2	342 ±16	0.968 <0.01	1.060	1.24
10 mg GAA	6	262 ± 4.0	262 ± 8.7	284 ±10	346 ± 9.8	0.936 <0.01	1.080	1.21
25 Mg GAA	3	218 ±11	235 ±12	237 ±13	302 ±11	-0.181 >0.10	1.009	1.27

Note: A = start of experiment; B = start of treatment; C = termination of treatment; and D = day before birth.

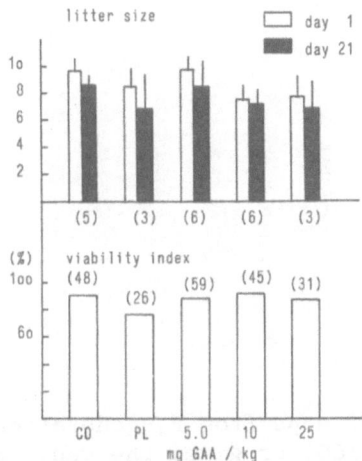

Fig. 1. Litter size (upper panel) and viability index on day 21
         (lower panel) of pups from F_1-generation. Mothers were
         left untreated (CO) or given the vehicle (PL) or gossypol
         acetic acid (GAA). Differences are not significant (p >
         0.10). Number of mothers per group (upper panel) and
         number of pups (lower panel) is put in parentheses.

tendency (r_s = -0.142, p < 0.05 and r_s = -0.640, p < 0.01 respectively). Within the group receiving 5 mg/kg of GAA, one female was
not pregnant. This animal displayed positive weight tendency (r_s =
0.540, p < 0.01).

    The body weight curves of pregnant females were characterized
by a sharp increase with day 15 of gestation. The gestational period was 21-22 days. During the treatment period (days 5-15), body
weight responses were positively correlated with time (r_s = 0.886-
0.986, p < 0.01) except for the 25 mg/kg dose group (r_s = -0.181,
p < 0.01, Table 2). In the last week of pregnancy, weight was increased for all groups with a body weight ratio between days 21-
22:15 ranging from 1.21-1.27 as can be seen in Table 2. This is
suggestive of normal fetal weight gain.

F₁-Generation

    Seventy-four pups were born to control females of which 7 (9%)
were found dead. One hundred and thirty-five pups were born from
GAA-treated females of which 13 (10%) were stillborn (p > 0.10₀.

    The litter size/female/group (Fig. 1) varied from 7.5 ± 1.3 to
9.8 ± 1.0 (p > 0.10) at birth and from 6.7 ± 2.4 to 8.6 ± 2.8 (p >
0.10) at weaning (21 days after birth). The viability index (%)

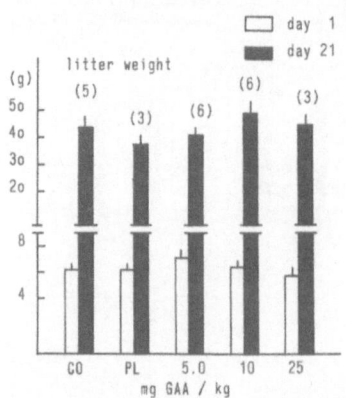

Fig. 2. Litter weight of pups from F_1-generation. Mothers were
         left untreated (CO) or given the vehicle (PL) or gossypol
         acetic acid (GAA). Differences are not significant (p >
         0.10). Number of mothers per group is put in parentheses.

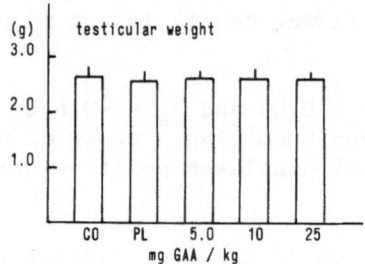

Fig. 3. Testicular weight of rats (5 per group) 50-55 days after
         birth. Mothers were left untreated (CO) or were given the
         vehicle (PL) or gossypol acetic acid (GAA). Differences
         are not significant (p > 0.10).

calculated for day 21 [(number of pups alive on day 21/number of
pups born alive) × 100] was 85.3% for pups from control and 90.3%
for pups from GAA-treated females (p > 0.10).

    Figure 2 shows that the litter weight/female/group ranged from
6.0 ± 0.6 g to 6.7 ± 0.6 g (p > 0.10) on day 1, and from 35.5 ± 3.0
g to 50 ± 7.2 g (p > 0.10) on day 21. This indicates normal weaning
growth. Testicular weight (g) of animals 50-55 days old did not differ significantly (p > 0.10), as Fig. 3 shows. Similarly, the relative testis weight (mg/100 g body weight) was unaltered (p > 0.05,
data not shown).

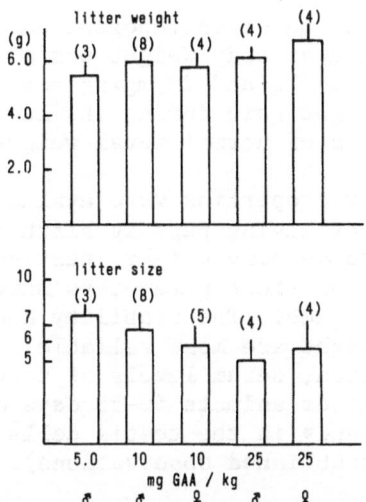

Fig. 4. Litter weight (upper panel) and litter size (lower panel)
        of pups from F_2-generation. Parents were born to gossypol
        acetic acid (GAA)-treated mothers. Differences are not
        significant (p > 0.10). Number of mated animals is put in
        parentheses.

     No alterations of main organs and viscera were macroscopically
visible. The sex ratio (female:male) at weaning was between 1.07
and 1:1 except for the 5 mg/kg GAA-group where it was 1.4. All
males and females randomly selected from GAA-treated mothers (3-8
per sex) and mated with offspring of control mothers were fertile,
as seen from resulting births. From the 5 mg/kg group only male
animals were allowed to breed.

F_2-Generation

     Figure 4 shows that the litter size/female/group varied between
5.2 ± 0.8 and 7.0 ± 0.4 at birth (p > 0.10). The litter weight/
female/group ranged from 5.6 ± 0.5 g to 6.8 ± 0.6 g (p > 0.10).
Matured offspring (3-5 per sex) were fertile, as proven by parturition.

DISCUSSION

     Consecutive, oral GAA-administration to adult female rats at
dosages of 10 mg/kg and 25 mg/kg for 10 days provoked some weight
loss which was less evident in the pregnant animals. Compared to
our data from male rats [8] (and unpublished observations), the
female seems to be less sensitive to the weight reducing effect of

GAA. An identical finding has been reported earlier [9]. In the female hamster, a decrease of body weight was observed with daily GAA-concentrations of 10 mg/kg and 20 mg/kg for 20 days [10]. The similar relative body weight gain during the last trimester of pregnancy is considered a sign of normal fetal weight development.

The following litter properties were evaluated: percentage of still-born pups, number of living pups at birth and at weaning time (viability), neonatal and weaning weight, testicular weight, and overall fecundity. None of these parameters showed any significant deviation from control values. The viability and the weaning weight as well as the testis weight are most reliable indices of drug toxicity [11]. In addition, serum levels of testosterone, LH and FSH, testicular histology of animals 50–55 days old, and the chromosomal aberration frequency in the testis cells were not altered due to GAA-treatment (unpublished observations).

Male and female offspring were raised to maturity and mated. The number and weight of the neonates (F_2-generation) were comparable among the groups. All animals mated were fertile. Thus GAA demonstrated no toxic action on the embryonic development as revealed from the litter characteristics measured.

In a previous study [12], male and female rats were fed a diet containing 0.028–0.084% free gossypol for 420 days. During this period the animals were bred six times. There was no effect on weaning and reproductive performance. Weight and histology of heart, liver, kidney, lung, spleen, and adrenal were normal. Similarly, dietary gossypol treatment of both males and females with 3.3–3.8 mg/kg/day for 3 weeks prior to breeding and identical treatment of the offspring for 24 weeks did not affect spermatogenesis and fertility [13].

The question might be raised as to whether the GAA-concentrations (maximal 25 mg/kg by the oral route) used provided adequate accumulation of GAA in the blood and quantitative diffusion through the placental barrier. Due to the lipophilic and acidic properties of gossypol [14], it should be highly absorbed from the rat stomach [15]. About 3 days might be necessary to establish a steady state concentration of gossypol in blood [16]. On the other hand, it is well known that lipophilic and non- or only slightly ionized compounds pass easily through the placenta and enter the fetal circulation [17, 18]. Therefore, it can be assumed that sufficient quantities of GAA have reached the embryo.

These observations notwithstanding, gossypol should undergo more detailed and exhaustive toxicology tests while it is under consideration for male fertility control.

AKNOWLEDGMENTS

Financial support was provided by The Rockefeller Foundation, New York, N. Y.

REFERENCES

1. A. dePeyster, Y. Y. Wang, Gossypol - proposed contraceptive for men passes the AMES test, New Engl. J. Med., 301:275 (1979).
2. N. Colman, Non-mutagenicity of gossypol in the Salmonella/ mammalian - microsome plate assay, Environ. Mutagen., 35:315 (1979).
3. S. K. Majumdar, J. D. Thatcher, E. H. Dennis, A. Cutrone, M. Stockage, and M. Hammond, Mutagenic evaluation of 2 male contraceptives: 5-thio-glucose and gossypol acetic acid, J. Hered., 73:76 (1982).
4. R. Reiser and H. C. Fu, The mechanism of gossypol detoxification by ruminant animals, J. Nutr., 76:215 (1962).
5. D. W. Gaylor, Methods and concepts of biometrics applied to teratology, in: "Handbook of Teratology" (J. G. Wilson and F. C. Fraser, eds.), Plenum Press, New York, Vol. 4, p. 429 (1977).
6. A. K. Palmer, The design of subprimate animal studies, in: "Handbook of Teratology" (J. G. Wilson and F. C. Fraser, eds.), Plenum Press, New York, Vol. 4, p. 215 (1977).
7. R. Langley, "Practical statistics," Pan Books Ltd., London, p. 199 (1979).
8. G. F. Weinbauer, E. Rovan, and J. Frick, Toxicity of gossypol at antifertility dosages in male rats: statistical analysis of lethal rates and body weight responses, Andrologia, 15, p. 213 (1983).
9. A. M. Ambrose and D. J. Robbins, Studies on the chronic oral toxicity of cottonseed meal and cottonseed pigment glands, J. Nutr., 43:357 (1951).
10. Y. M. Wu, S. C. Chappel, and G. L. Flickinger, Effects of gossypol on pituitary - ovarian endocrine function, ovulation and fertility in female hamsters, Contraception, 24:259 (1981).
11. B. A. Schwetz, K. S. Rao, and C. N. Park, Insensitivity of tests for reproductive problems, J. Environ. Pathol. Toxicol., 3:81 (1980).
12. R. Bressani, L. G. Elias, J. E. Braham, and M. Erales, Long term rat feeding studies with vegetable mixtures containing cotton flour prepared by different processing techniques, prepress solvent and screw press, J. Agr. Food Chem., 17:1135 (1969).
13. E. F. Reber and L. P. Jones, Effect of gossypol on rat fertility, Fed. Proc., 40:474, Abstr. 1386 (1981).

14. M. B. Abour-Donia, Physiological effects and metabolism of
     gossypol, Res. Rev., 61:125 (1976).
15. L. S. Schanker, P. A. Shore, B. B. Brodie, and C. A. M. Hogben,
     Absorption of drugs from the stomach. 1. The Rat, J. Pharmacol.
     Exp. Therap., 120:528 (1957).
16. Y. B. Ke and W. W. Tso, Variations of gossypol susceptibility
     in rat spermatozoa during spermatogenesis, Int. J. Fertil., 27:
     42 (1982).
17. H. Tuchmann-Duplessis, Teratogenic screening methods and their
     application to contraceptive products, meeting on Pharmacologi-
     cal Models to Assess Toxicity and Side Effects of Fertility
     Regulating Agents, Genea, September 17-20 (1973).
18. J. R. Gillette, Factors that affect drug concentration in
     maternal plasma, in: "Handbook of Teratology" (J. G. Wilson
     and F. C. Fraser, eds.), Plenum Press, New York, Vol. 3, p. 35
     (1977).

A REPRODUCTION AND TERATOLOGY STUDY WITH GOSSYPOL

Allan R. Beaudoin

Department of Anatomy and Cell Biology
University of Michigan
Ann Arbor, Michigan

INTRODUCTION

Following the initial report from China in 1978 of the antifertility effect of gossypol in human males [1], antifertility
studies have been conducted in various species: rats [2, 3, 4, 5],
mice [6], hamsters [7, 8, 9], rabbits [10, 11], and monkeys [12].
Differential susceptibility among species exist: hamsters appear
to be the most susceptible and mice and rabbits the least susceptible to the antifertility effects of gossypol [13, 14, 15]. The
physiological and medical aspects of gossypol have been reviewed
[16].

Gossypol causes deterioration of sperm culminating in the loss
of motility and often a separation of sperm head from sperm tail.
Studies of sperm ultrastructure have revealed abnormalities, especially in the mitochondrial sheath of the midpiece [17, 18, 19].
Gossypol has been shown to interfere with several biochemical events
in spermatozoa [e.g., uncouples oxidative phosphorylation and reduces ATP concentration in vivo and in vitro [20, 21]], inhibit the
activity of various enzymes [22, 23, 24, 25], and reduce steroidogenesis [26, 27, 28].

Considerable attention has been paid to the effects of gossypol
on the morphology and biochemistry of the testes and spermatozoa,
but relatively little information is available about the consequence
of fertilization with gossypol-treated sperm. This study was designed to investigate fertilization and subsequent embryonic development from matings in which the male was undergoing gossypol treatment. Of special interest was the period during which the sperm
were becoming abnormal and losing their capacity to fertilize, and

the period during which normal sperm were reappearing and fertility
returned. The effect of gossypol on the pregnant rat was also investigated.

MATERIALS AND METHODS

     Sprague Dawley rats, purchased from Charles River (Kingston,
N.Y.), were used in this study. Rats were acclimatized for one
week prior to placement in the experiment. The animal rooms were
maintained at a relatively constant temperature (72°F) with a 12-h
light/dark cycle. The rats were fed Purina Rodent Lab Chow 5001 and
water ad libitum.

     Gossypol acetic acid was obtained from Dr. Sheldon Segal of
The Rockefeller Foundation, New York. Gossypol was prepared from
its acetic acid according to the procedure described by Pons et al.
[29]. A mixture of gossypol in sesame oil containing 0.5% gum
tragacanth was prepared twice each week. The mixture was stored
in the refrigerator in brown bottles.

1. Reproduction and Teratology Study Following
    Treatment of Male Rats with Gossypol

     Male rats were kept in individual cages, except when breeding.
Female rats were kept in groups of five or six until they were bred.
For breeding, a male was caged overnight with three females. Pregnancy was determined in the morning by the presence of sperm in the
vaginal smear. The gossypol-sesame oil-gum tragacanth mixture was
prepared so that the appropriate dose was contained in approximately
0.5 ml. Male rats were gavaged under light ether anesthesia with
either 10 or 20 mg gossypol/kg body weight/day. Males were started
on gossypol shortly after puberty and following one successful
mating. The males were treated for five or six weeks with the
20 mg/kg dise and for 7-16 weeks with the 10 mg/kg dose. The
experimental and control males were treated by gavage six days
each week. Control males received 0.5 ml of the sesame oil-gum
tragacanth mixture. Throughout the experiment, each male was placed
with females each week until a successful copulation was achieved.
Rarely did a male fail to achieve copulation (determined by presence
of sperm in the vaginal smear). The experiment was continued until
each male had recovered his fertility and impregnated four females.

     Pregnant female rats were kept in individual cages and observed
daily for any change in behavior or appearance. Females were weighed
on gestation days 0, 6, 9, 12, 15, and 20. At day 20 the female rats
were given an overdose of ether, and the uteri exposed and examined
for resorption sites. The fetuses were recovered, weighed, and fixed
in Bouin's fluid or 95% alcohol. The fetuses fixed in Bouin's fluid
were subsequently examined for external malformations and then free-

hand sectioned with a razor blade. These sections were used to detect gross malformations in the palate, brain, eyes, heart, kidneys,
and sex organs. Abnormalities in other organs are not identified
easily. Fetuses fixed in alcohol were prepared for staining with
alizarin red S for visualization of the skeleton. The Student's "t"
test was used for statistical analyses of the results.

Four gossypol-treated males (20 mg/kg) and two sesame oil-
treated males were randomly selected to mate with females who were
allowed to deliver and rear their pups. There were eight such matings in the gossypol group and 10 matings in the sesame oil group.
Ninety viable pups (11.2/liter) were delivered from the gossypol
matings and 115 pups (11.5/liter) from the sesame oil matings, two
of which died. Each litter was culled to three male pups and three
female pups, except in two litters, one of which had no male pups
and the other in which four pups of each sex were reared. The pups
in each litter were tested for postnatal maturation using procedures
suggested by Zbinden [30].

2. Teratology Study Following Treatment of Pregnant Female Rats with Gossypol

Gossypol was prepared so that the appropriate dose was contained
in approximately 0.5 ml. Pregnant females were gavaged under light
ether anesthesia with a dose of either 10 mg or 20 mg gossypol/kg
maternal body weight. Control animals received 0.5 ml of the seame
oil-gum tragacanth mixture. Some pregnant rats received a gavage
treatment at one day of pregnancy, either day 6, 8, 10, 12, 14, or
16, while others were gavaged daily from day 6 through day 15. Some
rats in the latter group received a dose of 5 mg/kg. All rats were
observed daily for signs of drug-induced toxicity. Body weights
were taken at days 0, 6, 9, 12, 15, 20, and the day of single treatment gavage. Pregnancy was terminated at day 20, resorption sites
were counted, and the fetuses recovered and weighed. Three fetuses
from each litter were fixed in 95% alcohol for subsequent bone staining with alizarin red S. The remaining fetuses in each litter were
fixed in Bouin's fluid for subsequent examination for external malformations followed by free-hand sectioning with a razor blade, as
in the previous study (vide supra). The Student's "t" test was used
for statistical analysis of the results.

RESULTS

Table 1 summarizes the weight gain of male rats treated with
20 mg/kg gossypol. Twenty-one male rats were gavaged with the
gossypol mixture daily, except Sunday, for 5 or 6 weeks. Two males
died from complications resulting from the procedure, not because
of the gossypol. Three males became sick during treatment (list-
less, rough coat, anorexic) but recovered completely following cessa-

TABLE 1. Weight Gain in Male Rats

Duration of treatment	Dosage of gossypol	Number males treated/ survived	Weight gain (g ± SD)		
			during treatment period	following treatment period	throughout experiment
Experiment No. 1 6 weeks	20 mg/kg/day	6/5	2.4 ± 39.5 (P = 0.001)	120.4 ± 35.3 (P = 0.02)	122 ± 39.5 (P = 0.01)
	0 mg/kg/day	5/5	101.0 ± 16.7	77.6 ± 8.4	176.4 ± 13.3
Experiment No. 2 5 weeks	20 mg/kg/day	7/7	2.5 ± 42.3 (P = 0.001)	114.2 ± 41.8 (P = 0.2)	114.1 ± 33.3 (P = 0.05)
	0 mg/kg/day	3/3	77.3 ± 12.2	88.3 ± 22.1	165.7 ± 16.8
Experiment No. 3 5 weeks	20 mg/kg/day	8/7	41.1 ± 26.1 (P = 0.005)	89.8 ± 13.4 (P = 0.1)	131.0 ± 28.5 (P = 0.3)
	0 mg/kg/day	5/5	80.8 ± 12.2	73.0 ± 29.2	141.8 ± 40.3

TABLE 2. Gossypol and Fertility

Gossypol treatment	Week of last fertile mating*	Week fertility returned*	Duration of infertility*
19 males 20 mg/kg/day	3rd – 3 males	9th – 1 male	3 weeks – 1 male
	4th – 9 males	10th – 8 males	4 weeks – 4 males
	5th – 5 males	11th – 8 males	5 weeks – 8 males
	6th – 2 males	12th – 1 male	6 weeks – 4 males
		18th – 1 male†	7 weeks – 1 male
			13 weeks – 1 male†
16 males 10 mg/kg/day	4th – 2 males	12th – 1 male	2 weeks – 1 male
	5th – 6 males	13th – 6 males	3 weeks – 1 male
	6th – 4 males	15th – 6 males	4 weeks – 7 males
	8th – 1 male	16th – 4 males	5 weeks – 2 males
		18th – 1 male†	7 weeks – 2 males‡
	3 males did not lose fertility		

*Times for some males can only be approximate because some males failed to mate each week.
†Inadvertently, male was not bred in weeks 8–12.
‡Both males failed to breed during week 5 and 6.

A. R. BEAUDOIN

TABLE 3. Gossypol-Treated Males and the Outcome of Pregnancy

Treat-ment	No. of fe-males preg-nant	Fetal weight (g ± SD)	No. of im-planta-tion sites	Sites/litter	% Re-sorbed	% Sur-vivors mal-formed	% Fe-males	% Males
Pretreatment								
GP-20	21	3.65 ± 0.38	270	12.8	3.7	0	39.3	60.7
Sesame	11	3.58 ± 0.20	144	13.1	5.5	0	44.4	55.6
GP-10	20	3.67 ± 0.30	260	13.0	5.3	0.4	44.7	55.3
Sesame	8	3.51 ± 0.21	105	13.1	5.6	0	43.8	56.2
During treatment								
GP-20	72	3.72 ± 0.27	920	12.7	4.0	0	45.4	54.6
Sesame	59	3.81 ± 0.49	783	13.2	7.4	0.1	45.1	54.9
GP-10	83	3.64 ± 0.50	954	11.5†	7.0	0.2	47.1	52.9
Sesame	37	3.52 ± 0.31	525	14.1	9.0	0.4	50.0	50.0
Posttreatment								
GP-20	91	3.72 ± 0.53	1125	12.3	7.3	0.3	45.9	54.1
Sesame	64	3.62 ± 0.40	870	13.5	4.5	0	45.4	54.6
GP-10	76	3.58 ± 0.33	937	12.3	4.6	0.4	46.7	53.3
Sesame	20	3.52 ± 0.27	270	13.5	4.8	0	52.9	47.1

*GP-20 = 19 males treated with gossypol 20 mg/kg/day for 5 or 6 weeks; GP-10 = 16 males treated with gossypol 10 mg/kg/day for 7 to 16 weeks; Sesame = 20 males treated with seame oil (13 for GP, 20, 7 for GP 10).

†P = 0.001.

tion of treatment. The remaining males appeared healthy throughout the experiment. Thirteen males were used as controls and received the sesame oil and gum tragacanth mixture for five or six weeks. These males were healthy throughout the experiment. In each experiment, weight loss was marked during the period of gossypol treatment. In the period following treatment, the gossypol-treated males resumed their weight gain, at times exceeding the weight gained by the controls. For the duration of the experiment, gossypol-treated males tended to gain less weight than their control counterparts. It is not known why the males in experiment No. 3 experienced less weight loss than the males of experiment No. 1 or No. 2.

Seventeen males were gavaged daily, except Sunday, with 10 mg/kg gossypol. One male died from complications of the procedure. One male became sick during treatment, but recovered when the treatment was discontinued. The remaining males appeared healthy throughout the experiment. Eight males were gavaged with sesame oil and served as controls. The results with the 10 mg dose paralleled those with the 20 mg/kg dose. There was a statistically significant (P = 0.02) reduction in weight gain by the experimental males only during treatment. Following treatment there was a catch-up period so that at the end of the experiment there was no significant difference in weight gain between experimental and control males.

Table 2 catalogs the onset of infertility and the resumption of fertility for the treated males. Sesame oil did not interfere with fertility. The high dose of gossypol induced infertility in all treated males, as early as the third week of treatment, and as late as the sixth week. Infertility usually lasted five weeks, although there were exceptions. The low dose of gossypol induced infertility in the majority of males, but not in all. Three males continued to have fertile matings throughout the experiment. Infertility was induced as early as the fourth week and as late as the ninth week. The duration of infertility was variable, from two to seven weeks, with the majority at four weeks. It must be noted, however, that these figures are not exact because, for one reason or another, males occasionally failed to mate during a given week.

Table 3 summarizes the results of breeding males prior to, during, and following treatment with gossypol. There were 19 males treated with 20 mg/kg/day gossypol and 16 males treated with 10 mg/kg/day gossypol. Twenty males received sesame oil. An analysis of the table reveals that gossypol administered to males had no effect on the fetal weight of their offspring or the number of implantation sites, with the possible exception of implantations in pregnancies resulting from matings during the treatment period with males treated with 10 mg/kg/day. There was no increase in resorptions following gossypol treatment of males when compared with the sesame oil-treated males. In five of the six groupings there were more resorptions in the sesame oil groups than in the gossypol

TABLE 4. Malformations in Fetuses from Matings with Gossypol-Treated Males

Treatment	Dosage	Male No.	Malformation	Time of occurrence
Gossypol	20 mg/kg/day	23	one fetus: hydronephrosis	7 weeks after cessation of treatment
		27	one fetus: tailless, imperforate anus, fused kidneys	8 weeks after cessation of treatment
		32	one fetus: right-sided aortic arches	6 weeks after cessation of treatment
	10 mg/kg/day	43	one fetus: right-sided aortic arches	8 weeks after cessation of treatment
		46	one fetus: gastrochschisis	3 weeks after cessation of treatment
		58	one fetus: right-sided aortic arches	1st week of treatment
			one fetus: tailless, imperforate anus,	6 weeks after cessation of treatment
		60	one fetus: hydronephrosis	6 weeks after cessation of treatment
		62	one fetus: hydronephrosis	1 week before treatment
			one fetus: hydronephrosis	3rd week of treatment
		10 fetuses malformed of 4213 surviving fetus (0.20%)		
Sesame Oil		28	one fetus: anophthalmia	5th week of treatment
		45	one fetus: cleft palate	4th week of treatment
		54	one fetus: microphtalmia	9th week of treatment
		3 fetuses malformed of 2524 surviving fetuses (0.1%)		

TABLE 5. Gossypol-Treated Males (20 mg/kg) and Fetal Skeletal Development

	Pretreatment		During treatment		Posttreatment	
	gossypol	sesame oil	gossypol	sesame oil	gossypol	sesame oil
Number of fetuses examined	60	39	216	166	265	193
MISSING OSSIFICATION CENTERS (%)						
1. Centra of cervical vertebrae						
C1-6	95.8	97.0	94.1	89.7	91.3	94.6
C7	71.6	56.4	55.0	53.6	57.3	55.4
2. Sternebrae						
No. 5	28.3	30.7	28.2	16.2	25.6	25.9
No. 6	13.3	15.3	13.4	9.6	13.5	22.7
3. Forelimb phalanges						
No. 1-5	68.4	64.1	67.5	63.2	73.9	81.3
Nos. 1, 2, 4, 5	1.6	12.8	6.0	10.8	10.9	8.8
Nos. 1, 2, 5	20.0	33.3	27.3	27.1	17.3	17.0
metacarpals						
No. 1	85.0	76.9	75.4	85.5	70.1	65.8
Nos. 1, 5	16.6	25.6	29.6	13.8	29.0	36.7
4. Hindlimb phalanges						
No. 1-5	98.3	100	99.0	96.3	96.2	99.4
metatarsals						
No. 1	98.3	100	99.0	96.3	93.9	97.4
5. Basioccipital bone	71.6	84.6	73.6	64.4	76.9	65.8
6. Hyoid bone	10.0	0	7.8	3.0	7.1	6.7
REDUCED OSSIFICATION CENTERS (%)						
1. 13th rib	1.6	7.6	2.7	1.8	1.5	3.1
2. Double centra	3.3	0	0.9	6.6	2.6	1.0
3. Sternebrae						
No. 5	70.0	64.1	58.3	71.6	68.3	62.1
No. 6	41.6	41.0	25.9	30.7	43.0	29.5
4. Supraoccipital bone	11.6	15.2	11.4	3.6	12.6	9.7
5. Interparietal bone	20.0	15.3	11.5	10.2	12.8	11.9
6. Basioccipital bone	28.3	15.3	26.8	34.9	21.8	33.0
7. Hyoid bone	6.6	15.3	11.0	12.6	4.4	7.2
EXTRA 14th RIB	0	0	0.9	0.6	1.8	1.5
WAVY RIBS	0	2.5	0.4	0	0.3	1.5

groups.   In only one group was the incidence higher in the treated
pregnancies (posttreatment GP-20).   The incidence of resorption in
Sprague Dawley untreated rats can be expected to be around 6% (based
on observations of 1758 litters at a commercial laboratory).   There
were 2524 fetuses in pregnancies from sesame oil-treated males examined for soft tissue defects.   Three of these (0.1%) were malformed.   Ten malformed fetuses were found in 4231 fetuses examined.
for soft tissue defects in matings from gossypol-treated males (0.2%).
The incidence in untreated Sprague Dawley rats can be expected to be
about 0.5% (based on observations of 21,186 fetuses at a commercial
laboratory).   There was no significant alteration in the sex ratio
of the fetuses following treatment of the male parent with gossypol.

Table 4 lists the malformations observed.   In the gossypol-
treated groups, one malformed fetus occurred in a litter from a
mating prior to treatment and two malformed fetuses occurred in
litters from matings during treatment.   The remaining seven malformed fetuses were found in litters from matings after treatment.
No single abnormality was common to all malformed fetuses.   In the
sesame oil-treated matings, all malformations occurred in litters
from matings during the treatment period.

Table 5 compares the appearance of certain skeletal features
in fetuses from dams mated with 20 mg/kg gossypol-treated or sesame
oil-treated males.   Matings occurred prior to treatment, during
treatment, and following treatment.   A total of 541 fetuses from the
experimental matings and 398 fetuses from the control matings were
examined.   The percentages given in the table for each observation
will not always total 100% because not all categories are listed
for each observation, and sometimes a portion of a fetus was lost
during preparation.

Cervical Vertebral Centra.   The ossification centers of the
cervical vertebral centra are among the last vertebral ossification
centers to appear.   Relatively few are present in the day 20 fetus.
Gossypol had no effect on ossification in the cervical vertebrae.

Sternebrae.   The ossification centers for sternebrae 5 and 6
are the last to appear.   Gossypol had no apparent affect on their
ossification.

Forelimbs.   The ossification centers in the phalanges begin to
appear around day 20.   All phalangeal ossification centers were
missing in about 70% of both experimental and control fetuses.   There
was no consistent effect of gossypol on the appearance of the phalangeal ossification centers.   About 70-80% of all fetuses lacked
only the ossification center in the first metacarpal.   The more
primitive condition, absence of both the No. 1 and No. 5 ossification center, appeared to be more prevalent in the fetuses from sesame
oil-treated matings.

Hindlimbs. Nearly 100% of all fetuses from both experimental
and control matings lacked the ossification centers in all phalanges
and the ossification center in the first metatarsal.

Head. There was no marked difference between experimental and
control fetuses in the absence of the ossification center for the
basioccipital bone, it was absent in approximately 70% of all fetuses.
The hyoid bone, on the other hand, was present in almost all fetuses.

Another way to attempt to quantify effects on ossification is
to look for reductions in the size of the ossification centers.

13th Rib. Occasionally the extent of ossification of the 13th
rib was reduced, but, as the table shows, this was a rare occurrence.

Double Centra. Double centra indicate a delay in maturation,
but relatively few were seen in this study, and, during treatment,
greater numbers were found in fetuses from sesame oil-treated matings.

Sternebrae. The ossification centers of the fifth and sixth
sternebrae were often found to be quite small, but there was no
marked difference between experimental and control fetuses.

Head. The supraoccipital bone was sometimes found to be deficient in its ossification. The numbers deficient were rather
uniform in fetuses from gossypol-treated matings. There was a
greater variation in the control fetuses. The interparietal, basioccipital, and hyoid bones were sometimes deficient in their ossification, but there were no marked differences between the control and
experimental fetuses.

Extra Rib. Rarely, an extra rib was found, but there was no
difference between gossypol and sesame oil fetuses.

Wavy Rib. Wavy ribs were found in greater numbers in fetuses
from sesame oil-treated matings than in fetuses from gossypol-treated
matings.

Skeletal features were also examined in fetuses from dams mated
with 10 mg/kg gossypol-treated males. A total of 466 fetuses were
examined from the experimental matings and 188 fetuses from the control matings. The results did not differ significantly from those
observed in the 20 mg/kg group. There were minor differences between
ossification in the experimental and control fetuses, but no trend
was established and no dose response was demonstrated.

Table 6 presents the results observed in behavioral tests of
the offspring from matings between untreated females and either

TABLE 6. Behavioral Studies, F1 Generation

Test	Day of occurrence	Percent positive	
		gossypol*	sesame oil†
Righting reflex	1	95	100
	2	5	0
Pina detachment	2	9	60
	3	73	40
	4	18	0
Negative geotaxis	4	58	30
	5	27	52
	6	15	14
	7	0	4
Downy hair present	5	86	100
	6	14	0
Palmar grasp	6	89	88
	7	11	12
Fur present	9	100	100
Auditory startle reflex	11	38	52
	12	47	43
	13	15	5
Full eye opening	14	36	48
	15	30	35
	16	34	17
Free-fall righting reflex	17	77	100
	18	23	0
Testes descent	24	20	35
	25	60	61
	26	20	4
Vaginal opening	30	25	25
	31	0	38
	32	25	13
	33	50	12
	34	0	12

*50 pups tested.
†61 pups tested.

gossypol-treated or sesame oil-treated males. The events occurring during the first week of postnatal life (righting reflex, pina detachment, negative geotaxis, presence of downy hair and attainment of the palmar grasp) had relatively little variation between the experimental group and the control group. During the second week of postnatal life observations were made on the presence of fur, auditory startle reflex, full eye opening, and the free-fall righting reflex. The final two events evaluated, descent of the testes and opening of the vagina, occur during the fifth and sixth postnatal week. Minor discrepancies were found between experimental and control pups, but they could be accounted for by age differences at

TABLE 7. Pregnancy Outcome Following Maternal Treatment with Gossypol

Day of treatment	Dosage	No. of females gavaged/survived	No. of implantation sites	Sites/liter	% Re-sorbed	% Survivors mal-formed	Fetal weight (g) mean ± SD
6	10 mg/kg	3/3	41	13.6	2.4	0	3.62 ± 0.25
	20 mg/kg	15/15	206	13.7	8.2	0	3.75 ± 0.25
	0	10/10	107	10.7	11.2	0	3.64 ± 0.42
8	10 mg/kg	3/3	39	13.0	5.1	0	3.77 ± 0.30
	20 mg/kg	14/14	194	13.8	3.1	0	3.71 ± 0.24
	0	10/10	126	12.6	9.5	0	3.49 ± 0.53
10	10 mg/kg	3/3	41	13.6	4.8	0	3.42 ± 0.15
	20 mg/kg	17/17	225	13.2	4.4	0.4*	3.75 ± 0.49
	0	10/10	141	14.1	6.3	0	3.87 ± 0.33
12	10 mg/kg	3/3	43	14.3	0	0	3.62 ± 0.07
	20 mg/kg	16/16	224	14.0	9.8	0	3.79 ± 0.40
	0	10/10	118	11.8	7.6	1.8†	3.73 ± 0.31
14	10 mg/kg	3/3	32	10.6	6.2	3.1‡	3.73 ± 0.43
	20 mg/kg	10/10	112	11.2	3.5	0.9**	4.05 ± 0.38
	0	9/9	104	11.5	4.8	0	3.77 ± 0.36
16	10 mg/kg	3/3	36	12.0	5.5	0	3.19 ± 0.71
	20 mg/kg	12/12	152	12.7	7.2	0	3.67 ± 0.27
	0	8/8	98	12.2	4.0	0	3.68 ± 0.23

*One fetus with anophthalmia and cleft plate.
†One fetus with agnathia, one fetus with right-sided aortic arches.
‡One fetus with microphthalmia.
**One fetus with microphthalmia.

TABLE 8. Pregnancy Outcome Following Maternal Treatment with Gossypol

Day of treatment	Dosage	No. of females injected/survived	No. of implantation sites	Sites/liter	% Re-sorbed	% Survivors malformed	Fetal weight mean ± SD
6-15	5 mg/kg	15/15	213	14.2	7.0	0.5*	3.48 ± 0.67
	10 mg/kg	15/15	213	14.2	6.5	0	3.83 ± 0.36
	20 mg/kg	15/15	188	12.5	3.7	1.1†	3.65 ± 0.30
	0	24/24	342	14.2	4.9	0.3‡	3.71 ± 0.30

*One fetus with agnathia.
†One fetus with anophthalmia and micrognathia; one fetus with anophthalmia, exencephaly, and umbilical hernia.
‡One fetus with umbilical hernia.

the time of testing. Deliveries were not always observed, especially at night and during weekends and, therefore, the exact age
of the pups was sometimes unknown.

Table 7 summarizes the effects of gossypol when administered
to pregnant dams as a single gavage dose during one day of pregnancy.
The days of treatment were gestation days 6, 8, 10, 12, 14, or 16.
Neither the 10 mg/kg dose nor the 20 mg/kg dose had any adverse
affect in the dams. Their pregnancies were uneventful and the dams
remained healthy throughout the experiment. Gossypol had no significant affect on the number of implantation sites in each litter
or on the number of resorptions. During the first half of gestation, there were more resorptions in the sesame-oil controls than
in the gossypol-treated animals. In the second half of pregnancy,
treatment could be expected to cause the presence of a dead and perhaps partially resorbed fetus, but not a resorption site. Fetal
weight was unaffected by gossypol treatment. There were very few
malformations seen in either the experimental or control fetuses.
Of 1268 fetuses examined from gossypol-treated dams, only three
fetuses were abnormal (0.2%). One fetus from a dam treated at day
10 had anophthalmia and cleft palate and one fetus from a dam treated
at day 14 had microphthalmia and another fetus had anophthalmia. Of
643 fetuses examined from sesame oil-treated dams, two were abnormal (0.3%). Both abnormal fetuses were found in litters of dams
treated with sesame oil at day 12. One fetus was agnathic and the
other had right-sided aortic arches. The incidence of malformations
was very low in both experimental and control litters, less than the
expected spontaneous incidence for the Sprague Dawley rat (0.5%).
No dose response was demonstrated.

Table 8 gives the results of the effect of gossypol on pregnancy when administered throughout the period of organogenesis (day
6-15). There was no adverse affect of gossypol on the health of the
pregnant dam. The number of implantation sites were somewhat reduced in litters of dams receiving the highest dose of gossypol.
It is unlikely that this reduction was caused by the gossypol treatment. Implantation is probably complete at the time of the first
treatment at day 6, therefore, any reduction in implantation sites
should be reflected in a corresponding increase in resorptions.
This was not observed. The incidence of resorption in the 20 mg/kg
group was less than in the two other gossypol groups, and also less
than in the sesame oil control group. Therefore, it is unlikely
that a causal relationship exists between the administration of
gossypol and the incidence of resorption. The weight of the day 20
fetus was unaffected by gossypol treatment. Of 578 fetuses examined
from gossypol-treated dams, three were malformed (0.5%). One fetus
in the 5 mg/kg group was agnathic. One fetus in the 20 mg/kg group
had anophthalmia and micrognathia and one fetus had anophthalmia,
exencephaly, and umbilical hernia. Of 325 fetuses examined from
dams treated with sesame oil, one was malformed (0.3%). The ab-

TABLE 9.   Fetal Skeletal Development Following Maternal
            Gossypol Treatment.   Combined Results
            of Treatment at Day 6, 8, 10, 12, 14, or 16

	Sesame oil	Gossypol	
		10 mg/kg	20 mg/kg
Number of fetuses examined	466	158	648
MISSING OSSIFICATION CENTERS (% ± SD)			
1. Centra of cervical vertebrae			
C 1-6	97 ± 1	97 ± 4	94 ± 2
C 7	53 ± 13	58 ± 20	53 ± 10
2. Sternebrae			
5	28 ± 9	23 ± 10	29 ± 7
6	22 ± 1	15 ± 17	24 ± 5
3. Forelimb phalanges			
1-5	81 ± 5	90 ± 14	79 ± 6
1, 2, 4, 5	7 ± 3	6 ± 5	9 ± 4
1, 2, 5	14 ± 5 ·	15 ± 11	13 ± 4
4. Forelimb metacarpals			
1	61 ± 17	74 ± 14	66 ± 4
1, 5	40 ± 17	35 ± 21	39 ± 14
5. Basioccipital bone	69 ± 9	75 ± 14	60 ± 13
6. Hyoid bone	7 ± 5	6 ± 8	5 ± 2
REDUCED OSSIFICATION CENTERS (% ± SD)			
1. Sternebrae			
5	54 ± 8	68 ± 16	63 ± 13
6	29 ± 4	43 ± 15	37 ± 5
2. Supraoccipital bone	10 ± 4	23 ± 15	14 ± 5
3. Interparietal bone	23 ± 5	29 ± 13	23 ± 7
4. Basioccipital bone	28 ± 11	17 ± 11	34 ± 21
5. Hyoid bone	7 ± 2	17 ± 17	5 ± 4
EXTRA RIB	1 ± 2	2 ± 4	6 ± 3
WAVY RIBS	0.8 ± 1	0	3 ± 3

normal fetus had an umbilical hernia. The incidence of malformations was very low in both experimental and control fetuses, no
higher than the expected spontaneous incidence for the Sprague Dawley
rat.

Table 9 summarizes the results of the study of the skeleton in
fetuses from dams treated with gossypol or sesame oil at one day of
pregnancy, day 6, 8, 10, 12, 14, or 16. A total of 466 fetuses were
examined from sesame oil-treated dams, 645 fetuses were examined
from dams treated with 20 mg/kg gossypol, and 158 fetuses examined
from dams treated with 10 mg/kg gossypol. The results from each
day of treatment have been combined into a single table because
there was little or no difference in ossification between experimental and control fetuses at any day examined.

Table 10 contains the results of examinations of skeletons of
fetuses from dams treated daily throughout the organogenetic period

TABLE 10.   Fetal Skeletal Development Following Maternal Gossypol Treatment Days 6-15

	Sesame oil	Gossypol		
		5 mg/kg	10 mg/kg	20 mg/kg
Number of fetuses examined	60	66	51	84
MISSING OSSIFICATION CENTERS (%)				
1. Centra of cervical vertebrae				
C1-7	98.0	98.0	90.8	90.1
C7	45.0	57.6	41.2	30.9
2. Sternebrae				
No. 5	30.0	9.1	25.5	27.4
No. 6	10.0	3.0	13.7	4.8
3. Forelimb phalanges				
No. 1-5	86.7	89.4	96.1	85.7
Nos. 1, 2, 4, 5	3.3	4.5	2.0	8.3
Nos. 1, 2, 5	10.0	4.5	2.0	8.3
metacarpals				
No. 1	85.0	60.1	78.4	95.2
Nos. 1 and 5	21.6	45.4	23.5	8.3
4. Hindlimb phalanges				
No. 1-5	100	100	100	100
metatarsals				
No. 1	100	100	96.1	100
5. Basioccipital bone	55.0	86.4	47.0	67.8
6. Hyoid bone	13.3	21.2	5.9	9.5
REDUCED OSSIFICATION CENTERS (%)				
1. 13th Rib	3.3	0	9.8	3.6
2. Double centra	1.6	1.5	2.0	0
3. Sternebrae				
No. 5	46.7	59.1	66.7	67.8
No. 6	31.7	50.0	27.4	30.9
4. Supraoccipital bone	9.9	21.2	21.6	11.9
5. Interparietal bone	40.0	30.3	35.2	19.0
6. Basioccipital bone	44.9	12.1	49.0	28.6
7. Hyoid bone	13.3	16.6	9.8	6.0
EXTRA 14th RIB	0	1.5	9.8	3.6
WAVY RIBS	1.6	0	7.8*	0

*All in one liter.

(days 6-15). There were no significant differences in skeletal development between the experimental and control fetuses.

DISCUSSION

Gossypol can induce both morphological and biochemical alterations in spermatozoa. As long as spermatozoa retain the ability to fertilize, however, these alterations have no effect on the outcome of that fertilization, as shown by the results of the present study.

The high dose of gossypol (20 mg/kg/day) used in this experiment markedly interfered with weight gain during the period of treatment. Subsequently, the gossypol-treated males resumed weight gain, but at the termination of the experiment they still had not always caught up with the sesame oil-treated controls. The low dose of gossypol (10 mg/kg/day) had a much less dramatic effect on weight gain in the treated males. A dose-correlated suppression of weight gain is a common finding with gossypol treatment.

Based on the results obtained, it can be concluded that gossypol treatment of male rats had no adverse effect on the outcome of pregnancies resulting from conception during the treatment period, or after the treatment period when fertility returned. There were no observable effects on fetal weight or the incidence of resorption at day 20 of gestation. The number of implantation sites was largely unaffected, except that there seemed to be a reduction in implantation sites in litters sired by males treated with 10 mg/kg/ day. Inspection of the raw data, however, revealed that matings with one male in this group produced consistently fewer fetuses than matings with any other male in the group. The significance of this observation is not known. The results also indicate that there are individual variations in the response of males to the gossypol treatment with respect to the time of onset of infertility, the duration of infertility subsequent to treatment, and the success of the recovered fertility, as measured by the number of implantation sites. This experiment did not permit the distinction between variations inherent in the male and variations induced by gossypol. The antifertility effect of gossypol was obtained without any marked toxicity to the males, in contrast to a previous report [31].

The incidence of malformations was very low in this experiment, lower than expected to occur spontaneously in a colony of untreated Sprague Dawley rats. Regardless of treatment, there was never more than one malformed fetus in any given litter. Each malformation observed in both experimental and control fetuses has previously been described as a spontaneous malformation in these rats [32]. A dose response was not demonstrated, and there was no distinct or reproducible syndrome of malformations. These observations suggest that the malformations are not due to the treatment of males with gossypol.

A comparison of the results of the skeletal studies reveals no significant pattern to the variation in ossification between fetuses from gossypol-treated matings and fetuses from sesame oil-treated matings. There was no consistent dose response demonstrated. In many cases, there was little or no change in ossification within each dose group when the results were compared between pretreatment, treatment, and posttreatment periods. Overall, there is nothing in the results obtained to suggest gossypol-treatment of males has an adverse affect on the development of the fetal skeleton.

Minor variations in the timing of events associated with post-natal maturation occurred between pups from gossypol-treated matings and pups from sesame oil-treated matings. However, the variation in time rarely exceeded 24 h and, therefore, could easily be caused by differences in age of the pups at the time of testing. The exact age of all the pups was not known because not all births were ob-served. Combining observations for a two-day period eliminates the differences between control and experimental animals for most events.

The effect of gossypol treatment of the female has not been studied extensively. One group of investigators found that doses of gossypol up to 80 mg/kg administered for the three consecutive days prior to ovulation had no effect on ovulation in the rat [33]. They also reported that treatment of pregnant mice from day 1-13 of pregnancy resulted in increased numbers of nonviable fetuses. However, the authors raised serious questions about the unhealthy condition of the mice used in their experiment. Another team ex-amined gossypol-treated hamsters for effects on endocrine function, ovulation, and fertility [34]. They reported a rise in serum FSH, a fall in pituitary FSH, and a higher serum and ovarian concentra-tion of estrone and estradiol in gossypol-treated hamsters compared with controls. The estrus cycle remained normal and there was no effect on ovulation. They also reported that gossypol failed to alter the pregnancy rate or affect the outcome of pregnancy: all fetuses appeared normal with no retardation of growth. However, only five pregnant hamsters were examined.

In the present experiment, gossypol administered to pregnant dams, either at a single day during gestation or throughout the organogenetic period, had little observable effect on the outcome of pregnancy. There was no effect on fetal weight at day 20 of gestation. The number of implantation sites/litter was unaffected, and there was no increase in resorptions. Examination of the fetal skeleton revealed little or no difference between experimental and control fetuses. Three fetuses from gossypol-treated dams were ab-normal (0.2%) and two fetuses from sesame oil-treated dams were ab-normal (0.3%). The incidence of malformations was lower than the spontaneous incidence expected in a colony of Sprague Dawley rats (0.5%). This observation together with the lack of a demonstrable dose response, and the lack of a distinct or reproducible syndrome of malformations, strongly favors the conclusion that gossypol is not teratogenic in the pregnant rat.

Under the conditions of these experiments, gossypol administered to either the breeding male rat or the pregnant female rat had no significant adverse effect on the outcome of conception.

REFERENCES

1. National Coordinating Group on Male Antifertility Agents, Gossypol, a new antifertility agent for males, Chinese Med. J., 4: 417 (1978).
2. M. C. Chang, Z. Gu, and S. K. Saksena, Effect of gossypol on the fertility of male rats, hamsters, and rabbits, Contraception, 21:461 (1980).
3. M. A. Hadley, Y. C. Lin, and M. Dym, Effects of gossypol on the reproductive system of male rats, J. Androl., 2:190 (1981).
4. D. W. Hahn, C. Rusticus, A. Probst, R. Homm, and A. N. Johnson, Antifertility and endocrine activities of gossypol in rodents, Contraception, 24:97 (1981).
5. G. F. Weinbauer, E. Rovan, and J. Frick, Antifertility efficacy of gossypol acetic acid in male rats, Andrologia, 14:270 (1982).
6. D. W. Hahn, et al., 1981, op. cit. (see Ref. 4).
7. M. C. Chang, et al., 1980, op. cit. (see Ref. 2).
8. D. W. Hahn, et al., 1981, op. cit. (see Ref. 4).
9. S. K. Saksena and R. A. Salmonsen, Antifertility effects of gossypol in male hamsters, Fertil. Steril., 37:686 (1982).
10. M. C. Chang, et al., 1980, op. cit. (see Ref. 2).
11. S. K. Saksena, R. Salmonsen, I. F. Lau, and M. C. Chang, Gossypol: Its toxicological and endocrinological effects in male rabbits, Contraception, 24:203 (1981).
12. L. Shandilya, T. B. Clarkson, M. R. Adams, and J. C. Lewis, Effects of gossypol on reproductive and endocrine functions of male cynomolgus monkeys (Macaca-Fascicularis), Biol. Reprod., 27:241 (1982).
13. M. C. Chang, et al., 1980, op. cit. (see Ref. 2).
14. D. W. Hahn, et al., 1981, op. cit. (see Ref. 4).
15. S. K. Saksena, et al., 1981, op. cit. (see Ref. 11).
16. M. R. N. Prasad and E. Diczfalusy, Gossypol, Int. J. Androl. Suppl. 5:53 (1982).
17. S. A. Bozek, D. R. Jensen, and J. M. Tone, Scanning electron microscopic study of spermatozoa from gossypol-treated rats, Cell Tissue Res., 219:659 (1981).
18. A. P. Hoffer, Ultrastructural studies of spermatozoa and the epithelial lining of the epididymis and vas deferens in rats treated with gossypol, Arch. Androl., 8:233 (1982).
19. R. Oko and F. Hrudka, Segmental aplasia of the mitochondrial sheath and sequelae induced by gossypol in rat spermatozoa, Biol. Reprod., 26:183 (1982).

20. Y.-B. Ke, and W. W. Tso, Variations of gossypol susceptibility in rat spermatozoa during spermatogenesis, Int. J. Fertil., 27:42 (1982).

21. W. W. Tso, C.-S. Lee, and M.-Y. W. Tso, Effect of gossypol on boar spermatozoal adenosine triphosphate metabolism, Arch. Androl., 9:319 (1982).

22. N. R. Kalla and M. Vasudev, Studies on the male antifertility agent-gossypol acetic acid. II. Effect of gossypol acetic acid on the motility and ATPase activity of human spermatozoa, Andrologia, 13:95 (1981).

23. W. P. Kennedy, H. H. Vand der Ven, J. W. Straus, A. K. Bhattacharyya, D. P. Waller, L. J. D. Zaneveld, and K. L. Polakoski, Gossypol inhibition of acrosin and proacrosin, and oocyte penetration by human spermatozoa, Biol. Reprod., 29:999 (1983).

24. C. Y. G. Lee, Y. S. Moon, J. H. Yuan, and A. F. Chen, Enzyme inactivation and inhibition by gossypol, Molec. Cell. Biochem., 47:65 (1982).

25. W. W. Tso and C.-S. Lee, Gossypol: An effective acrosin blocker, Arch. Androl., 8:143 (1982).

26. M. A. Hadley, et al., 1981, op. cit. (see Ref. 3).

27. T. Lin, E. P. Murono, J. Osterman, H. R. Nankin, and P. B. Coulson, Gossypol inhibits testicular steroidogenesis, Fertil. Steril., 35:563 (1981).

28. S. K. Saksena and R. A. Salmonsen, 1982, op. cit. (see Ref. 9).

29. W. A. Pons, J. Pominski, W. H. King, J. A. Harris, and T. H. Hopper, Recovery of gossypol from cottonseed gums, J. Amer. Oil Chemists Soc., 36:328 (1959).

30. G. Zbinden, Experimental methods in behavorial teratology, Arch. Toxicol., 48:69 (1981).

31. G. F. Weinbauer, E. Rovan, and J. Frick, Toxicity of gossypol at antifertility dosages in male rats: Statistical analysis of lethal rates and body weight responses, Andrologia, 15:213 (1983).

32. J. L. Schardein, March, 1984, personal communication.

33. D. W. Hahn, et al., 1981, op. cit. (see Ref. 4).

34. Y.-M. Wu, S. C. Chappel, and G. L. Flickinger, Effects of gossypol on pituitary-ovarian endocrine function, ovulation and fertility in female hamsters, Contraception, 24:259 (1981).

EFFECT OF GOSSYPOL ON PROSTATIC ANDROGEN

RECEPTORS IN MALE RATS

Natwar R. Kalla,* Erwin Rovan,†
Gerhard F. Weinbauer,† and Julian Frick‡

*Department of Biophysics
 Panjab University
 Chandigarh, India

†Institute of Zoology
 University of Salzburg
 Salzburg, Austria

‡Urology Department
 General Hospital
 Salzburg, Austria

INTRODUCTION

In China, gossypol has been given to more than 8000 human volunteers over a period of three years without any overt toxicity; the drug has been reported to be 98.4% effective [1]. Apart from some preliminary observations, the precise mechanism of action of gossypol is not clear. It has been reported that it inhibits testosterone production in the rats [2] and impairs accessory sex organs function in mice and rats [3, 4]. Chinese researchers have reported a decrease in the weight of the ventral prostate after gossypol treatment [6], and these same investigators have further observed that the weight of the ventral prostate can be restored to normal after testosterone administration [5]. The impairment of prostate function after gossypol treatment could be due to inhibition in testosterone release/synthesis or to the direct effect of gossypol on the prostate. Coulson and his associates have suggested that gossypol might act as an antiandrogen [6]. The present investigations have been designed to examine the direct effect of gossypol on prostate androgen receptors.

MATERIAL AND METHODS

Chemicals

Tris, dithiothreitol, EDTA, and non-labelled dihydrotestosterone were purchased from Sigma Chemical Company; sodium molybdate,
from Fischer Chemical Company; and ^{3}H-d-dihydrotestosterone (^{3}H-DHT
190 Ci/mmol), from Amersham.

Preparation of Cytosol

The prostate was placed in ice-cold buffer consisting of 10 mM
Tris HCl, 1.5 mM EDTA, 1.0 mM dithiothreitol, 10 mM sodium molybdate
(TED.Mo) pH 7.4 [7]. All subsequent steps were carried out in a
cold room (4°C). The tissue was homogenized in 6 volumes of Tris-
HCl buffer (TED-Mo) with a Brinkman polytron. The homogenate was
centrifuged at 105,000 xg for one hour at 2°C. The supernatant
(cytosol) was used for the analysis of androgen receptors [8]. An
aliquot of the cytosol was assayed for protein concentration by the
method of Lowry [9].

Receptor Binding Assay

Aliquots of the cytosol (200 μl) containing approximately 260
to 400 μg protein were incubated in the presence of ^{3}H DHT for 18
hours at 0°C in 12 × 75 culture tubes. The nonspecific binding was
determined by parallaled incubation of cytosol with 1000-fold excess of radioinert dihydrotestosterone (DHT). Removal of the free
from the bound was achieved by adding 500 μl of dextran charcoal
buffer (1% charcoal, 0.05% dextran) at 0 to 4°C for 15 minutes,
vortexing every 5 minutes. The tubes were then centrifuged (4°C)
at 6000 rpm for 10 minutes, and the 500 μl aliquot of the supernatant
was transferred to the scintillation vials containing 10 ml of aqueous scintillation fluid.

Measurement of Radioactivity and Expression of Data

The specific binding ^{3}H DHT to the androgen receptor was calculated from the difference between the binding to the labelled
hormone alone, and the labelled hormone plus the thousand-fold excess of radioinert hormone. Androgen receptor binding is expressed
as cpm (the mean, X ± the standard error S.E.).

Experiment No. 1: Effect of Gossypol on Prostate
Androgen Receptors in vitro

The ventral prostates were removed from 270 gram Wistar rats
48 hours after orchiectomy. The cytosol was prepared by the method
described above. The cytosol was incubated in the presence of different amounts of gossypol (100 ng, 1 μg, 10 μg, and 100 μg) and
binding assays were done by the method described above.

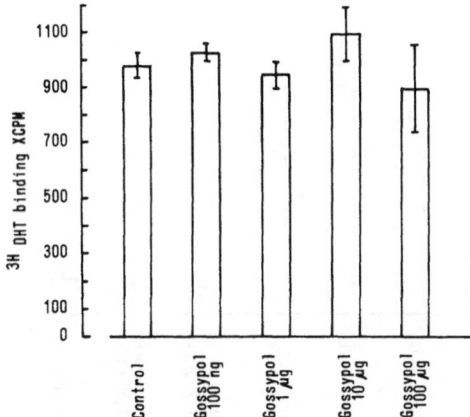

Fig. 1. Effect of gossypol on androgen receptor binding in the rat
prostate cytosol. The androgen receptor binding was calculated by incubating the cytosol with ^{3}H–DHT in the
presence/absence of 1000–fold excess of radioinert DHT.
Each point is the mean of 3 samples ± S.E. Binding in
the gossypol–treated samples was not different from that
of the control.

Experiment No. 2: Effect of Gossypol on Prostate Androgen Receptors in Immature Rats Treated with Different Dosages of Gossypol and Testosterone Propionate

Eight groups of immature (30 day–old) male rats were exposed to
different dosages of gossypol and/or testosterone propionate. Group
I served as the control, whereas animals in groups II–IV were given
gossypol (4.0, 8.0, and 40 mg/kg/day) respectively. Animals in
groups V and VII as well as VI and VIII were given testosterone
propionate (20 μg and 50 μg/rate/day respectively). Animals in
groups V and VI received 8 mg/kg of gossypol in addition to testosterone propionate. The drug treatment was given (subcutaneously)
for four weeks to all the animals; 24 hours after the last dose of
gossypol and/or testosterone propionate, the animals were sacrificed and the ventral prostate removed. Cytosol was prepared by the
method described above and the binding assay was done in the pres-
ence/absence of radioinert DHT.

Experiment No. 3: Effect of Gossypol on Prostate Androgen Receptors of Mature Rats

Gossypol, 15 mg/kg body weight, was administered orally to male
adult rats for 12 weeks. In another group, gossypol 40 mg/kg was
given orally to male adult rats for 30 days. After the last dose

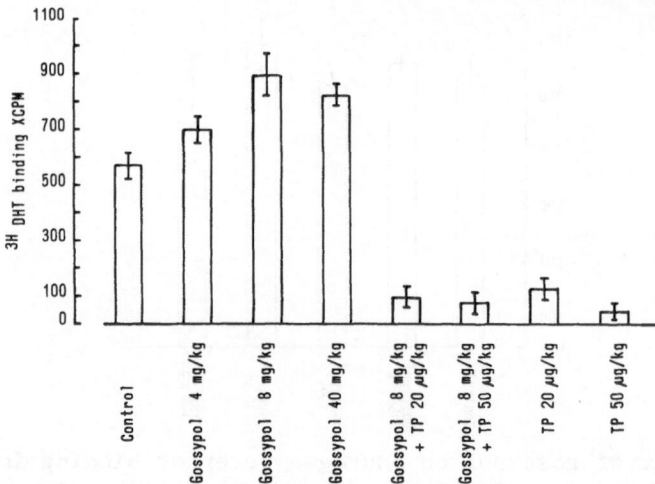

Fig. 2.   Effect of different doses of gossypol on the androgen re-
           ceptor binding in the rat prostate cytosol. The binding
           in the gossypol-treated cytosol samples was not different
           from that of the controls. In animals treated with testo-
           sterone propionate all the binding sites were saturated.
           Each point is the mean of six samples ± S.E.

of gossypol, the animals were sacrificed and the ventral prostate
was immediately transferred to liquid nitrogen and then stored at
-40°C until used. The cytosol was prepared and the binding assay
was done in the presence/absence of radioinert DHT.

OBSERVATIONS

     Figure 1 summarizes the effect of gossypol on the binding of
^{3}H-DHT to rat ventral prostate cytosol; gossypol did not inhibit the
binding of ^{3}H-DHT to prostate androgen receptors. The binding of
^{3}H-DHT to androgen receptors in gossypol treated animals was not
significantly different from that of the controls. However, all
the binding sites were occupied after testosterone proprionate (TP)
treatment (Fig. 2). Similarly, gossypol treatment, 15 mg/kg body
weight and 40 mg/kg, also did not have any effect on ^{3}H-DHT binding
to ventral prostate androgen receptors (Fig. 3).

DISCUSSION

     It is now generally accepted that prostatic function is di-
recently related to the androgenic status of the animal [10]. The

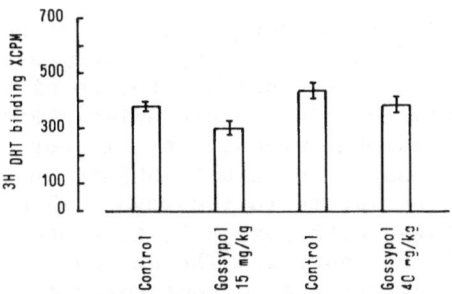

Fig. 3.   Effect of high doses of gossypol on the androgen receptor
          binding in the rate prostate cytosol. The binding in the
          gossypol treated cytosol samples was not different from
          that of the control.   Each value is the mean ± S.E. of 7
          rats (15 mg/kg) and 6 rats (40 mg/kg).

impairment of prostate function after the administration of any antispermatogenic agent may be due to: i) effects at the hypothalamic-
pituitary level causing suppression or release of luteinizing hormone which, in turn, inhibits the testosterone synthesis; ii) direct inhibition of testicular androgen synthesis either by inhibiting the binding of LH/hCG at the receptor level or by inhibiting the
enzymes involved in the biosynthesis of testosterone; or iii) inhibition of the action of testosterone or dihydrotestosterone at the
target tissue level. We have reported earlier that gossypol does
not suppress the release of gonadotropins from the pituitary in the
mature animals [11, 12]. Similar observations have been made by
others [13].

        We have also shown that gossypol neither affects the binding
of LH/hCG to Leydig cell receptors nor the androgen biosynthesis
in vitro (Kalla, Weinbauer, Rovan, and Frick, unpublished). Shi
and Yingong have reported that with subcutaneous injection of gossypol to male infantile mice and rats every other day at a dosage of
8.3 mg/kg for 4 weeks, the antispermatogenic effects were accompanied by significant decreases in the weight of the seminal vesicle,
ventral prostate and levator ani [14]. In the same report, these
authors noted that when gossypol was injected subcutaneously with
the same schedule and in combination with 20 µg/kg of TP similar results were obtained. However, they found that the effect of TP was
not suppressed when the dosage of TP was increased from 20 µg/kg to
50 µg/kg. We have not observed any effect on the weights of accessory sex organs after gossypol treatment nor have we observed any
effect of gossypol on androgen function, as has been reported previously [15, 16]. The levels of citric acid and fructose (both in-
dicators of androgenic status in the semen) are also not affected
by gossypol treatment [17, 18].

Our present investigations suggest that gossypol does not compete for the binding of ^{3}H-DHT to androgen receptors of the prostate. It is pertinent to mention here that the testes of immature animals respond differently from those of mature animals after gossypol treatment in terms of androgen production. In our unpublished study, we have observed that gossypol does not inhibit testosterone production in the testis of the mature rat; however, when testes from immature rats were incubated with gossypol, testosterone production was lower than that of the control. The decrease in prostate weight in the Chinese studies may be due to some toxic effect of gossypol on the infantile rats and mice used in their studies. The dose used by them might have some deleterious effects on the metabolic systems, thus reducing the weight of the vital body organs.

REFERENCES

1. G. Z. Liu, Clinical study of gossypol as a male contraceptive, Reproduction, 5:189 (1981).
2. M. K. Hadley, Y. C. Lim, and M. Dym, Effect of gossypol in the reproductive system of male rats, J. Andrology, 2:190 (1981).
3. P. B. Coulson, R. L. Smell, and C. Parise, Short term metabolic effect of the antifertility agent. Gossypol on various reproductive organs of male mice, Int. J. Andról., 3:507 (1980).
4. Q. X. Shi and Z. C. Yingong, Studies on antifertility effect of gossypol. I. Effect of gossypol on androgen dependent organs in mice and rats, Acta Zool. Sinica, 26:311 (1980).
5. Ibid.
6. P. B. Coulson, op. cit. (see Ref. 3).
7. W. W. Wright, K. C. Cham, and C. W. Bardin, Characterization of the stabilizing effect of sodium molybdate on the androgen receptor present in mouse kidney, Endocrinology, 108:2210 (1981).
8. J. L. S. Barano, M. Tesone, R. Oliveriera-Fieho, V. A. Chiauzzi, J. C. Calvo, E. H. Charreau, and R. S. Calandra, Effect of prolactin on prostate androgen receptors in male rats, J. Andrology, 3:281 (1982).
9. O. H. Lowry, N. J. Rosebrough, A. L. Rarr, and R. J. Randall, Protein measurement with the folin phenol reagent, J. Biol. Chem., 193:265 (1951).
10. K. B. Eik-Nes, Biosynthesis and secretion of testicular steroids, in: "Handbook of Physiology" (D. W. Hamilton and R. O. Greep, eds.), Section 7, Endocrinology, Vol. 5, American Physiol. Soc. Washington, p. 95 (1975).
11. N. R. Kalla, J. Foor, T. W. and A. R. Sheth, Studies on the male antifertility agent-gossypol acetic acid. V. Effect of gossypol acetic acid on the fertility of male rats, Andrologia, 14:492 (1982).

12. G. F. Weinbaurer, E. Rovan, and J. Frick, Toxicity of gossypol at antifertility dosages in male rats: Statistical analysis of lethal rates and body weight responses, Andrologiya, 15(3): 213 (1983).
13. Y. Wong, Y. Lous, and X. Tang, Studies on the antifertility actions of cottonseed meal and gossypol, Acta Pharm. Sinica, 14:662 (1979).
14. Q. X. Shi and Z. C. Yingong, op. cit. (see Ref. 4).
15. N. R. Kalla, et al., op. cit. (see Ref. 11).
16. Y. Wong, et al., op. cit. (see Ref. 13).
17. N. R. Kalla, J. Foo, K. S. Hurkadli, and A. R. Sheth, Studies on the male antifertility agent-gossypol acetic acid. VI. Effect of Gossypol on the fertility of bonnet monkey, Andrologia (1983).
18. J. Frick, Ch. Danner, R. Köhle, and G. Kunit, Male fertility regulation, in: "Research in Fertility and Sterility" (J. Cortes-Prieto, A. Campos-da-pax, and M. Neves-e-Castro, eds.), M.T.P. Press, Lancaster (1981), p. 291.

EFFECT OF GOSSYPOL ON ACCUMULATION OF RHODAMINE-123

BY SERTOLI CELL MITOCHONDRIA

Nongnuj Tanphaichitr and Anthony R. Bellvé

Department of Physiology and Biophysics
and the Laboratory of Human Reproduction
and Reproductive Biology
Harvard Medical School
Boston, Massachusetts

INTRODUCTION

General Antifertility Effects of Gossypol

Clinical application of gossypol as an antifertility agent in Chinese men has demonstrated that the drug is not only >99% efficient, but that its antifertility effect is reversible and reportedly not detrimental to nonreproductive organs, providing the subjects' protein and iron intake are adequate [1, 2, 3, 4]. Gossypol is neither mutagenic when assessed by the Ames test [5], nor does it cause chromosomal aberrations [6, 7].

The drug's antifertility effects have been studied primarily in rats [8, 9]; but mice, hamsters, and the stumptail and cynomolgus monkeys also are sensitive [10, 11]. Early research on rats sought evidence for an endocrine imbalance. These studies, however, did not detect any changes in the serum concentrations of FSH, LH, and testosterone [12, 13, 14, 15], or in the levels of microsomal steroidogenic enzymes in the testes [16], following gossypol treatment. Furthermore, Leydig cells cultured in the presence of gossypol secrete normal levels of testosterone [17]. But, reductions in serum levels of LH and/or testosterone levels have been reported [18, 19].

Deleterious Effects on Spermatozoa and the Differentiating Spermatogenic Cells

Gossypol appears to act at multiple sites in spermatozoa in vitro, and several investigators have reported a rapid cessation of sperm motility [20, 21, 22], an effect most likely due to a per-

turbation of the cells' mitochondrial functions. Several mitochondrial enzymes have been shown to exhibit decreased activities,
including sperm-specific LDH-C_4 (LDH-X) [23, 24, 25, 26], malate
dehydrogenase, glutathione-S-transferase [27], NAD-isocitrate dehydrogenase, succinyl CoA synthetase, fumarase [28, 29], pyruvate
dehydrogenase, and Mg^{2+}-, Na^+-, and K^+-dependent ATPases [30].
Sperm also show a reduced conversion of fructose to CO_2 [31]. Gossypol also inhibits sperm capacitation and fertilizing capability [32,
33], decreases the activity of acrosin [34, 35], and enhances the
production of superoxide, a substance toxic to sperm [36].

    Both testicular and epididymal germ cells exhibit morphologi-
cal defects after gossypol is administered to rats daily for three
weeks. These abnormalities include structural defects of the sperm
head [37, 38], degeneration of the cells' plasma membrane and mitochondria, and derangements and/or absence of one or more of the
tails' outer dense fibers [39, 40, 41]. In Stage VII pachytene
spermatocytes and spermatids (steps 7 to 9 and 18 to 19) the detrimental effects of gossypol are evident in the form of nuclear vacu-
olation, mitochondrial swelling, demembranation, and, in maturing
spermatids, detachment of the acrosome [42, 43, 44, 45]. However,
it is not clear whether the sensitivity of these particular cells
is due to their higher permeability to gossypol or to the sensitivity of processes unique to their stage of differentiation. The
Stage-VII pachytene spermatocytes and spermatids are also among the
most sensitive to the depletion of FSH and LH [46, 47, 48].

    Following chronic exposure to gossypol, the cellular damage ex-
tends to most other stages of spermiogenesis, presumably as a consequence of effects incurred at earlier stages of spermatocyte and
spermatid development. Formation of multinucleated cells, cyto-
lysis, pycnosis, asynchronous cellular associations, and exfolia-
tion of germ cells into the tubular lumen have been observed. The
prematurely exfoliated spermatogenic cells and abnormal sperm, with
morphologically deranged nuclei, mitochondria, acrosome and plasma
membranes, gradually accumulate in the epididymis. Eventually, only
Leydig cells, Sertoli cells and spermatogonia may remain in the
testis [49, 50, 51].

Direct Effects on Sertoli Cells

    Gossypol could have a detrimental effect on Sertoli cells.
These sustentacular cells develop numerous intra- and intercellular
vacuoles in rats given 10-30 mg gossypol/kg body weight for three
weeks or more [52, 53, 54]. The origin of these intracellular
vacuoles is unknown; they could be derived from phagosomes or other
distended organelles. By contrast, the intercellular vacuoles probably reflect damage to the Sertoli cell tight junctions [55]. Such
deleterious effects on Sertoli cells could modify the microenviron-
ment of the developing germ cells [56, 57, 58], and thereby disrupt
spermatogenesis [59, 60].

OBSERVATIONS

Cell Proliferation and Protein Synthesis in Gossypol-Treated TR-ST Cultures

Current efforts have focused on defining the primary mechanism(s) involved in the antispermatogenic action of gossypol, with an emphasis on Sertoli cells, for two reasons. First, recent biochemical evidence suggests that these sustentacular cells play a major role in sustaining and regulating mammalian spermatogenesis [61, 62]. Second, serum gossypol must traverse the Sertoli cells in order to reach the differentiating spermatogenic cells.

A "Sertoli cell" line derived from a rat testicular tumor, the TR-ST cells produce ABP and possess other properties characteristic of Sertoli cells [63]. These cells culture as a monolayer in a 1:1 mixture of Ham's F12 and Dulbecco's Minimal Eagle's medium supplemented with fetal calf serum (FCS, 0.5%), Hepes (15 mM), sodium bicarbonate (1.2 gm/l), gentamycin (10 mg/l), insulin (10 µg/ml), transferrin (5 µg/ml) and epidermal growth factor (EGF, 10 ng/ml) [64]. Confluent cells in cobblestone conformation are used for most experiments. Usually, prior to the addition of gossypol, the depleted culture medium is replaced with fresh medium containing all supplements, except FCS. Gossypol is dissolved in ethanol and then added directly to the cultures (1:100; vol/vol).

After adding fresh medium, confluent TR-ST cells proliferate rapidly, increasing 2.6-fold in number within 48 hours as can be seen in Fig. 1. By contrast, in the presence of gossypol (5 µg/ml) the addition of fresh culture medium promotes only a 1.6-fold increase. The reduced response is due partly to a morphological transformation of the TR-ST cells from a cobblestone to a rounded conformation, which causes some cells to slough into the medium (Fig. 1, inset). However, the total number of gossypol-treated cells, including the detached cells, is only ~72% of control. Thus, gossypol causes a real decrease in the rate of cell proliferation.

The effect of gossypol on protein synthesis can be assessed by measuring the radioactivity incorporated by the cells into TCA-precipitable material during a 1-hour pulse with an [^{3}H]amino acid mixture. By comparison to control cells, those exposed to gossypol for 1 hour show a 33% reduction in their rate of protein synthesis (Fig. 2). This synthetic rate decreases even further during prolonged treatment, reaching a level 60-75% below the control values at 12 to 24 hours. These results concur with the observed decrease in the rate of cell proliferation.

Effects of Gossypol on the Morphology of TR-ST Cells

Alterations in the morphology of confluent TR-ST cells can be observed within 3 hours of exposure to ≥5 µg gossypol/ml (wt:vol),

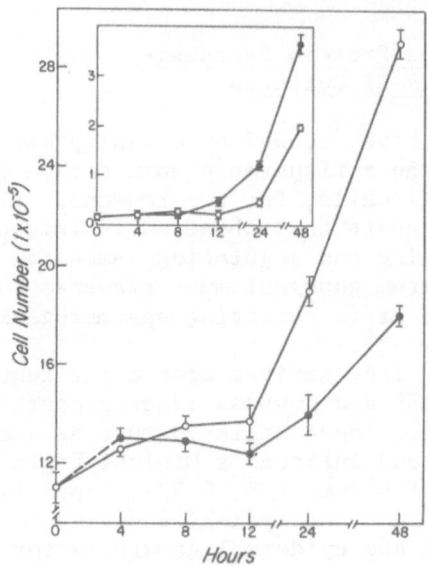

Fig. 1.   Proliferation of TR-ST cells during a prolonged exposure
           to gossypol. The TR-ST cells were seeded (2.5×10^5 cells/
           cm^2) in 1 ml of defined medium that was supplemented with
           Hepes (15 mM), FCS (0.5%), insulin (10 µg/ml), transferrin
           (5 µg/ml) and EGF (10 ng/ml). On reaching confluence the
           cells were given fresh medium containing all supplements
           except FCS. Half of these cultures were exposed to gossy-
           pol (5 µg/ml). At the end of the respective treatments,
           the culture medium containing detached cells was recovered
           and the wells were washed once with 200 µl PBS for combin-
           ing with the original medium. This combined sample was
           counted to quantify the number of detached cells (inset).
           Cells adhering to the plate were dissociated from the sub-
           stratum by a brief trypsin digestion and then the enzyme
           was neutralized by adding soybean trypsin inhibitor (1:1,
           wt/wt). The cells were quantified by using a Coulter
           counter Model ZB1. Data are expressed as mean ± S.E.
           Control (O), gossypol (●).

as Figs. 3 and 4 show. The cells form numerous vacuoles as they
retract their long cytoplasmic processes. Within 8 hours, many
cells assume rounded profiles and some detach from the substratum.
Repeated aspiration causes additional cells to detach, suggesting
that many are only loosely adherent. After a 24-hour exposure, the
nuclei of attached cells gradually translocate to the cell periphery

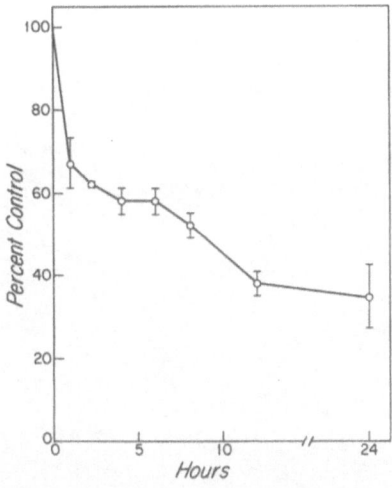

Fig. 2. Percent inhibition of protein synthesis during a 24-hour
         treatment with gossypol. TR-ST cells were seeded in 24-
         well microtiter plates and exposed to gossypol (5 μg/ml)
         as described (see Legend, Fig. 1). At the times indi-
         cated, control and gossypol-treated cells were incubated
         with 1 μCi of [³H]amino acid hydrolysate for 1 hour. The
         medium was removed and centrifuged (×1000 g) to pellet the
         detached cells. These were then treated with 5% TCA and
         solubilized with NaOH. Cells remaining attached to the
         substratum were washed once with 500 μl of PBS, fixed with
         1 ml of 5% TCA, washed again with 1 ml of PBS, and then dis-
         solved with 400 μl of 0.3 N NaOH. Aliquots of each sample
         were subjected to scintillation counting to quantify the
         incorporation of [³H]amino acids. Other aliquots were as-
         sayed for protein content for calculating the specific ac-
         tivity/μg protein At each time indicated, five samples
         of control and gossypol-treated cells were collected and
         the mean ± S.E. were computed. Experimental data are ex-
         pressed as a percent of control cells, derived by dividing
         mean ± S.E. of experimental values by those of control.
         Standard errors of specific activities of control cells are
         <10%. (Reproduced from Ref. 123 by permission, Biology of
         Reproduction).

(Fig. 5). Yet, the majority of cells (∿80%) remain viable during
this period (Fig. 6), as judged by their continued exclusion of
Trypan blue and their ability to hydrolyze fluorescein diacetate
[65]. The severity of the gossypol-induced damage appears to be inversely dependent on cell density and the concentration of FCS in
the medium, confirming an earlier report [66]. Primary cultures of

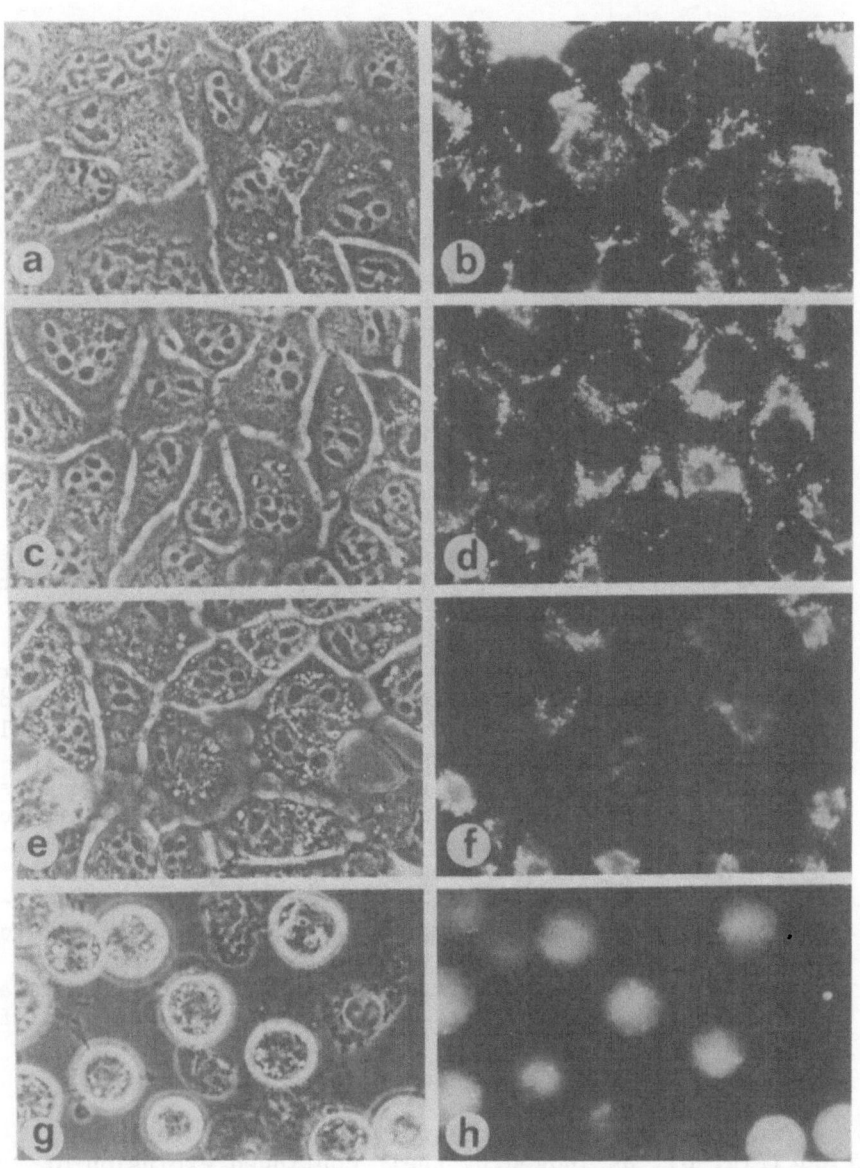

Fig. 3.   Effect of increasing concentrations of gossypol on the
          morphology and rhodamine-123 staining of TR-ST cells after
          a 3-hour treatment. TR-ST cells were seeded onto 1.2 mm
          diameter coverslips at densities of 2×10^5 cells/cm^2 and
          cultured to confluence in 5-ml petri dishes. After a 3-
          hour exposure to the various concentrations of gossypol
          the coverslips were removed and the cells were stained
          with rhodamine-123 (10 µg/ml) for 20 min at 37°C, followed
          by four changes of fresh culture medium. Each coverslip
          was placed in a microchamber and viewed with a Zeiss epi-
          fluorescent microscope using an excitation wavelength of
          485 nm. Note that gossypol caused the cells to retract
          their cytoplasmic processes, become rounded, form intra-
          cellular vacuoles, and exhibit reduced mitochondrial stain-
          ing with rhodamine-123. Cells are shown in phase contrast
          (a, c, e, g) and the corresponding rhodamine-123 fluores-
          cence (b, d, f, h). Treatments include control (a, b) and
          gossypol treatment at 3 µg (c, d), 5 µg (e, f), and 7 µg/ml
          (g, h). Bar = 30 µm. (Reproduced from Ref. 123 by permission,
          Biology of Reproduction.)

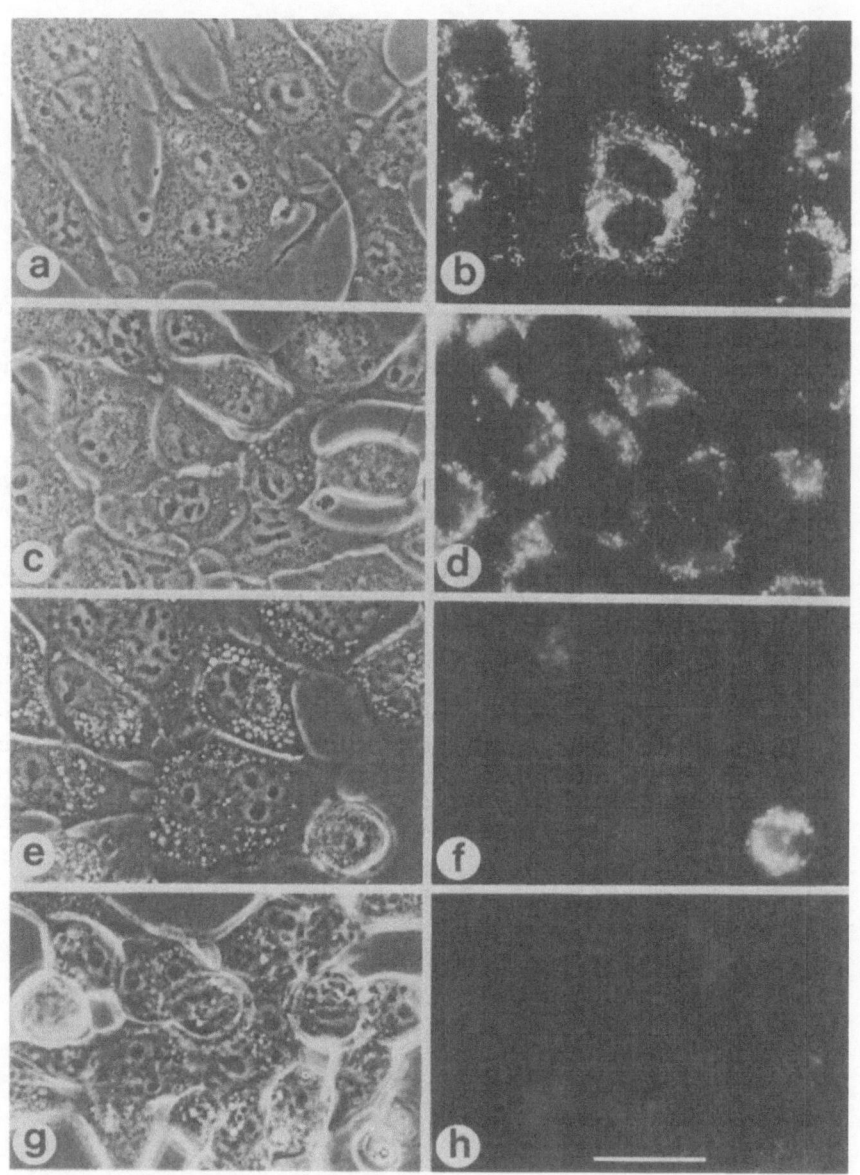

Fig. 4.   The morphology and rhodamine-123 staining patterns of TR-ST
          cells treated for increasing periods of time with gossypol
          (5 µg/ml). The cells were grown on coverslips, treated
          with gossypol and then stained with rhodamine-123 as de-
          scribed (see Legend, Fig. 3). In response to gossypol the
          cells' mitochondria first display a significant reduction
          in the accumulation of rhodamine-123 (1 hour) and then a
          progressive increase in the number and size of intra-
          cellular vacuoles (3 hour). The cells are shown in phase
          contrast (a, c, e, g) and the corresponding rhodamine-123
          fluorescence (b, d, f, h) following a 0-hour (a, b), a
          1-hour (c, d), 3-hour (e, f), and 24-hour (g, h) exposure
          to gossypol. Bar = 30 µm. (Reproduced from Ref. 123 by
          permission, Biology of Reproduction.)

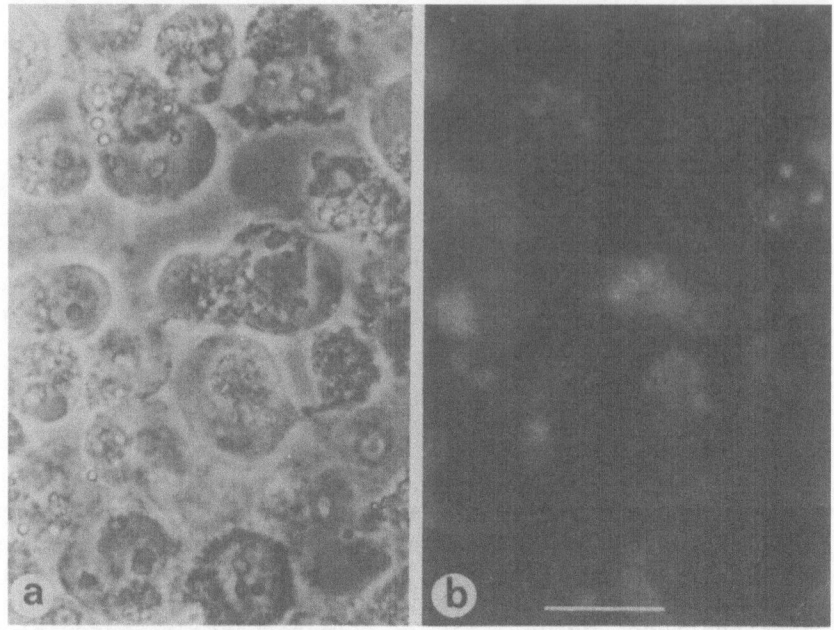

Fig. 5. Peripheral displacement of nuclei within TR-ST cells after
         a 24-hour treatment with gossypol (5 μg/ml). TR-ST cells
         were grown on coverslips, treated with gossypol and in-
         cubated with rhodamine-123 as described (see Legend, Fig.
         3). The cells became markedly swollen, displaying dis-
         tended plasma membranes, intracellular vacuoles, diffuse
         cytoplasmic labeling with rhodamine-123, and a peripherally
         displaced nucleus. Micrographs are shown in phase con-
         trast (a) and the corresponding rhodamine-123 fluorescence
         (b). Bar = 20 μm.

mouse Sertoli cells are similarly affected by gossypol at concentrations at or above 5 μg/ml.

    At lower doses of gossypol (3 μg/ml, wt:vol) the TR-ST cells
appear to be less severely affected, since the morphological changes
are not apparent until after 3 hours (Figs. 3 and 7). Even following an 8-hour exposure to 3 μg gossypol/ml, only 25% of the TR-ST
cells show damage comparable to those treated with 5 μg/ml for 3
hours. By 24 hours, the proportion of damaged cells increases to
50% of the total population (Fig. 7), with the affected cells usually
being grouped in clusters. At lower concentrations (<1 μg/ml) gossypol does not cause any apparent morphological defects in TR-ST cells,
even following 24 hours of treatment.

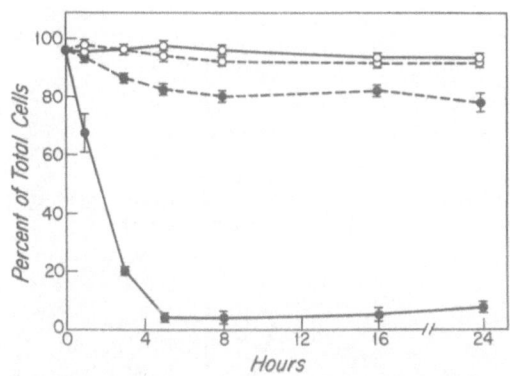

Fig. 6.   Percentage of TR-ST cells hydrolyzing fluorescein di-
          acetate or staining with rhodamine-123 following exposure
          to gossypol for the designated periods of time. The cells
          were grown to confluence on coverslips, treated with gossy-
          pol (5 µg/ml), and then stained with either fluorescein di-
          acetate (1 µg/ml) or rhodamine-123 (10 µg/ml) for 10 min
          at 37°C. Following a wash with fresh medium, the cells
          were examined to assess their ability to hydrolyze fluores-
          cein diacetate and to accumulate rhodamine-123 into their
          mitochondria. The percentage of cells hydrolyzing fluores-
          cein diacetate (-----) and staining with rhodamine-123
          (———) was determined in at least five counting areas.
          Data are expressed as a percent of control cells, derived
          by dividing mean ± S.E. of fluorescent cells by mean of
          total number of cells in the counting areas. Control (O),
          gossypol-treated (●). (Reproduced from Ref. 123 by permis-
          sion, Biology of Reproduction.)

Effect of Gossypol on the Accumulation of Rhodamine-123 by Sertoli Cell Mitochondria

     Several research teams have shown that rhodamine-123 and other
cationic, fluorescent dyes specifically stain mitochondria that are
actively engaged in oxidative phosphorylation and have an outside-
positive and inside-negative transmembrane potential [67, 68, 69].
These same investigators have also found that mitochondria in which
the normal transmembrane potential is perturbed fail to accumulate
the dye, and so it remains diffusely distributed in the cell cytoplasm.

     Mitochondria of TR-ST cells grown to confluence also avidly
accumulate rhodamine-123, thereby dramatically revealing the round
and tubular conformations of these organelles (Figs. 3a, b and 4a,
b). By contrast, after exposure to gossypol for 3 hours (5-7 µg/
ml), most of the TR-ST cells fail to retain any rhodamine-123 (Figs.

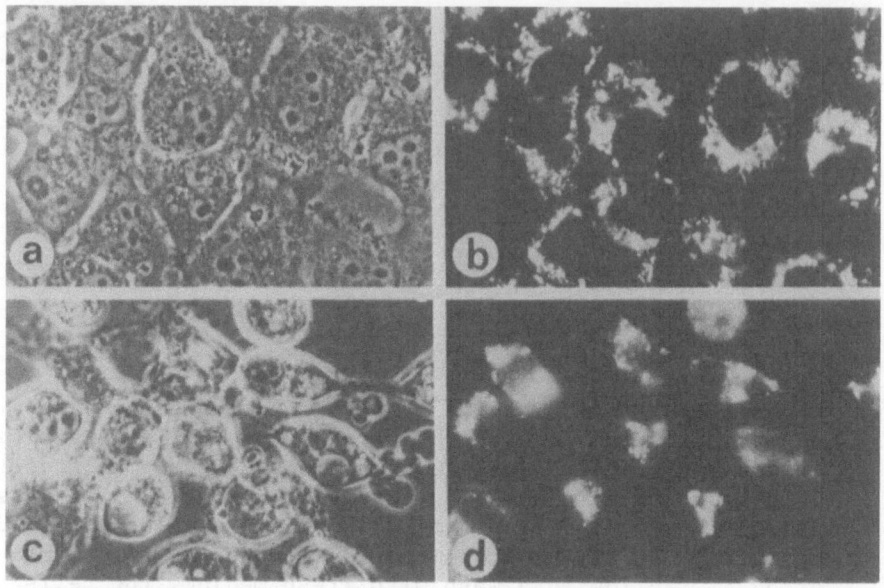

Fig. 7.   Morphology and rhodamine-123 staining pattern of TR-ST
           cells after a 24-hour treatment with gossypol (3 µg/ml).
           The conditions of cell culture, drug treatment and epi-
           fluorescence microscopy were as described previously (see
           Legend, Fig. 3).   The extent of cell damage varies sub-
           stantially in different areas of the cultures.   Micrographs
           include phase contrast (a, c) and the corresponding rhodam-
           ine-123 fluorescent (b, d) images.   Bar = 30 µm.   (Repro-
           duced from Ref. 123 by permission, Biology of Reproduction.)

3f, h).   Even the rounded, rhodamine-123-positive cells show only a
diffuse distribution of the probe throughout the cytoplasm.   At
lower concentrations (3 µg/ml)   the drug has less pronounced effects
(Fig. 3e, f), since only 50% of the cells show reduced mitochondrial
staining even after a 24-hour treatment (Fig. 7b, d).   No effects
are evident in Sertoli cells exposed to 1 µg gossypol/ml of medium.

        A considerable number of TR-ST cells show a reduced mitochon-
drial staining within 1 hour of exposure to 5 µg of gossypol/ml
(Fig. 4), although they still retain their cobblestone conformation
and have few intracellular vacuoles.   After longer treatment (>5
hour) with the drug virtually all of the TR-ST cells fail to accumulate the fluorescent dye (Fig. 4).   Yet, on removing gossypol,
most of the cells quickly resume incorporating rhodamine-123 into
their mitochondria (Fig. 8).   At this time the organelles still show
an asymmetric distribution due to their displacement by the peripherally located nucleus (cf. Fig. 5).   Eventually the cells extend new
cytoplasmic processes and return to a cobblestone-like conformation.

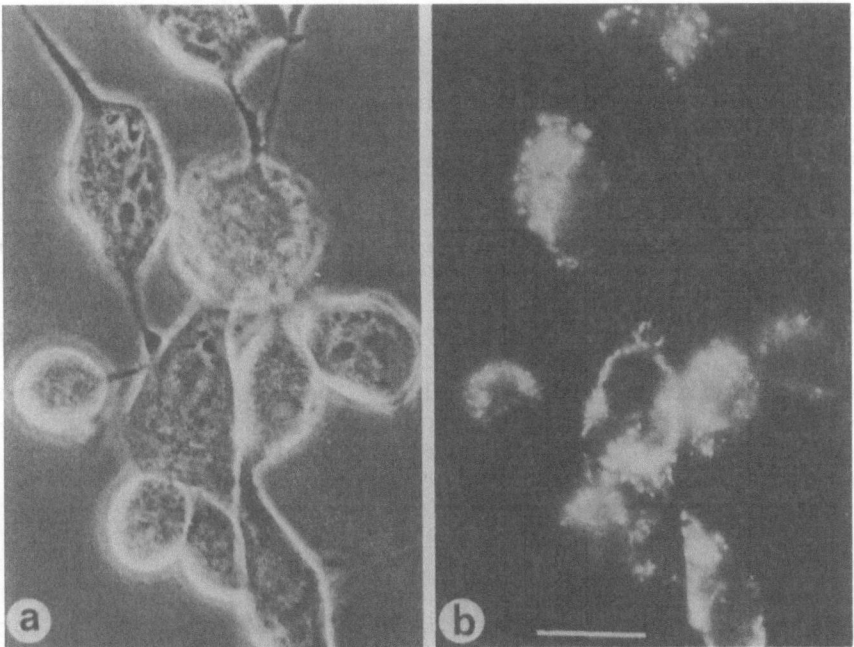

Fig. 8.   Recovery of "normal" morphology and mitochondrial function
          of TR-ST cells after the removal of gossypol. The cells
          were grown to confluency on coverslips, treated with gossy-
          pol (5 µg/ml) for 5 hours, and then transferred to fresh
          medium. After a 3-hour recovery period, most cells were
          reattaching to the substrate, actively extending cyto-
          plasmic processes, and again able to accumulate rhodamine-
          123 into their mitochondria. However, the fluorescent
          staining patterns in the cells were spatially asymmetric,
          suggesting that the nuclei were still displaced toward
          the cell periphery (arrow heads). The few remaining
          rounded cells were not able to incorporate rhodamine-
          123. Micrographs shown are phase-contrast (a) and rhodam-
          ine-123 fluorescence (b). Bar = 20 µm.

     The early onset of mitochondrial dysfunction, and their rapid
recovery after removing the drug, suggests that Sertoli cell mitochondria are primary targets for gossypol.

Effect of Gossypol on Germ Cells and Various
Somatic Cells

     The possible deleterious effect(s) of gossypol directly on
spermatogenesis can be examined by utilizing monodisperse suspensions of differentiating germ cells [70, 71, 72]. These sperma-

togenic cells, after incubating for 6 hours at 33°C in an enriched
Krebs Ringer bicarbonate medium (EKRB) supplemented with gossypol
(5 µg/ml), exhibit neither an altered morphology nor a change in
the mitochondrial accumulation of rhodamine-123. By contrast, when
epididymal spermatozoa are exposed to gossypol the cells show a
rapid and marked reduction of mitochondrial staining by the fluorescent cationic probe.

Gossypol has only minimal effects on the morphology and rhodam-
ine-123 staining of mitochondria in a variety of cultured cell lines,
even after a 48-hour exposure to 20 µg gossypol/ml. The cells
tested include rat and chick embryo fibroblasts, mouse BALB/c 3T3
fibroblasts, monkey and marsupial kidney epithelial cells, HeLa
cells and human breast carcinoma cells. Thus, based on rhodamine-
123 staining of mitochondria, gossypol appears to affect Sertoli
cells and epididymal spermatozoa preferentially. The reason for
this apparent selectivity remains to be determined.

DISCUSSION

This study demonstrates that TR-ST cells are directly and preferentially affected by gossypol. Within 3 to 5 hours of treatment
and at concentrations of 5 µg/ml or greater, gossypol causes marked
transformations in cell morphology. These changes include the re-
traction of cellular processes and a rounding in cell conformation,
the appearance of numerous intracellular vacuoles, displacement of
the nucleus to the cell periphery, and a gradual distension of the
plasma membrane. Comparable morphological changes occur in primary
Sertoli cells on exposure to gossypol. It is not clear whether the
newly-formed vacuoles in these cells are due to a distension of certain cellular organelles or to an increase in phagocytic activity.
The drug also causes a marked decrease in the mitochondrial transmembrane potential, as assessed by the diminished accumulation of
rhodamine-123 by these organelles. These various effects are accompanied by a decreased rate of TR-ST cell division during the first
24-48 hours of treatment. Moreover, the rate of protein synthesis
is reduced by 33% during the first hour and by 65-70% during longer
periods of exposure to gossypol.

Differentiated functions of Sertoli cells include the production of various secretory proteins, such as androgen binding protein
(ABP) [73, 74], plasminogen activator [75], transferrin [76, 77],
retinol-binding protein [78], and a potent mitogenic polypeptide,
the seminiferous growth factor (SGF) [79, 80]. A decrease in the
overall rate of protein synthesis after exposure to gossypol suggests a lower production of these particular proteins. In fact,
synthesis of ABP is known to be reduced in Sertoli cells cultured
in the presence of gossypol [81]. While ABP has no known effect
on germ cells, the many other Sertoli cell proteins probably have

important roles in promoting spermatogenesis [82, 83, 84, 85, 86].
For instance, FSH stimulates the synthesis and secretion of transferrin [87, 88], which is known to be essential for cells to progress through the G2 phase of the cell cycle [89, 90]. Therefore,
by extrapolation, an enhanced sensitivity of Sertoli cells in vivo
to gossypol presumably would perturb expression of their secretory
functions and hence, in turn, would have detrimental effects on the
differentiating germ cells.

The marked decrement in protein synthesis and proliferation by
TR-ST cells in response to gossypol could be mediated by the drugs'
action on mitochondria. The functional state of these organelles
can be assessed by using rhodamine-123 and other related fluorescent, cationic dyes. The staining specificity for mitochondria of
live cells is attributed to the positive charge of the dye at physiological pH and to the organelles' high transmembrane potential (inside-negative) [91, 92, 93]. Thus, the accumulation of these
fluorescent probes diminishes when the mitochondrial transmembrane
potential is decreased by uncoupling oxidative phosphorylation with
dinitrophenol (DNP) or with p-trifluoromethoxy-phenylhydrazone
(FCCP), by inhibiting electron transport with oligomycin or sodium
azide, or by treating the cells with the ionophore valinomycin. By
contrast, the ionophore nigericin enhances the accumulation of these
cationic dyes by mitochondria [94], presumably by increasing the
transmembrane potential through an electrically neutral exchange of
protons for K^+.

Rhodamine-123 was selected from among the fluorescent mitochondrial probes for the following reasons. First, a brief exposure to rhodamine-123 is not toxic to cells [95, 96]; although prolonged incubation with the probe may have cytostatic and cytotoxic
effects [97, 98, 99]. Second, this supravital dye has been used extensively to study the various structural and functional states of
mitochondria in different cells at successive stages of their proliferation and differentiation [100, 101, 102, 103, 104, 105, 106].
Finally, rhodamine-123 has been applied successfully to assess the
viability of leukemia cells after treatment with anticancer drugs
[107].

The decrease in the transmembrane potential of mitochondria is
an early event among the known responses of TR-ST cells to gossypol.
Moreover, on removing the drug from the cultured cells, the mitochondrial transmembrane potential appears to return to normal prior
to reformation of cellular morphology. These results suggest that
mitochondria may be the primary site of gossypol action in Sertoli
cells, an observation that concurs with previous reports of similar
effects on the mitochondria of advanced, differentiating spermatids
and maturing testicular and epididymal spermatozoa [108, 109, 110].
These deleterious effects could be mediated by gossypol's action as
an uncoupler of oxidative phosphorylation. The drug possesses three

functional groups typical of uncouplers [111], including an acid-
dissociable group (-OH) attached to an unsaturated ring structure,

an electron withdrawing moiety (H-C=O), and several hydrophobic groups
(-CH₃). Studies utilizing polarographic techniques suggest that
gossypol is an effective uncoupler of isolated rat liver mitochondria [112]. Alternatively, the drug may enhance other processes
that decrease the mitochondrial transmembrane potential. An example of this could be increased superoxide production as shown to occur in Arbacia sperm on exposure to gossypol [113].

The decrease in mitochondrial transmembrane potential during
gossypol treatment appears to be specific for Sertoli cells and
spermatozoa. Differentiating germ cells and several other cultured
somatic cells are considerably less sensitive to gossypol. Normally, a lipophilic uncoupler exerts its physiological effects after
binding to the plasma and/or mitochondrial membranes [114]. Therefore, the selective action of gossypol on Sertoli cells and spermatozoa could be due to their sharing unusual constituents in either
their mitochondrial or plasma membranes. For instance, these particular cells could be more permeable and therefore sequester higher
concentrations of gossypol. Such unusual membrane constituents also
could be responsible for the distinct conformation of sperm and Sertoli
cell mitochondria, which differ from those in germ cells at early
stages of differentiation. Sertoli cell mitochondria are orthodox
and frequently cup-shaped in conformation [115, 116], whereas those
of sperm are crescent-shaped and can appear in either orthodox or
condensed forms, depending on the osmolarity of the medium [117,
118]. By contrast, mitochondria of spermatocytes and early spermatids exist in a condensed form that appears to be resistant to
changes in media osmolarity [119]. These various conformations of
mitochondria could reflect differences in their levels of oxidative
phosphorylation [120]. It is feasible, therefore, that gossypol may
selectively affect mitochondria of a certain conformation or a particular state of oxidative phosphorylation. Consequently, studies
on the effect of gossypol on the structure and function of mitochondria in different conformational states, may help resolve these
questions [121, 122].

ACKNOWLEDGMENTS

The preparation of this article was funded by Rockefeller Foundation Grant RF 82014 and, in part, by Center Grant HD 06916 from the
National Institute of Child Health and Human Development.

The authors wish to acknowledge the scientific contributions
of Dr. Lan Bo Chen and Beth Shepherd, Dana Farber Cancer Institute,
Boston, Massachusetts. Appreciation is extended to Steven Borack for

providing photographic services and to Mrs. Barbara Lewis for pre-
paring the manuscript.

REFERENCES

1. N. R. Farnsworth and D. P. Waller, Current status of plant
    products reported to inhibit sperm, PARFR Research Frontiers
    in Fertility Regulation, 2:1 (1982), pp. 1-16.
2. M. R. N. Prasad and E. Diczfalusy, Gossypol, "Proc. Second
    International Congress Andrology," Tel Aviv, June 28-30
    (1981).
3. G. I. Zatuchni and C. K. Osborn, Gossypol: A possible male
    antifertility agent, PARFR Research Frontiers in Fertility
    Regulation, 1:4 (1981), pp. 1-16.
4. National Coordinating Group on Male Fertility, Gossypol - A
    new antifertility agent for males, Chinese Med. J., 4:417
    (1978).
5. A. De Peyster and Y. Y. Wang, Proposed contraceptive for men
    passes the Ames' test, New Eng. J. Med., 301:275 (1979).
6. Y. Cai, Y. Liu, G. Xu, S, Li, and S. Shieh, Effect of gossypol
    on the pregnancy of chromosomal aberrations and sister chro-
    matid exchanges in human peripheral lymphocyte in vitro, Acta
    Anat. Sin., 12:293 (1981).
7. W. S. Ye, J. C. Liang, and T. C. Hsu, Toxicity of a male con-
    traceptive, gossypol, in mammalian cell cultures, In vitro,
    19:53 (1983).
8. National Coordinating Group on Male Fertility, op. cit. (see
    Ref. 4).
9. S. Xue, S. Zong, S. Shuyun, W. Yanwan, Y. Liu, Z. Zhon, and
    X. Ma, Antispermatogenic effect of gossypol on the germinal
    epithelium of the rat testis. A cytological autoradiograph-
    ical and ultrastructural observation, Sci. Sin., 9:915 (Eng.
    ed.); 23:642 (1980).
10. M. C. Chang, Z. P. Gu, and S. K. Saksena, Effects of gossypol
    on the fertility of male rats, hamsters, and rabbits, Contra-
    ception, 21:461 (1980).
11. L. Shandilya, T. B. Clarkson, M. R. Adams, and J. C. Lewis,
    Effects of gossypol on reproductive and endocrine functions of
    male cynomolgus monkeys (Macaca fascicularis), Biol. Reprod.,
    27:241 (1982).
12. National Coordinating Group on Male Fertility, op. cit. (see
    Ref. 4).
13. A. P. Hoffer, Light and electron microscopic studies on the
    effects of gossypol in the male rat, Presented at PARFR Work-
    shop on Gossypol, Chicago (1980).
14. C. W. Bardin, U. S. Sundaram, and C. C. Chang, Toxicology,
    endocrine, and histopathologic studies in small animals and
    Rhesus monkeys administered gossypol, Presented at PARFR Work-
    shop on Gossypol, Chicago (1980).

15. M. C. Chang, Z. Gu, and Y. Y. Tsong, Studies on gossypol. I. Toxicity, antifertility and endocrine analyses in male rats, Int. J. Fert., 27:213 (1982).

16. A. P. Hoffer, S. J. Klein, S. Wesson, and J. Canick, Direct effects of gossypol on steroidogenic enzymes in rat and human testis nucleosomes. Abstracts, 65th Annual Meeting, The Endocrine Society, San Antonio, Texas, p. 104 (1983).

17. L. A. Zhuang, D. M. Phillips, G. L. Gunsalus, C. W. Bardin, and J. P. Mather, Effects of gossypol on rat Sertoli and Leydig cells in primary culture and established cell lines, J. Androl., 4:336 (1983).

18. M. A. Hadley, Y. C. Lin, and M. Dym, Effects of gossypol on the reproductive system of male rats, J. Androl., 2:190 (1981).

19. J. Lin, E. P. Morano, J. Osterman, H. Nankin, and P. Coulsen, Gossypol inhibits testicular steroidogenesis, Fertil. Steril., 35:563 (1981).

20. H. Poso, K. Wichmann, J. Janne, and T. Luukkainen, Gossypol: A powerful inhibitor of human spermatozoal metabolism, Lancet, 1980:885 (1980).

21. A. J. Ridley and L. Blasco, Testosterone and gossypol effects on human sperm motility, Fert. Steril., 36:638 (1981).

22. S. M. Cameron, D. P. Waller, and L. J. D. Zaneveld, Vaginal spermicidal activity of gossypol in the Macaca arctoides, Fertil. Steril., 37:273 (1982).

23. C. Y. Lee and H. Y. Malling, Selective inhibition of sperm-specific lactate dehydrogenase-X by an antifertility agent, Fed. Proc., 40:718 (1981).

24. C. Y. Lee, Y. S. Moon, and V. Gomel, Inactivation of acetate dehydrogenase-X by gossypol, Arch. Androl., 9:34 (1982).

25. W. W. Tso and C. S. Lee, Lactate dehydrogenase-X an isozyme particularly sensitive to gossypol inhibition, Int. J. Androl., 5:205 (1982).

26. W. W. Tso, C. S. Lee, and M. Y. W. Tso, Sensitivity of various spermatozoal enzymes to gossypol inhibitor, Arch. Androl., 9:31 (1982).

27. C. Y. G. Lee, Y. S. Moon, J. H. Yuan, and A. F. Chen, Enzyme inactivation and inhibition by gossypol, Mol. Cell Biochem., 47:65 (1982).

28. W. W. Tso and C. S. Lee, 1982, op. cit. (see Ref. 25).

29. W. W. Tso, C. S. Lee, and M. Y. W. Tso, 1982, op. cit. (see Ref. 26).

30. O. Adeyamo, C. Y. Chang, S. J. Segal, and S. S. Koide, Gossypol action on the production an utilization of ATP in sea urchin spermatozoa, Arch. Androl., 9:343 (1983).

31. Poso, et al., 1980, op. cit. (see Ref. 20).

32. M. Coburn, P. Sinsheimer, S. J. Segal, M. Burgos, and W. Troli, Oxygen free radical generation by gossypol: A possible mechanism of antifertility action in sea urchin sperm, Biol. Bull., 159:468 (1980).

33. H. H. Van der Ven, A. K. Bhattacharya, J. Karninski, Z. Bnior, L. Bauer, and L. J. D. Zaneveld, Inhibition of human sperm capacitiation by proteinase inhibitors and a high molecular weight factor from human seminal plasma, Biol. Reprod., 24: Suppl. 1, 38A (1981).

34. Ibid.

35. W. W. Tso and C. S. Lee, Gossypol: An effective acrosin blocker, Arch. Androl., 8:143 (1982).

36. Coburn et al., 1980, op. cit. (see Ref. 32).

37. R. Oko and F. Hrudka, Segmental aplasia of the mitochondrial sheath and sequelae induced by gossypol in rat spermatozoa, Biol. Reprod., 26:183 (1982).

38. R. Oko and F. Hrudka, Effect of gossypol on spermatozoa, Arch. Androl., 9:39 (1982).

39. R. Oko and F. Hrudka, 1982, op. cit. (see Ref. 37).

40. M. J. Nadakuvukaren, R. H. Sorensen, and J. M. Tone, Effect of gossypol on the ultrastructure of rat spermatozoa, Cell Tiss. Res., 204:293 (1979).

41. A. P. Hoffer, Ultrastructural studies of spermatozoa and the epithelial lining of the epididymis and vas deferens in rats treated with gossypol, Arch. Androl., 8:233 (1982). National Coordinating Group on Male Fertility, 1978, op. cit. (see Ref. 4).

43. R. Oko and F. Hrudka, 1982, op. cit. (see Ref. 37).

44. R. Oka and F. Hrudka, 1982, op. cit. (see Ref. 38).

45. A. P. Hoffer, Effects of gossypol on the seminiferous epithelium in the rat: A light and electron microscope study, Biol. Reprod., 28:1007 (1983).

46. Y. Clermont and H. Morgentaler, Quantitative study of spermatogenesis in the hypophysectomized rat, Endocrinology, 57:369 (1955).

47. L. Russell and Y. Clermont, Generation of germ cells in normal, hypophysectomized and hormone-treated hypophysectomized rats, Anat. Rec., 188:347 (1977).

48. M. Parvinen, Regulation of the seminiferous epithelium, Endocrine Rev., 3:404 (1982).

49. National Coordinating Group on Male Fertility, 1978, op. cit. (see Ref. 4).

50. M. C. Chang, et al., 1980, op. cit. (see Ref. 10).

51. A. P. Hoffer, 1983, op. cit. (see Ref. 45).

52. R. Oko and F. Hrudka, 1982, op. cit. (see Ref. 38).

53. Y. Clermont and H. Morgentaler, 1955, op. cit. (see Ref. 46).

54. R. M. Pelletier and D. S. Friend, Effects of the experimental contraceptive agent gossypol on guinea pig Sertoli cell junctions, J. Cell Biol., 87(1519a.

55. Ibid.

56. M. Dym and D. W. Fawcett, The blood testis barrier in the rat and the physiological compartmentation of the seminiferous epithelium, Biol. Reprod., 3:308 (1970).

57. L. Russell, Movement of spermatocytes from the basal to the
     adluminal compartment of the rat testis, Am. J. Anat., 148:
     313 (1977).
58. L. Russell, Sertoli-germ cell interrelations: A review.
     Gamete Res., 3:179 (1980).
59. D. W. Fawcett, in: "Regulation of mammalian reproduction"
     (S. Segal, ed.), Charles Thomas, Springfield (1973).
60. D. W. Fawcett, The ulstructure and functions of the Sertoli
     cell, in: "Frontiers in Reproduction and Fertility Control -
     A Review of the Reproductive Sciences and Contraceptive De-
     velopment" (R. O. Greep and M. A. Koblinsky, eds.), M.I.T.
     Press, Cambridge, p. 302 (1977).
61. M. Parvinen, 1982, op. cit. (see Ref. 48).
62. D. W. Fawcett, 1977, op. cit. (see Ref. 60).
63. J. P. Mather, L. Z. Zhuang, V. Perez-Infante, and D. M. Phillips,
     Culture of testicular cells in hormone-supplemented serum-free
     medium, Ann. NY Acad. Sci., 383:44 (1982).
64. Ibid.
65. B. B. Mishell, S. M. Shiigi, C. Henry, E. L. Chan, J. North,
     R. Gallily, M. Slomich, K. Miller, J. Marlbrook, D. Parks, and
     A. H. Good, in: "Selected Methods in Cellular Immunology,"
     W. H. Freeman and Company, San Francisco, pp. 3-27 (1980).
66. J. P. Mather, et al., 1982, op. cit. (see Ref. 63).
67. L. V. Johnson, M. L. Walsh, and L. B. Chen, Localization of
     mitochondria in living cells with rhodamine-123, Proc. Nat.
     Acad. Sci., 77:990 (1980).
68. L. V. Johnson, M. L. Walsh, B. J. Bockus, and L. B. Chen, Mon-
     itoring of relative mitochondrial membrane potential in living
     cells by fluorescence microscopy, J. Cell Biol., 88:526 (1981).
69. Z. Darzynkiewicz, F. Traganos, L. Staiano-Coico, J. Kapuscinski,
     and M. R. Melamed, Interactions of rhodamine-123 with living
     cells studied by flow cytometry, Cancer Res., 42:779 (1982).
70. A. R. Bellvé, C. F. Millette, Y. M. Bhatnagar, and D. A.
     O'Brien, Dissociation of the mammalian testis and character-
     ization of spermatogenic cells, J. Hist. Chem., 25:480 (1976).
71. A. R. Bellvé, J. C. Cavicchia, C. F. Millette, D. A. O'Brien,
     Y. M. Bhatnagar, and M. Dym, Spermatogenic cells of the pre-
     puberal mouse: Isolation and morphological characterization,
     J. Cell Biol., 74:68 (1977).
72. L. J. Romrell, A. R. Bellvé, and D. W. Fawcett, Separation of
     mouse spermatogenic cells by sedimentation velocity: A morph-
     ological characterization, Dev. Biol., 49:119 (1976).
73. C. W. Bardin, N. Musto, G. Gunsalus, N. Kotite, S. L. Cheng,
     F. Farrea, and R. Becker, Extracellular androgen binding
     proteins, Ann. Rev. Physiol., 43:189 (1981).
74. V. Hansson, S. C. Waddington, O. Naess, A. Altramadal, F. S.
     French, N. Kotite, S. M. Nayfeh, E. M. Ritzén, and L. Hagenäs,
     Testicular androgen-binding protein (ABP): A parameter of
     Sertoli cell secretory function, in: "Hormonal Regulation of
     Spermatogenesis" (F. J. French, V. Hansson, E. M. Ritzén, and
     S. N. Nayfek, eds.), Plenum Press, New York, p. 323 (1975).

75. M. Lacroix, M. Parvinen, and I. B. Fritz, Localization of testicular plasminogen activator in discrete portions (stages VII and VIII of the seminiferous tubule), Biol. Reprod., 25: 143 (1981).

76. M. K. Skinner and M. D. Griswold, Sertoli cells synthesize and secrete transferrin-like protein, J. Biol. Chem., 255:9523 (1980).

77. W. W. Wright, N. A. Musto, J. P. Mather, and C. W. Bardin, Sertoli cells secrete both testis-specific and serum proteins, Proc. Nat. Acad. Sci., 78:7565 (1981).

78. J. Huggenvik and M. D. Griswold, Retinol binding protein in rat testicular cells, J. Reprod. Fert., 61:403 (1981).

79. L. A. Feig, A. R. Bellvé, N. H. Erickson, and M. Klagsbrun, Sertoli cells contain a mitogenic polypeptide, Proc. Nat. Acad. Sci., 77:4774 (1980).

80. L. A. Feig, M. Klagsbrun, and A. R. Bellvé, Mitogenic peptide of the mammalian seminiferous epithelium: Biochemical characterization and partial purification, J. Cell Biol., Vol. 97: 1435 (1983).

81. L. A. Zhuang, et al., 1983, op. cit. (see Ref. 17).

82. M. Parvinen, 1982, op. cit. (see Ref. 48).

83. M. Lacroix, et al., 1981, op. cit. (see Ref. 75).

84. W. W. Wright, et al., 1981, op. cit. (see Ref. 77).

85. L. A. Feig, et al., 1980, op. cit. (see Ref. 79).

86. E. Steinberger, A. Steinberger, and B. Sanborn, in: "Recent Progress in Andrology" (A. Fabbrini and E. Steinberger, eds.), Academic Press, New York pp. 143-178 (1978).

87. M. K. Skinner, and M. D. Griswold, 1980, op. cit. (see Ref. 76).

88. M. K. Skinner and M. D. Griswold, Secretion of testicular transferrin by cultured Sertoli cells is regulated by hormones and retinoids, Biol. Reprod., 27:211 (1982).

89. P. S. Rudland, H. Durbin, D. Clingan, and L. J. de Asua, Iron salts and transferrin are specifically required for cell division of cultured 3T6 cells, Biochem. Biophys. Res. Commun., 75:556 (1977).

90. I. Bottenstein, I. Hayashi, S. Hurchinga, H. Masui, J. Mather, D. B. McClure, S. O'Hara, A. Rossino, G. Sato, G. Serrerq, R. Wulf, and R. Wu, The Growth of cells in serum-free hormone-supplemented media, in: "Methods in Enzymology" (W. B. Jakoby and I. N. Pastan, eds.), Academic Press, New York, 58:94 (1979).

91. L. V. Johnson, et al., 1980, op. cit. (see Ref. 67).

92. L. V. Johnson, et al., 1981, op. cit. (see Ref. 68).

93. Z. Darzynkiewicz, et al., 1982, op. cit. (see Ref. 69).

94. L. V. Johnson, et al., 1981, op. cit. (see Ref. 68).

95. L. B. Chen, I. C. Summerhayes, L. V. Johnson, M. L. Walsh, S. D. Bernal, and T. J. Lampides, Probing mitochondria in living cells with rhodamine-123, Cold Spring Harbor Symp. Quant. Biol., 56:141 (1982).

96.   A. R. L. Gear, Rhodamine 6G: A potent inhibitor of mito-
      chondrial oxidative phosphorylation, J. Biol. Chem., 249:3628
      (1974).
97.   Z. Darzynkiewicz et al., 1982 op. cit. (see Ref. 69).
98.   T. J. Lampidis, S. D. Bernal, I. C. Summerhayes, and L. B.
      Chen, Rhodamine-123 is selectively toxic and preferentially
      retained in carcinoma cells in vitro, Ann. New York Acad.
      Sci., 397:299 (1982).
99.   T. J. Lampidis, S. J. Bernal, I. C. Summerhayes, and L. B.
      Chen., Selective toxicity of rhodamine-123 in carcinoma cells
      in vitro, Cancer Res., 43:716 (1983).
100. L. V. Johnson, et al., 1981, op. cit. (see Ref. 68).
101. T. J. Lampidis, et al., 1982, op. cit. (see Ref. 98).
102. T. J. Lampidis, et al., 1983, op. cit. (see Ref. 99).
103. A. Darzynkiewicz, L. Staiano-Coico, and M. R. Melamed, In-
      creased mitochondrial uptake of rhodamine-123 during lympho-
      cytic stimulation, Proc. Nat. Acad. Sci., 78:2383 (1981).
104. R. L. Cohen, R. A. Muirhead, J. E. Gill, A. S. Waggoner, and
      P. U. Horan, A cyanine dye distinguishes between cycling and
      noncycling fibroblasts, Nature, 290:593 (1981).
105. S. Goldstein and L. B. Kroczack, Status of mitochondria in
      living human fibroblasts during growth and senescence in
      vitro: Use of the laser dye rhodamine-123, J. Cell Biol.,
      91:392 (1981).
106. R. Levenson, I. G. Macara, R. L. Smith, L. Cantley, and D.
      Housman, Role of mitochondrial membrane potential in the
      regulation of murine erythroleukemia cell differentiation,
      Cell, 28:855 (1982).
107. S. M. Bernal, H. M. Shapiro, and L. B. Chen, Monitoring the
      effect of anti-cancer drugs on L1210 cells by a mitochondrial
      probe, Rhodamine-123, Int. J. Cancer, 30:217 (1982).
108. R. Oko and F. Hrudka, 1982, op. cit. (see Ref. 37).
109. R. Oko and F. Hrudka, 1982, op. cit. (see Ref. 38).
110. A. P. Hoffer, 1983, op. cit. (See Ref. 45).
111. H. Terada, The interaction of highly active couplers with
      mitochondria, Biochem. Biophys. Acta, 639:225 (1981).
112. M. A. Abou-Donia and J. W. Dieckert, Gossypol: Uncoupling of
      respiratory chain and oxidative phosphorylation, Life Sciences,
      14:1955 (1974).
113. M. Coburn, et al., 1980, op. cit. (see Ref. 32).
114. N. V. Katre and D. F. Wilson, Interaction of uncouplers with
      the mitochondrial membrane: Identification of the high af-
      finity binding site, Arch. Biochem. Biophys., 191:647 (1978).
115. C. De Martino, A. Floridi, M. C. Marcante, W. Malorni, P. S.
      Barcellone, M. Bellocci, and B. Silvestrini, Morphological and
      histochemical and biochemical studies on germ cell mitochondria
      of normal rats, Cell Tiss. Res., 196:1 (1979).
116. C. De Martino, M. C. Marcante, A. Floridi, G. Citro, M.
      Bellocci, A. Cantafora, and P. G. Natali, Sertoli cells of
      adult rats in vitro, Cell Tiss. Res., 176:69 (1977).

117. Ibid.
118. F. Hrudka, A morphological and cytochemical study on isolated sperm mitochondria, J. Ultrastruct. Res., 63:1 (1978).
119. C. De Martino, et al., 1979, op. cit. (see Ref. 115).
120. C. R. Hackenbrock, Ultrastructural bases for metabolically linked mechanical activity in mitochondria, J. Cell Biol., 37:345 (1968).
121. Ibid.
122. P. L. Pederson, J. W. Greenawalt, B. Reynafarje, J. Hulliben, G. L. Decker, J. W. Soper, and E. Bustamente, Preparation and characterization of mitochondria and submitochondrial particles of rat liver and liver derived tissues, in: "Methods in Cell Biology," Vol. 20 (D. M. Prescott, ed.), Academic Press, New York, p. 411 (1978).
123. N. Tanphaichitr, L. B. Chen, and A. R. Bellvé, Accumulation of rhodamine-123 by mitochondria of TR-ST cells is perturbed by gossypol, Biol. Reprod. (1984).

ULTRASTRUCTURAL, BIOCHEMICAL, AND ENDOCRINE STUDIES ON
THE EFFECTS OF GOSSYPOL AND ITS ISOMERIC DERIVATIVES
ON THE MALE REPRODUCTIVE TRACT

Anita P. Hoffer

Harvard Program in Urology (Longwood Area)
and
The Department of Anatomy
Harvard Medical School
Brigham and Women's Hospital
Boston, Massachusetts, 02115, U.S.A.

INTRODUCTION

Chinese scientists have reported that in clinical trials in-
volving more than 8000 men tested over a four-year period gossypol
was found to be a 99.89% effective, safe, and reversible contraceptive [1]. Treatment for eight weeks with 20 mg of gossypol daily
decreases sperm counts to well below 4×10^6/ml; a maintenance dose
of 40 mg of gossypol/wk thereafter sustains infertility. Gossypol
does not appear to affect plasma testosterone levels in human subjects [2, 3] or in monkeys [4, 5], and the drug is without adverse
effects on sexual function. A few minor side effects occur but they
are transient and disappear spontaneously within the first few weeks
of treatment. Hypokalemic paralysis, a potentially serious side
effect reported by Chinese investigators in 66/8806 cases (0.75%)
[6], was not observed in Brazilian men treated with gossypol [7]
and it has since been suggested that the incidence of hypokalemia
in China may be related more to regional differences in dietary
intake than to effects of gossypol on serum potassium [8]. More
recently, double-blind studies in gossypol-treated men in China have
failed to confirm a causal relationship between gossypol and hypokalemia [9]. Interestingly, there is a high incidence of spontaneously occurring periodic hypokalemic paralysis in Oriental men
[10].

The specific mechanism of action of gossypol as a male contraceptive is not known. While it has become increasingly clear that

gossypol exerts multiple effects [11, 12, 13, 14, 15, 16], none of these explains the basis for the unique and selective effect which gossypol appears to have on the male reproductive tract. It has been shown that the concentration of gossypol in the testis is lower than that in many other organs [17, 18], suggesting that the selective action of gossypol on the testis and/or epididymis is due not to its concentration but to a greater sensitivity and vulnerability of the testis to the drug. Researchers have speculated that gossypol may selectively inhibit an as yet unknown function specific to testicular tissues [19]. Evidence which suggests but does not prove that epididymal spermatozoa may be directly affected in the lumen of the epididymis has also been reported [20, 21, 22, 23], but this intriguing hypothesis remains to be demonstrated conclusively. The possibility that gossypol produces a single molecular lesion with multiple sequelae also can not be excluded.

It is essential that we understand the exact mechanism of action of gossypol in order to (1) determine conclusively whether it is safe, effective and reversible as a human antifertility agent, and (2) develop, if necessary, chemical modifications or alternative approaches based on thorough investigation of gossypol as a representative of a new and unique class of non-steroidal male contraceptives. The purpose of the present paper will be to summarize our efforts to date to analyze the mechanisms of action of gossypol at the systemic, cellular, and subcellular level and to study the in vitro effects of several isomeric derivatives of gossypol on sperm.

MORPHOLOGICAL STUDIES

It is well known from serial mating studies in the rat that fertility defects are inversely related in time to the phase of spermatogenesis or epididymal sperm maturation affected by drugs or other experimental manipulations; damage to epididymal sperm is indicated by defects which appear within 1-2 weeks of treatment whereas damage to testicular sperm and spermatids is indicated within 3-5 weeks of treatment [24]. The possibility that epididymal sperm or the processes involved in their maturation are directly affected by gossypol was suggested by reports that mice exhibit a significant decrease in sperm count within 10 days of gossypol treatment [25]; injection of gossypol into the epididymal fat pad of rats causes a decline in sperm motility within 24 h [26]; and distal migration of the cytoplasmic droplet from the neck of the sperm of the distal end of the midpiece, a phenomenon generally viewed as a function of epididymal sperm maturation, is impaired in gossypol-treated rats [27]. Because a contraceptive which interferes with the complex post-testicular events in the epididymis would carry with it the least risk of mutagenesis and provide for both rapid onset and reversal of the antifertility effect, the possibility that gossypol has a direct effect on epididymal sperm warrants careful attention.

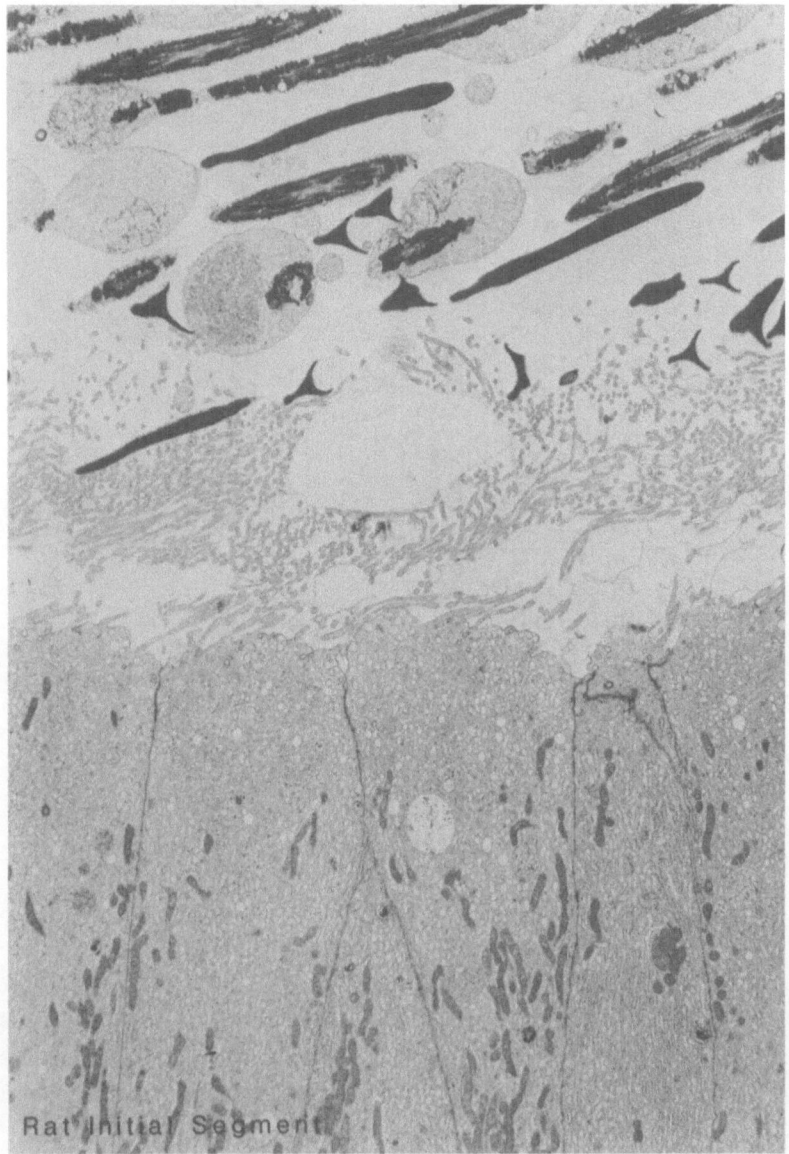

Fig. 1. Electron micrograph of the apical cytoplasm of principal
cells of the initial segment of a rat treated with 30 mg/
kg/day of gossypol for 3 weeks. Endoplasmic reticulum,
Golgi apparatus, vesicular and vacuolar elements are present
and normal in their appearance; mitochondria also exhibit
normal ultrastructural features. By contrast, the sperm in
the lumen exhibit the mitochondrial sheath defects which are
pathognomonic for gossypol treatment.

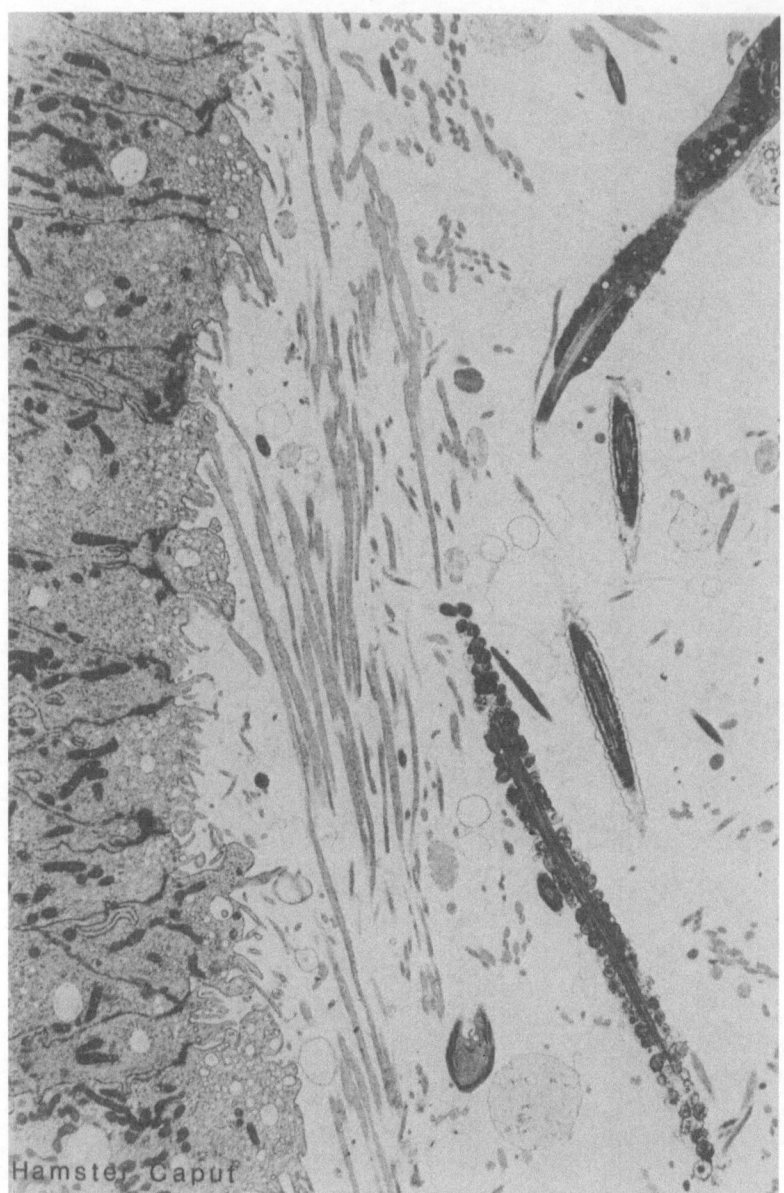

Fig. 2.   Electron micrograph of hamster caput epididymidis after
          treatment with 15 mg/kg/day of gossypol for 9 weeks. The
          epididymal epithelium appears normal in all respects; nu-
          merous multivesicular bodies in the apical cytoplasm are
          characteristically found in this region of the epididymal
          duct.   Mitochondrial sheath defects similar to those seen
          in rat epididymal sperm are also observed in the hamster.
          The hamster, as well as the rat shown in the preceeding
          micrograph, were infertile.

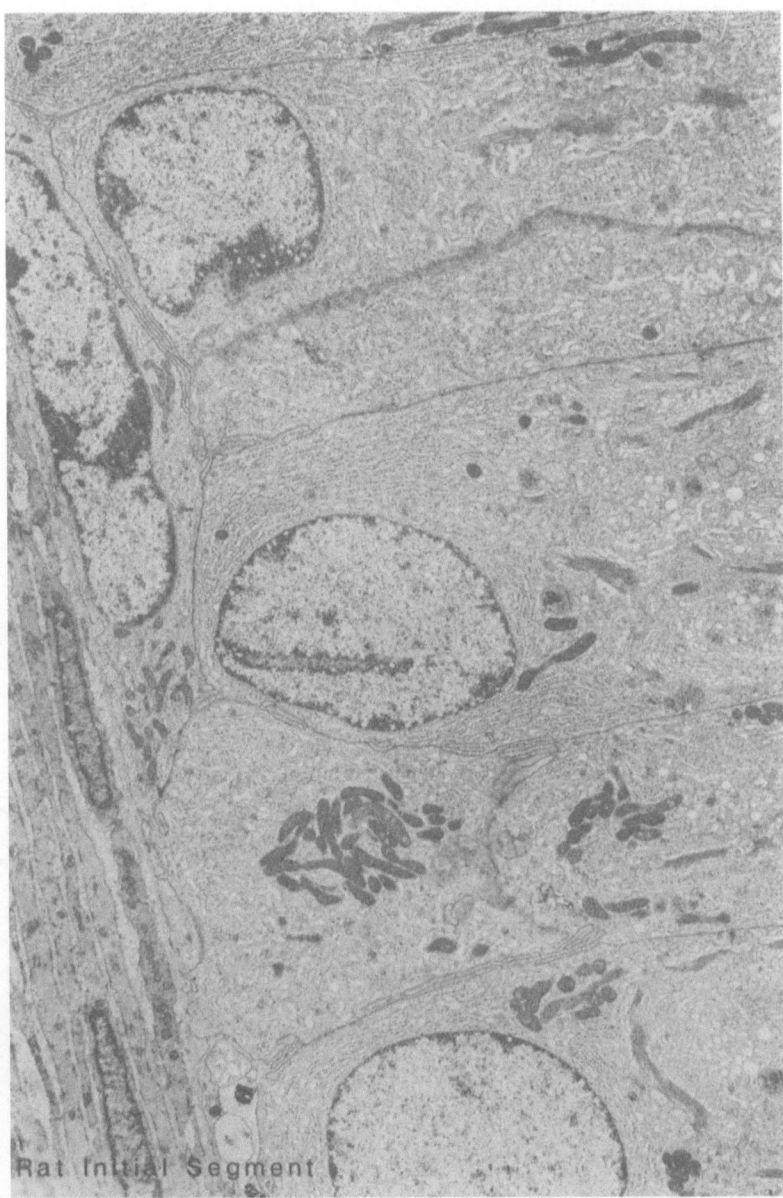

Fig. 3. A basal cell and the basal cytoplasm of several principal
cells are shown in this electron micrograph of the rat
initial segment following daily treatment with 30 mg/kg of
gossypol for 3 weeks.

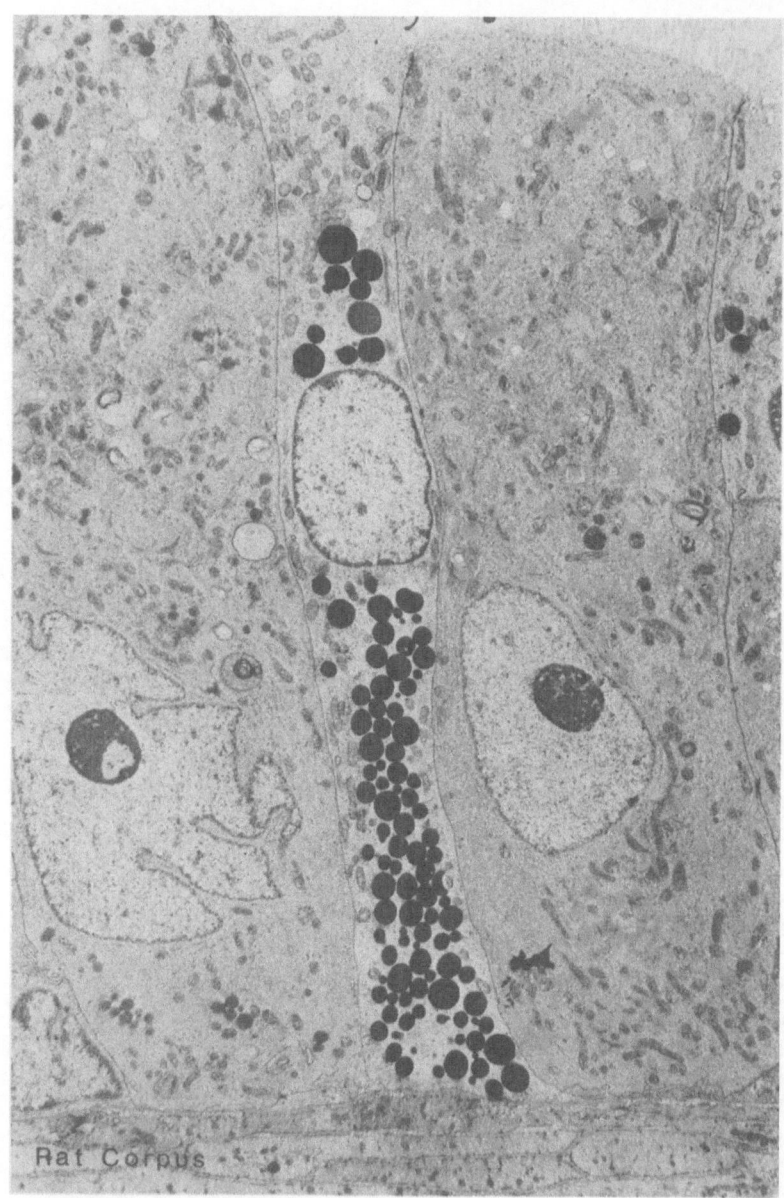

Fig. 4.   The corpus epididymidis of a rat treated with 20 mg/kg/day
          of gossypol for 5 weeks. Principal cells as well as an
          apical cell with numerous dark granules in the infra- and
          supranuclear cytoplasm exhibit normal ultrastructural fea-
          tures. A portion of a normal appearing basal cell is
          visible at the left.

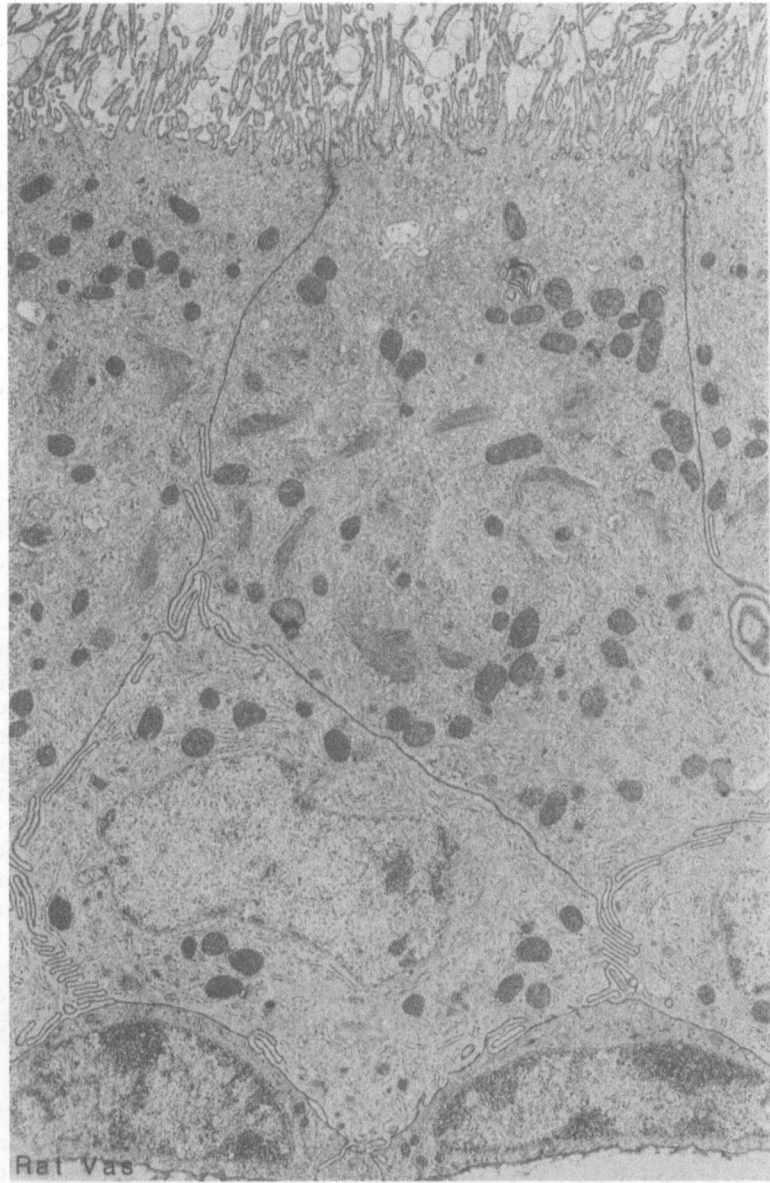

Fig. 5. Electron micrograph showing the epithelium of the vas
deferens of a rat treated daily with 10 mg/kg for 9 weeks.
The pseudostratified columnar epithelium in this region of
the excurrent ducts consists only of principal cells, basal
cells and an occasional pencil cell (not shown here). No
differences between vasa of control and gossypol-treated
rats can be detected with the electron microscope.

In analyzing the antifertility effect of gossypol, we first set out to determine whether gossypol exerts a direct effect on the ultrastructure of epididymal sperm and/or the epididymal and vasal epithelium in rats and hamsters; the effect of gossypol on sperm motility was also studied. In rats (1) epididymal sperm were examined at early time intervals (2 and 3 weeks) after 20 or 30 mg/kg/day of gossypol, (2) the extent of cellular damage at two dose levels over a 7-week period was compared to determine whether the effects of gossypol treatment are time and dose related (3) sperm were examined at different points along the length of epididymis to determine the stage of spermatogenesis or sperm maturation initially affected, and (4) the epithelial lining of the epididymis and vas were studied with the electron microscope for evidence of drug-related damage [28]. In hamsters, epididymal spermatozoa and the epididymal and vasal epithelia were examined in animals made infertile with 15 mg/kg/day of gossypol for 9 weeks.

In all rats and hamsters examined, no ultrastructural differences between gossypol-treated and control animals were observed in the epididymal epithelium at any of the doses or time intervals examined. The tall principal cells of the initial segment and caput were entirely normal in their appearance (Figs. 1 and 2). The apical cells, basal cells and agranular leucocytes were also morphologically normal in every respect (Fig. 3). In the corpus and cauda (Fig. 4), apical cells, as well as all other cell types were unaffected by the contraceptive. In contrasts to the findings of Gu and co-investigators [29], we were unable to detect degenerating mitochondria or abnormal granular and vesicular elements throughout the epididymal epithelium of gossypol-treated hamsters or rats. Recently, another team of researchers was also unable to detect an effect of gossypol on epididymal epithelium using methods for determination of Na^+ and potassium concentrations and protein patterns in fluids flushed from the cauda epididymidis of gossypol-treated rats [30]. Finally, in the vas deferens, where the pseudostratified columnar epithelium consists only of principal cells, basal cells and an occasional pencil cell, no differences between control and gossypol-treated rats could be detected with the electron microscope (Fig. 5).

The first detectable ultrastructural effects of gossypol treatment were observed in the flagella of the epididymal sperm. In order of their frequency, the types of flagellar defects observed were (a) degeneration of the midpiece mitochondria, (b) absence of one or more outer dense fibers (ODF) and/or axonemal doublets in the principal piece, (c) supernumerary or displaced outer dense fibers, (d) constriction or indentation of the mitochondrial sheath at ODF 1, 2, and 9 resulting in a separation of these three ODF's from the others, (e) profiles consisting only of outer dense fibers but devoid of mitochondria or fibrous sheath, and (f) spermatozoa with double tails (Figs. 6a, b, c). These ultrastructural defects oc-

curred regularly in the initial segment of the caput as early as 3
weeks after either 20 or 30 mg/kg/day, although minor degenerative
changes in a few sperm were observed as early as 2 weeks after treatment. Severity and frequency of the drug-induced defects increased
with dose and duration of treatment. By the fifth week at either
20 or 30 mg/kg/day, significant damage to virtually all sperm flagella
was observed throughout the epididymal duct of all treated rats.

Sperm motility was also affected in each of these experimental
groups. At 20 mg/kg/daily, a slight decline in sperm motility occurred in all the rats within the first 3 weeks of treatment followed by total inhibition after 5 weeks of treatment. At 30 mg/kg/
daily a slight decrease in sperm motility was already evident after
only 2 weeks of treatment; after 3 weeks, the decline in motility
was more severe and by the fifth week motility was completely inhibited.

Similar effects were observed in hamsters [31]. Electron micrographs reveal mitochondrial sheath defects, identical to those
found in the rat, in sperm throughout the epididymis (Fig. 6d). In
addition, motility of sperm from the cauda epididymis was totally
inhibited. These observations confirm the antifertility effect of
gossypol in hamsters previously demonstrated in mating studies
[32, 33, 34], and show that the ultrastructural basis of epididymal
sperm motility inhibition is the same in these species.

Because the time of appearance of ultrastructural defects in
epididymal sperm is consistent with a deleterious effect of gossypol
on late spermatids and testicular sperm, we next undertook a detailed
analysis of the ultrastructural effects of this contraceptive on the
rat and hamster testis [35, 36]. The doses used in each species are
those reported to produce infertility within the time period being
studied and are said to produce no pathological changes detectable
with the light microscope in organs other than the testis. In the
testis of the rat, the electron microscope reveals that gossypol
produces specific ultrastructural defects in the mitochondrial sheath
of virtually all stage 18 and 19 spermatids (Fig. 7); similar defects in midpiece mitochondria are never observed in normal rats.
As in the epididymal sperm of gossypol-fed rats, the drug-induced
defects in late spermatids are time and dose-related. They occur
as early as two weeks after 20 mg/kg/day of gossypol and increase
with time. In contrast, neither the ultrastructure nor the distribution of mitochondria in the cytoplasm of earlier elongating or
round spermatids appear to be affected (Fig. 8). Spermatocyte and
spermatogonial mitochondria are also undamaged by gossypol treatment. No other significant differences between germ cells of control and gossypol-treated rats can be observed under the conditions
employed in our study. Similar results were obtained in the testes
of hamsters treated with gossypol (Fig. 9).

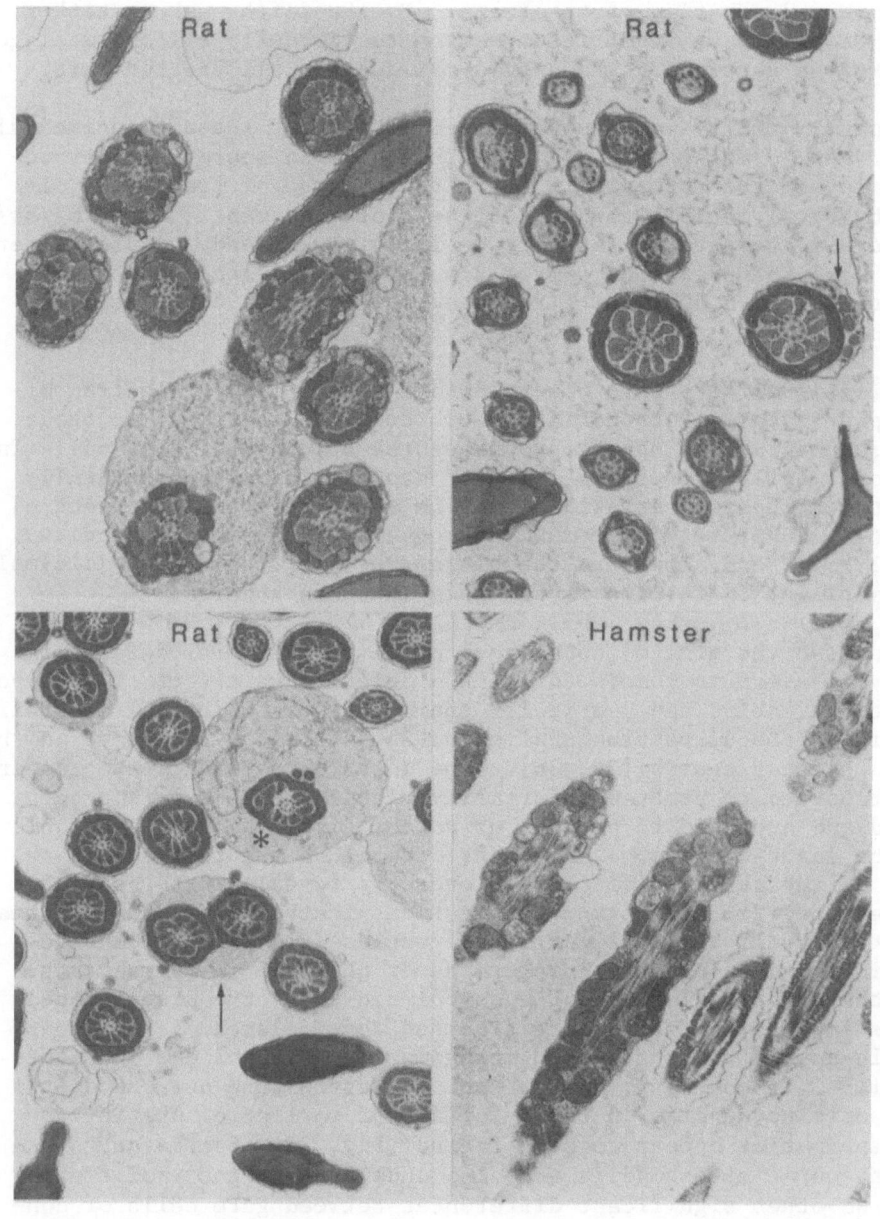

Fig. 6. Ultrastructural defects in the flagella of rat and hamster
         epididymal sperm are shown in this plate. a) In the rat,
         evidence of damage in corpus sperm is seen here after 3
         weeks of treatment with 20 mg/kg/day of gossypol; be-
         ginning degenerative changes are also visible in a few
         flagella after only 2 weeks of treatment (not shown). b)
         This electron micrograph shows sperm in the corpus epi-
         didymidis after 20 mg/kg/day of gossypol for 3 weeks.
         In several profiles, outer dense fibers and axonemal doub-
         lets are missing; supernumery and displaced outer dense
         fibers can also be seen (arrow). c) Electron micrograph
         from the lumen of the initial segment of a gossypol-
         treated rat showing a spermatozoan with a double tail
         (arrow) and a flagellum with a constriction of the mito-
         chondrial sheath at outer dense fibers 1, 2, and 9, re-
         sulting in a separation of these three outer dense fibers
         from the others (asterisk). d) Epididymal sperm from
         gossypol-treated hamsters exhibit the same mitochondrial
         sheath defects as those found in rat epididymal sperm.

154

A. P. HOFFER

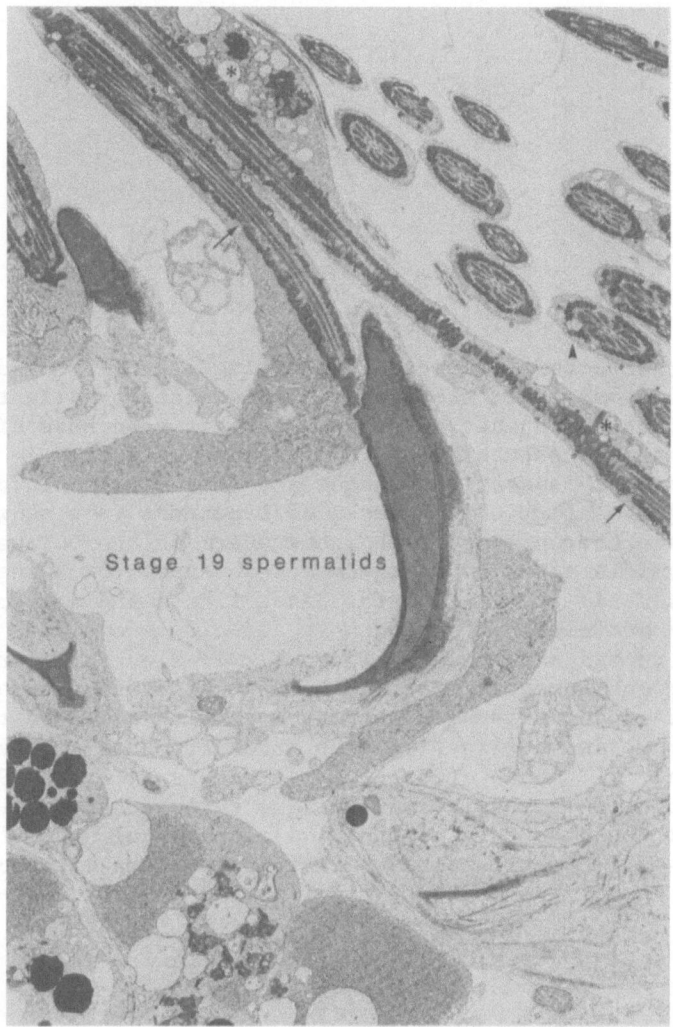

Fig. 7.   Electron micrograph of stage 19 spermatids from a stage VII
         seminiferous tubule of a rat treated with 10 mg/kg/day of
         gossypol for 9 weeks. Gossypol produces a pathognomonic
         defect in the mitochondrial sheath of late (stage 18 and
         19) spermatids. Abnormal mitochondria (arrowhead), inter-
         ruptions in the continuity of the mitochondrial sheath
         (arrows) and foci of disoriented mitochondria (asterisks)
         can be recognized along the length of the midpiece in sev-
         eral of the stage 19 spermatid tails. Similar defects in
         midpiece mitochondria are never observed in normal rats
         (not shown).

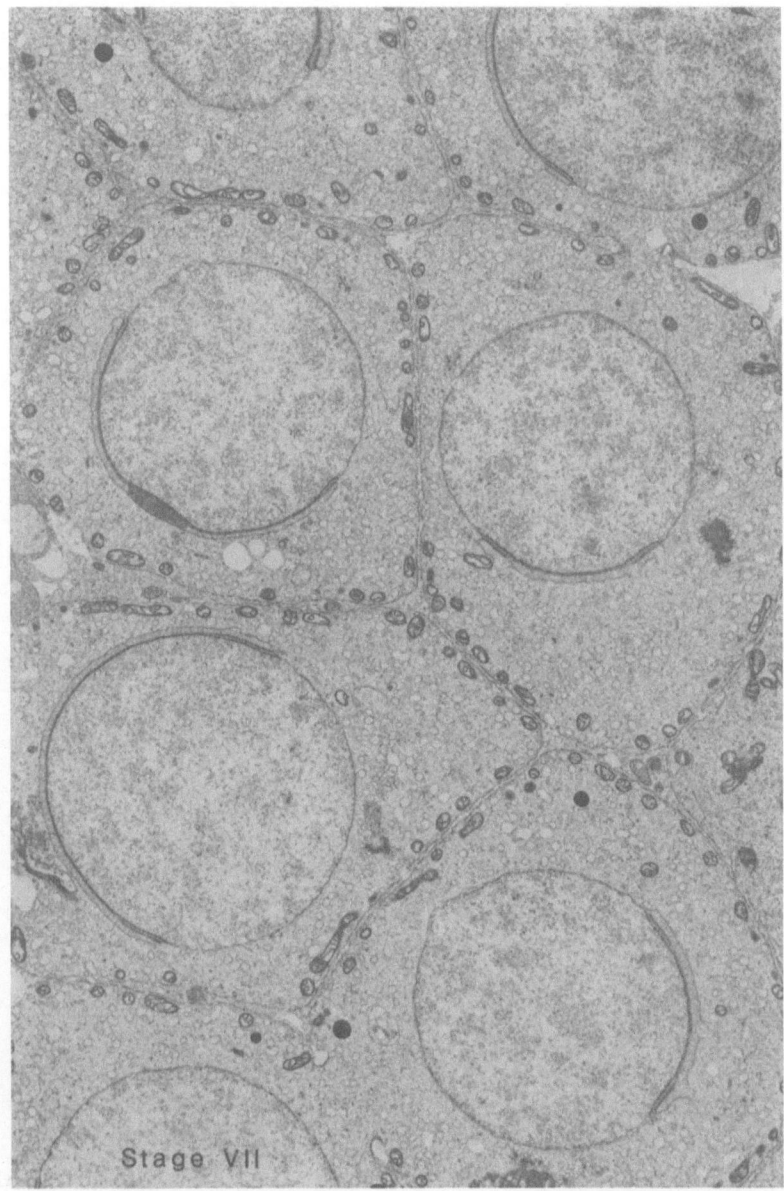

Fig. 8. Electron micrograph of a stage VII seminiferous tubule of a rat treated with 20 mg/kg/day of gossypol for 11 weeks showing portions of seven normal round spermatids with peripherally arranged mitochondria and normal chromatoid body and nuclear structure. This rat was infertile and its sperm were 100% immotile; nevertheless, the germ cells at this stage of maturation show no evidence of ultrastructural damage due to gossypol.

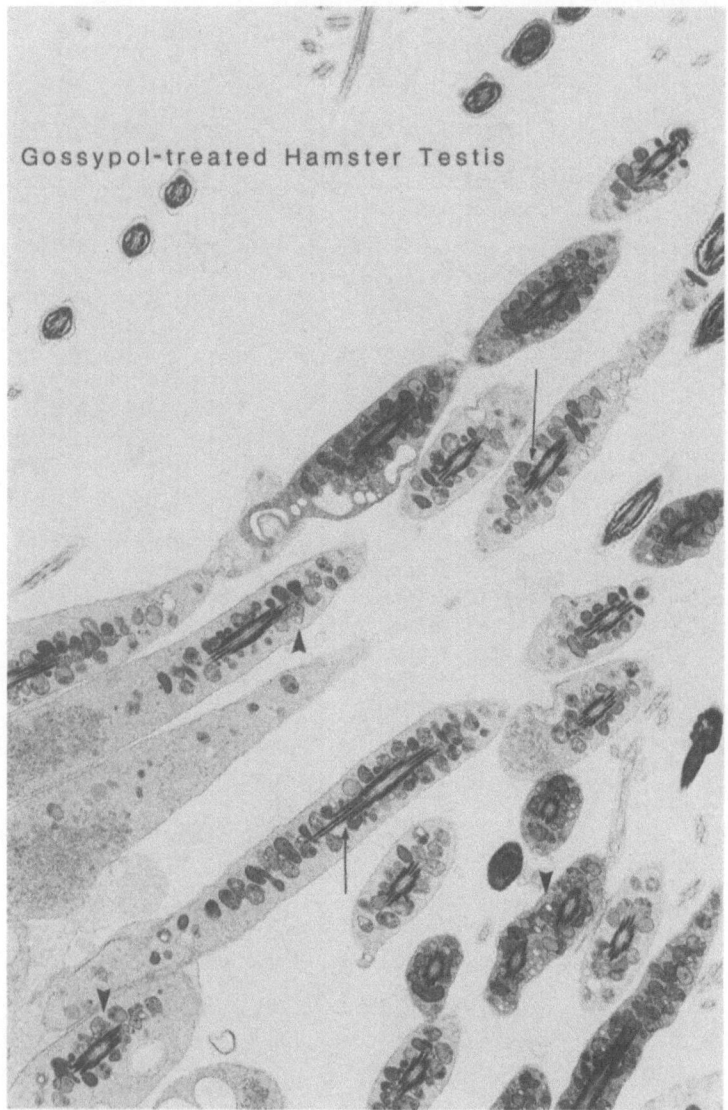

Fig. 9.   Electron micrograph of the testis of a hamster made infertile
          with 15 mg/kg/day of gossypol for 9 weeks. Defects in the
          midpiece of the flagellum of late spermatids, similar to
          those seen in the rat testis, can be observed here; these
          include severely vacuolated mitochondria (arrowheads), in-
          terruptions in the continuity of the mitochondrial sheath
          (arrows), and numerous foci of disoriented mitochondria.
          Similar defects in midpiece mitochondria are never observed
          in late spermatids of normal hamsters.

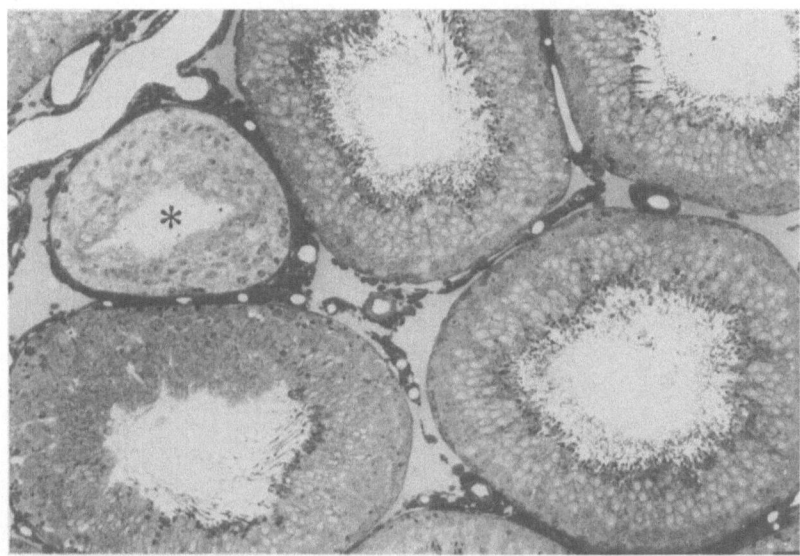

Fig. 10. Light micrograph of the testis of a rat treated with 30 mg/kg/day of gossypol for 5 weeks. Notice the presence of a severely damaged tubule (asterisk) among entirely normal seminiferous tubules. The occurrence of normal and abnormal tubular profiles in the same testis was common at doses ranging from 10-30 mg/kg/day of gossypol for 3-11 weeks. (Reproduced with the permission of Biology of Reproduction, 28:1007, 1983.)

The basis for this pathognomonic effect of gossypol in late spermatids is not known. Similar ultrastructural defects in the mitochondrial sheath of testicular sperm in gossypol-treated rats have been noted recently [37], but no data on the specific stages of germ cell differentiation which were affected by the drug were included. Other male antifertility agents are known to produce specific ultrastructural changes in the sperm head and axial fiber bundle [38, 39, 40], but to date, none have been reported which exclusively damage the mitochondria in post-meiotic germ cells.

In addition to the pathognomonic mitochondrial defects in late spermatids, another consequence of gossypol treatment in rat testes, visible at the light microscope level, is a random distribution of normal and occasional abnormal seminiferous tubules in the same section (Fig. 10) at all dose and time intervals examined [41]. The frequency and severity of damage in the seminiferous tubules varies directly with time and dose but the frequency never exceeded 46%, even in animals treated at 30 mg/kg/day for 11 weeks, the highest dose and time interval used in our study. In rats made infertile

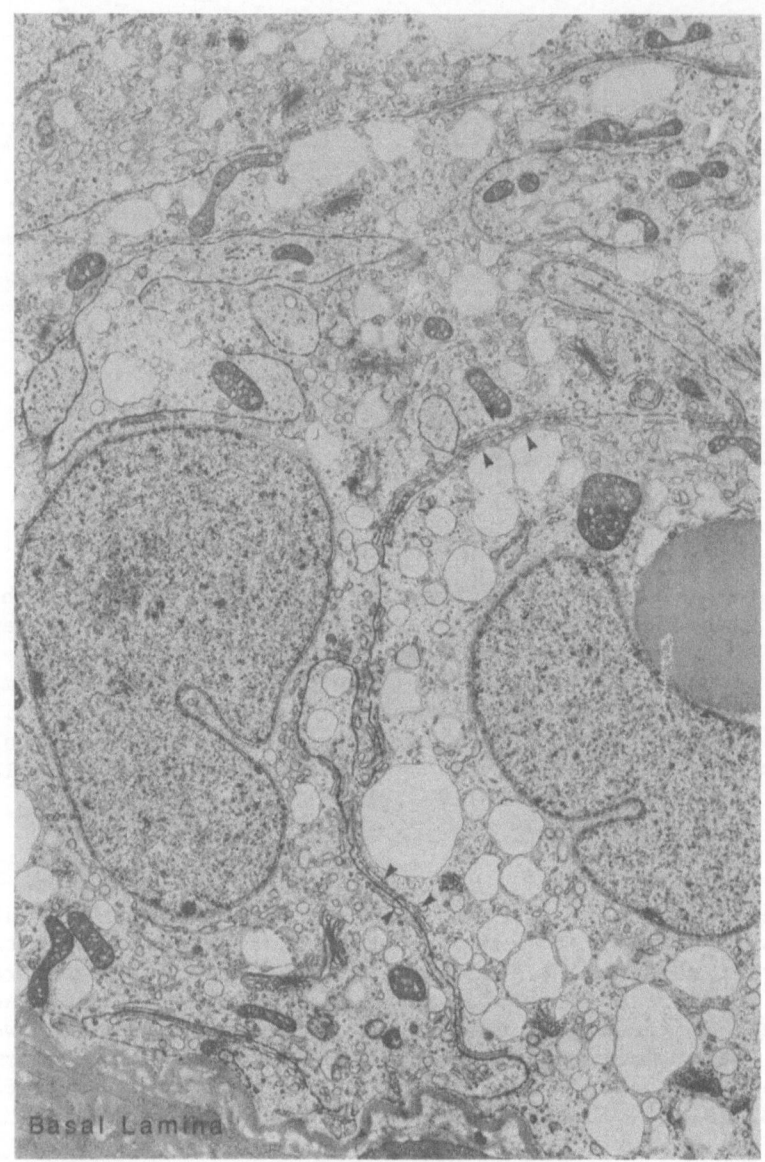

Fig. 11.   Electron micrograph of a severely damaged seminiferous
           tubule of a rat treated with 20 mg/kg/day of gossypol for
           5 weeks.   The Sertoli cells shown here exhibit large intra-
           cellular vacuoles and an overall decrease in cytoplasmic
           ground substance, endoplasmic reticulum and Golgi ele-
           ments.   Sertoli cell mitochondria, lipid droplets and nu-
           clear morphology are not significantly changed.   Interest-
           ingly, the Sertoli-Sertoli cell junctions are intact in
           several regions along the cell surface (arrowheads).

with 20 mg/kg/day of gossypol, only 10-20% of the seminiferous tubules appeared abnormal. Ultrastructural examination demonstrates that the cellular basis of this damage to the seminiferous tubules is the presence of inter- and intraepithelial vacuoles occurring primarily though not exclusively in the Sertoli cells. In electron micrographs, Sertoli cells which are damaged exhibit many large vacuoles and an overall decrease in cytoplasmic ground substance, rought and smooth endoplasmic reticulum and Golgi elements (Fig. 11). Although in general, vacuolization is a well-documented non-specific reaction of Sertoli cells to injury and several unrelated forms of male infertility [42, 43, 44, 45, 46], the significance of the response of Sertoli cells to gossypol treatment in our rat studies is unclear. The extreme focal nature and the limited extent of Sertoli cell damage is puzzling since it is reasonable to assume that blood-borne gossypol is present in equal concentration throughout the microvascular bed of the testis. The question as to whether or not the pathognomonic effect of gossypol on all late spermatids is related to or mediated through the Sertoli cells is extremely important, however. The possibility that biochemical damage to Sertoli cells underlies the spermatid defect cannot be excluded entirely although the fact that, in vivo, the mitochondrial sheath abnormalities and the decrease in sperm motility occur well in advance of the Sertoli cell changes argues against this interpretation. In addition, the frequency of vacuolated and/or atrophic seminiferous tubules in hamsters made infertile with 15 mg/kg/day of gossypol for 9 weeks is extremely low [47, 48]. An effect of gossypol on Sertoli cells of immature (20 day old) rats has been demonstrated in vitro by a decrease in androgen-binding protein production [49] but a significant direct effect of the contraceptive on Sertoli cells in vivo remains to be demonstrated.

Ultrastructural differences between the Leydig cells of control and gossypol-treated hamsters and rats were not observed at any of the dose and time intervals in our studies (Fig. 12a, b). These results are consistent with our findings on the absence of a statistically significant difference in serum testosterone levels between control and gossypol-fed rats at 5, 9, and 11 weeks [50] and with other studies reporting unchanged testosterone levels in several gossypol-treated laboratory rodents, monkeys, and man [51, 52, 53, 54, 55, 56]. In the 20 and 30 mg treatment groups, no ultrastructural differences could be detected by routine inspection at the 7 week time interval, although a statistically significant increase in testosterone production was observed at this time period (vide infra); stereological methods of analysis were not utilized.

In order to determine whether the antifertility effect of gossypol is related to a breakdown of the blood-testis (BTB) or blood-epididymis barriers (BEB), their permeability to small electron dense tracers such as lanthanum or macromolecules such as inulin was evaluated in gossypol-treated rats by electron microscope and micro-

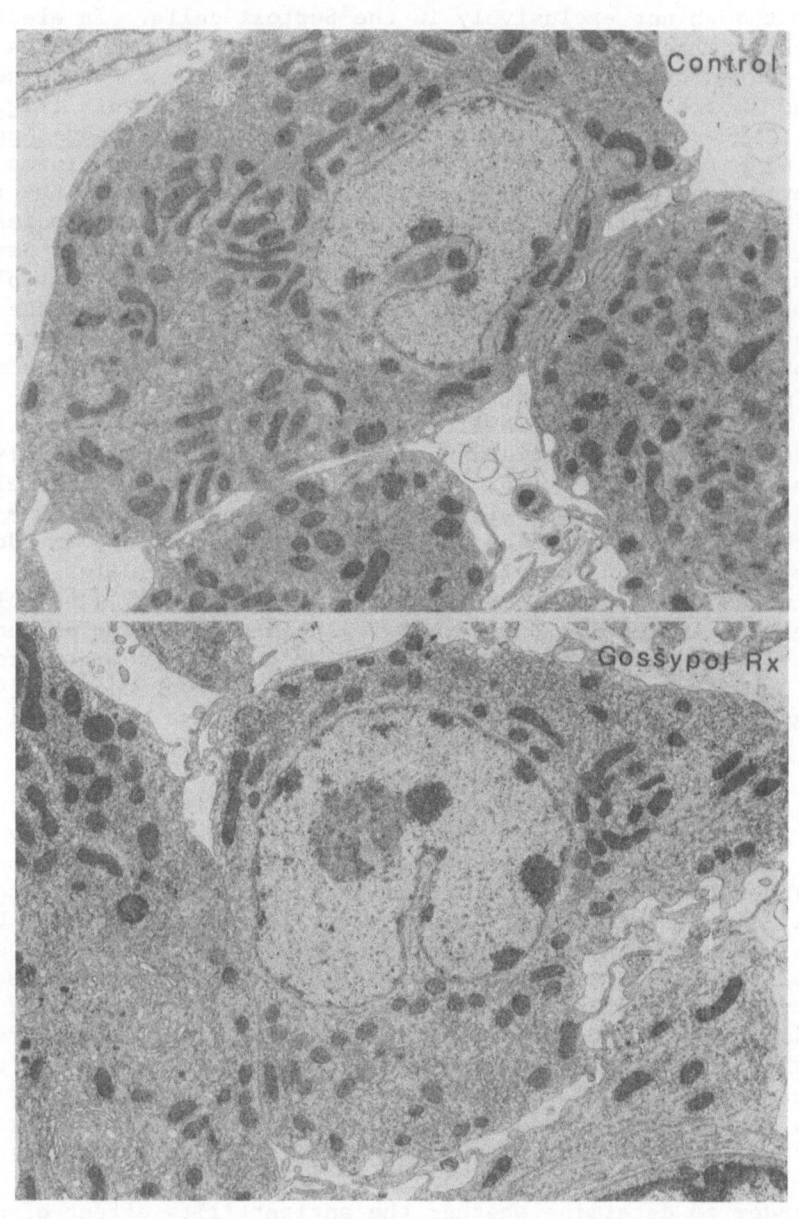

Fig. 12.   Electron micrographs showing Leydig cells from the inter-
            stitium of control and gossypol-treated rat testes. a)
            In the control testis, the Leydig cell agranular reticulum
            is extremely well-developed and consists of an elaborately
            anastomosing meshwork of smooth-surfaced tubules; numerous
            mitochondria with lamellar cristae, occasional mitochon-
            drial granules and a dense matrix are randomly distributed
            throughout the cytoplasm. b) In the testis of a rat treated
            daily with 20 mg/kg of gossypol for 7 weeks, the ultra-
            structural features are similar to those of control Leydig
            cells in all respects. Well-developed agranular reticulum,
            mitochondria and normal nuclear ultastructure are easily
            recognized.

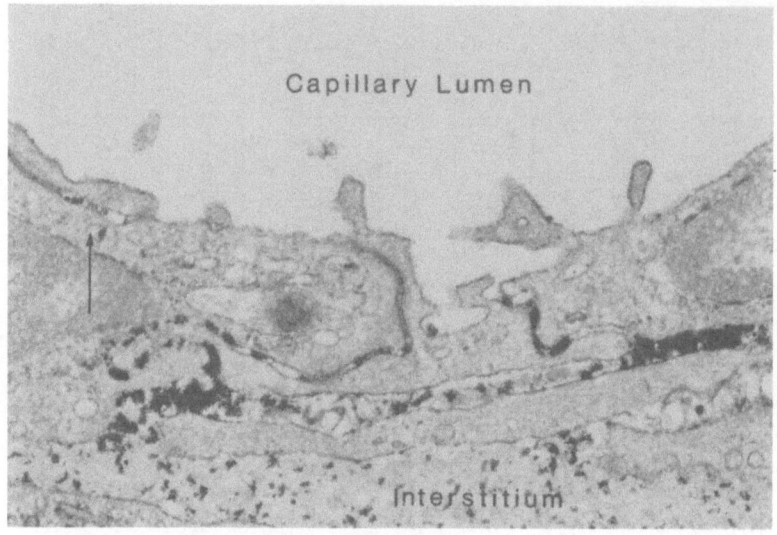

Fig. 13.   Electron micrograph showing a portion of capillary endo-
           thelium from the epididymis of a gossypol-treated rat
           which was intravascularly perfused with lanthanum.
           Throughout the epididymis of both control and gossypol-
           treated rats, lanthanum is observed between neighboring
           endothelial cells, in micropinocytosis vesicles (arrow),
           as deposits in the basal lamina and throughout the inter-
           stitium.

puncture techniques [59, 60]. No permeability differences in either
the blood-testis or blood-epididymis barrier were found to lanthanum
in control or gossypol-treated rats. Throughout the epididymis of
adult control rats or rats made infertile with 20 mg/kg/day for 6
weeks, lanthanum is observed between endothelial cells and throughout the interstitium (Fig. 13). Similarly, the cell contacts between myoid cells offer little resistance to penetration of tracer
and the increasing thickness of the peritubular myoid layer in the
distal regions of the duct has little effect on the amount of lanthanum which gains access to the base of the epithelial compartment.
Within the intercellular compartment of the epididymal epithelium,
lanthanum encounters little resistance along the basal and mid-
portions of the lateral cell surface (Fig. 14). Although the depth
of penetration may vary somewhat from one specimen to another,
tracer is readily found surrounding the basal cells and in the
lateral and extracellular space up to and including the macula and
zonula adhaerentes of the junctional complex (Fig. 15). Although
the vast majority of tracer particles is stopped at the level of
the zonula occludens (z.o.), limited penetration can occasionally
be recognized beyond the first or second point of fusion in the z.o.

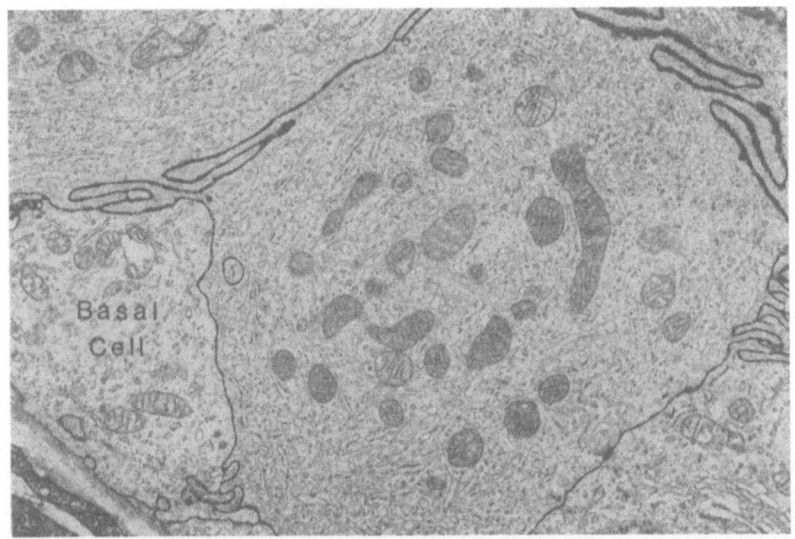

Fig. 14. Following extravasation, lanthanum is readily found along
the basement membrane (lower left hand corner) and within
the intercellular compartment throughout the epididymal
epithelium. Lanthanum encounters little resistance along
the basal and mid-portions of the lateral cell surface.
This is an electron micrograph of the cauda epididymidis
of a rat made infertile with gossypol; tracer can be observed surrounding the basal cell and in the intercellular spaces near the bases of the principal cells. A similar distribution of lanthanum is seen in the epididymal
epithelium of control rats.

as (1) a limited linear series of dense patches which delineates
the sites of fusion of the outer leaflets of the unit membranes or
as (2) negatively stained thread-like contact areas which are rendered visible in oblique view (Figs. 15, 16). In all cases, however, tracer is prevented from reaching the epididymal lumen without exception.

In the testes of both control and gossypol-treated rats, lanthanum escapes from the blood vessels, crosses the myoid layer and
enters the intercellular spaces of the seminiferous epithelium where
it is consistently prevented from reaching the adluminal compartment by the Sertoli-Sertoli cell junctions (Fig. 17). Finally, no
statistically significant differences between tritiated inulin in
the blood and luminal fluid of testes or epididymes of control and
gossypol-treated rats can be observed by micropuncture studies in
sexually mature rats fed daily with 20 mg/kg/day for 6 weeks (Table
1). We conclude that gossypol does not alter the permeability of

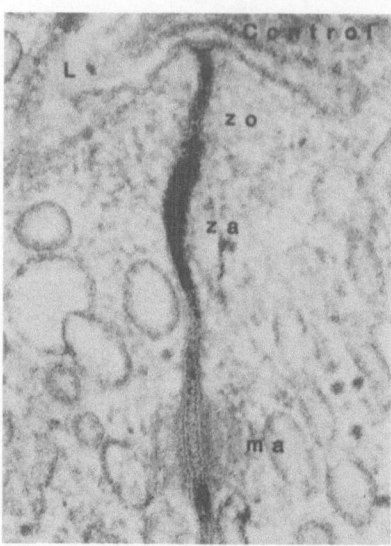

Fig. 15.   Electron micrograph of the caput epididymidis of a control
           rat showing lanthanum in the lateral intercellular space
           up to an including the macula (ma) and zonula adhaerentes
           (za) of the junctional complex. Between the principal
           cells shown here, a few particles of tracer have penetrated
           beyond the first or second point of fusion in the zonula
           occludens and are visible as a limited linear series of
           dense patches which delineate the sites of fusion of the
           outer leaflets of the opposing unit membranes but which
           fail to enter the epididymal lumen (L).

TABLE 1.   Micropuncture Studies on the Effects of
           Gossypol on the Amount[a] of ^{3}H-Inulin Which
           Penetrates the Blood-Testis and Blood-
           Epididymis Barriers in Rats After
           Intravenous Injection

	STF	CAPUT	CAUDA
Control (n = 5)	3.1 ± 1.2[c]	1.2 ± 0.5	1.7 ± 0.6
Gossypol[b]	1.9 ± 0.7	1.4 ± 0.2	2.1[d]

[a]Expressed as % plasma isotope appearing in luminal fluid.
[b]Administered by gavage at 20 mg/kg/day for 7 weeks.
[c]Values are mean ± s.e.m. for the No. of rats (n) indicated.
[d]Value of luminal fluid obtained from one rat.

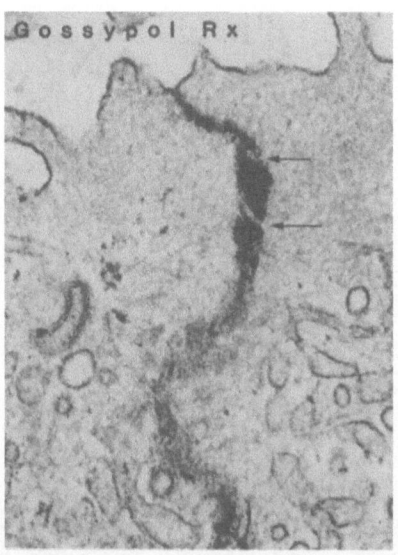

Fig. 16. Electron micrograph of the cauda epididymidis of a gossy-
          pol-treated rat showing lanthanum in the apico-lateral
          intercellular space. Between the principal cells shown
          here, as in the controls, tracer has penetrated beyond
          the first or second point of fusion in the zonula oc-
          cludens (z.o.) and is visible as thread-like contact
          areas which are negatively stained and rendered visible
          in oblique view (arrows). Regardless of the extent of
          lanthanum penetration into the z.o., however, tracer is
          prevented from entering the epididymal lumen without ex-
          ception.

the BEB or BTB to lanthanum or inulin and that damage to these barriers is not a prerequisite to its mechanism of antifertility activity in the rat.

     Finally, there has been concern that the contraceptive benefits
of gossypol may be accompanied by irreversible deleterious effects
which have escaped detection heretofore. Previous morphological
investigations to determine the reversibility of the effects of
gossypol on the rat testis have been limited to one light microscope study using significantly higher dose and time intervals than
those necessary to induce infertility [61]. Therefore, we undertook a study with the electron microscope of the nature and extent
of recovery of the rat testis from gossypol-induced damage [62].

     The results of this investigation demonstrated that rats made
infertile with low doses of gossypol (10 mg/kg, 6 days/week for 12

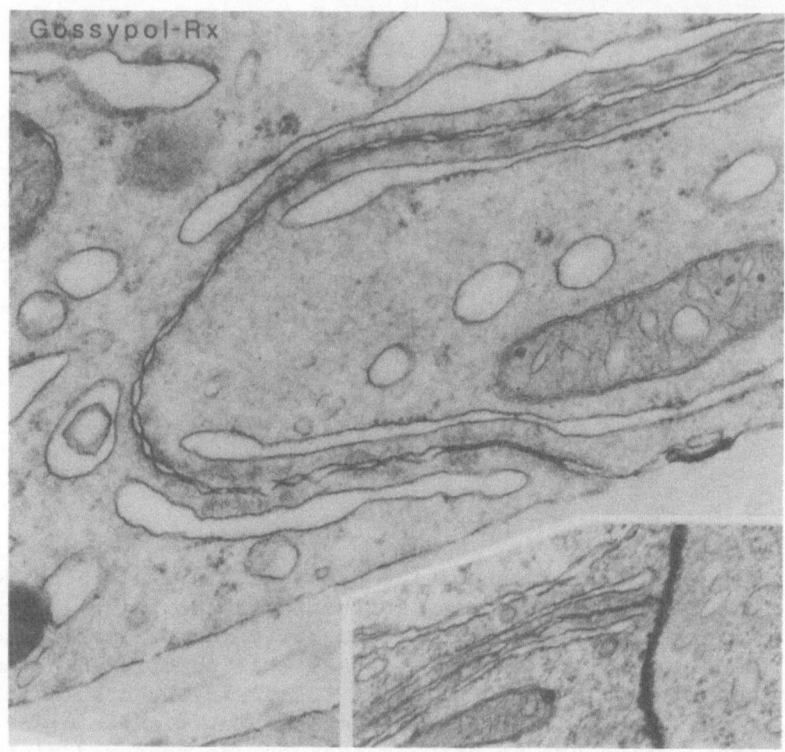

Fig. 17.   Two adjacent Sertoli cells in the testis of a rat made
           infertile with 20 mg/kg/day of gossypol for 6 weeks are
           shown in this electron micrograph. The ultrastructural
           features of the Sertoli-Sertoli cell junction seen here
           are the same as those found in control rat testes. The
           inset shows lanthanum in the intercellular space sur-
           rounding a spermatogonium of a gossypol-treated rat; the
           tracer has entered the space between the Sertoli cells
           but is prevented from permeating the cleft for more than
           250-300 nm. Intravascularly perfused lanthanum con-
           sistently failed to reach the adluminal compartment of
           the seminiferous epithelium in the gossypol-treated
           testes.

weeks) recovered completely within 6 weeks after cessation of treatment. No persisting defects could be detected with the electron
microscope in late spermatids (stages 18 and 19) or other cell types
of the seminiferous epithelium and no residual decrease in sperm motility was observed (data not shown). In rats made infertile with
a higher dose of gossypol (20 mg/kg, 6 days/week for 12 weeks), recovery was somewhat slower, requiring between 6 and 12 weeks. The

TABLE 2. In vivo Effects of Gossypol on Serum Levels of Testosterone and Gonadotrophins[a,b]

Species	Dose	Daily treatment regimen		Changes in hormone levels			Reference
		time	route of adminis.	FSH	LH	I	
Rat	7.5 mg/kg	12 wks	p.o.	none	none	none	Chang et al., 1982[1]
	15 mg/kg	12 wks	p.o.	none	none	none	
	30 mg/kg	6 wks	p.o.	none	↓	↓	
	30 mg/kg	5 wks	p.o.	none	↓	↓	Hadley et al., 1981[2]
	1.0 mg/kg	1 wk	s.c.	-	-	↓	Lin et al., 1981[3]
	5.0 mg/kg	1 wk	s.c.	-	-	↓	
	10.0 mg/kg	1 wk	s.c.	-	-	↓	
Hamster	10 mg/kg	5 wks	p.o.	-	none	none	Saksena and Salmonsen, 1982[4]
	15 mg/kg	5 wks	p.o.	-	none	none	
	10 mg/kg	10 wks	p.o.	-	none	↓	
Monkey	10 mg/kg	6 mos.	p.o.	-	-	none	L. Shandilya et al., 1982 (see Ref. 5)
Man[d]	20 mg/day	2 mos.	p.o.	-	none	none	National Coordinating Group, 1978 (see Ref. 1)
			p.o.	none	none	none	E. Coutinho et al., 1983 (see Ref. 3)
	20 mg/day	2-2½ mos.	p.o.	-	none	↓	Z. Liu et al., 1981 (see Ref. 54)
	20 mg/day	2 mos.	p.o.	none	none	none	Xue, 1981 (see Ref. 52)

[a] All data were evaluated for statistical significance by Student's T-test and were reported as statistically significant by the respective authors.

[b] Abbreviations and symbols: p.o., per os; s.c., subcutaneous; ↓ significantly lowered.

[c] In each case, RIA was performed only at the time indicated; hormone determinations were not reported at intermediate time points.

[d] In all human studies, the loading dose, 20 mg/day is followed by a weakly or biweekly maintenance dose ranging from 150-220 mg.

[1] C. C. Chang, Z. Gu, and Y. Y. Tsong, Studies on Gossypol. I. Toxicity antifertility and endocrine analyses in male rats, Int. J. Fertil., 27:213-218 (1982).

[2] The Hadley reference is No. 57 in the references.

[3] T. Lin, E. Murono, J. Osterman, H. Nankin, and P. Coulson, Gossypol inhibits testicular steroidogenesis, Fert. Steril., 35:563-566 (1981).

[4] S. K. Saksena and R. Salmonsen, Antifertility effects of gossypol in the male hamster, Fert. Steril., 37:311 (Abstract) (1982).

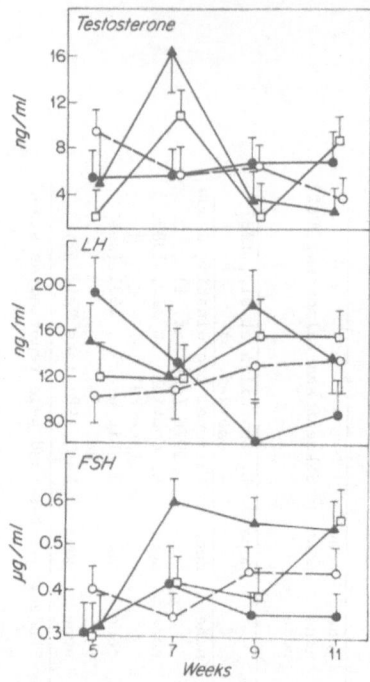

Fig. 18. Effects of varying doses of gossypol for 5, 7, 9, and 11
          weeks on serum testosterone, LH, and FSH in adult rats.
          Control group, o–o; 10 mg/kg/day gosssypol ●–●; 20 mg/
          kg/day gossypol, □–□; 30 mg/kg/day gossypol, Δ–Δ. All
          data were evaluated by two–way analysis of variance (ANOVA)
          with contrasts; see text for discussion of methodology and
          results.

exact time between the 6th and 12th weeks at which ultrastructural
evidence of gossypol treatment disappeared was not determined. The
observations do not support the concern that use of gossypol at
doses required for a contraceptive effect leads to irreversible
damage in the rat which has previously escaped detection.

ENDOCRINE STUDIES

      There has been considerable interest in the in vivo effects of
gossypol on the pituitary–gonadal axis. To date, observations on
whether gossypol affects serum concentrations of testosterone and
gonadotropins have been in conflict, with inconsistencies between
species and in the same species being reported. Nonetheless there
seems to be general agreement, at least in human and subhuman pri–
mates, that no changes in circulating levels of testosterone, LH,

FSH, and PRL ensue from gossypol treatment. A summary according to hormone and species of all the data presently available on this subject is shown in Table 2.

In our laboratory, the effects of gossypol on serum testosterone (T), luteinizing hormone (LH) and follicle-stimulating hormone (FSH) were analyzed in rats fed 0, 10, 20, or 30 mg/kg/day for 5, 7, 9, and 11 weeks [63]. Previous studies on the effects of gossypol on circulating FSH, LH, and T levels (Table 2) have focussed on variations in dose at a single time point but none have examined changes in serum testosterone and gonadotrophins as a function of both parameters. The results of our study are shown in Fig. 18; all data were evaluated by a two-way analysis of variance (ANOVA) with contrasts. Significance levels reported have not been adjusted for multiple comparisons. These methods of statistical analysis best evaluate the effects of two variables, namely time and dose. For a discussion of the methodology, please see [64].

Our results show no significant differences in serum LH levels regardless of dose ($p = 0.55$) or time ($p = 0.86$) and there is no significant time-dose interaction ($p = 0.13$). For testosterone, however, there is a significant dose-time interaction ($p = 0.02$). Because of this interaction we tested for dose differences at each time point. There are no significant differences among doses at times 5, 9, and 11 ($p \geq 0.10$ at each time) but there is a significant difference among doses at time 7 ($p = 0.05$). Closer scrutiny of these findings shows that the difference appears to be due to the effects of 20 and 30 mg/kg/day in causing increased serum testosterone levels at the 7 week interval compared to weeks 5, 9, and 11 ($p = 0.002$). By the 9th and 11th weeks of treatment, significant time-related differences in serum testosterone concentrations, as compared to the 5th week, have disappeared ($p = 0.10$). Interestingly, no significant differences in serum testosterone with respect to time are seen in animals rendered infertile with 10 mg/kg/day of gossypol ($p = 0.96$).

Circulating levels of FSH are not significantly altered with respect to dose ($p = 0.09$) and there is no interaction between time and dose ($p = 0.27$). By contrast, a definite effect over time of gossypol treatment on serum FSH levels can be seen ($p = 0.03$). Although there was no significant interaction between time and dose, inspection of the data suggests that most of the differences are a consequence of high serum FSH levels at 11 weeks in the 20 mg/kg/day group and at 7, 9, and 11 weeks in the 30 mg/kg/day group.

Our LH levels confirm those of one team of researchers who found no significant changes in serum LH in rats made infertile with 7.5-15 mg/kg/day of gossypol for 12 weeks [65]. Higher doses (30 mg/kg daily) were unable to cause a statistically significant change in serum LH concentrations in our study although others have reported

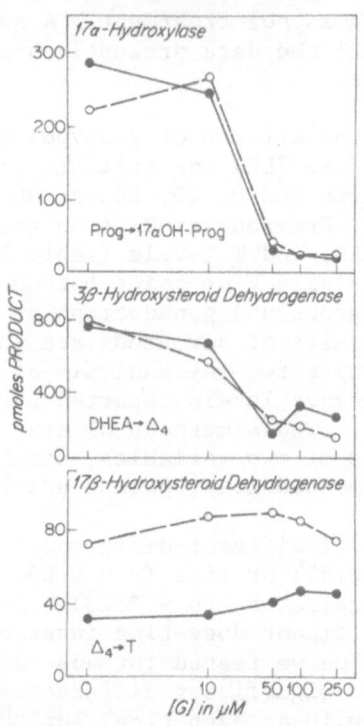

Fig. 19. <u>In vitro</u> effects of gossypol on steroidogenic enzymes of
the Δ_4 and Δ_5 pathways for androgen biosynthesis in rat
testicular microsomes. Inhibition of 17 α-hydroxylase,
3β-hydrosysteroid dehydrogenase and 17β-hydroxysteroid
dehydrogenase was evaluated at concentrations of gossypol
varying from 0-250 μM. Silica gel thin layer chromatography was used to determine conversion of radiolabeled
substrates to metabolites as shown. Abbreviations: PROG,
progesterone; 17α-OH-PROG, 17α-hydroxyprogesterone; DHEA,
dehydroepiandrosterone; Δ_4, androstenedione; T, testosterone. The activities of 17α-hydroxylase and 3β-HSD
were strongly inhibited by gossypol whereas 17β-HDS was
moderately stimulated by gossypol at all inhibitor concentrations examined.

a decline in LH after 30 mg/kg/day for 5 weeks [66, 67]. The possibility that this difference is a consequence of the different statistical methods used to evaluate the results or differences in
sample size cannot be excluded. Although we found no significant
differences in serum testosterone with respect to dose alone, we
did observe an increase in circulating T at higher doses at 7 weeks.
At lower doses (10-15 mg/kg/day) for 11-12 weeks, neither we nor
others [68] observed any effects of gossypol on serum testosterone. A

significant effect of time of gossypol treatment on circulating levels of FSH was observed; this effect was primarily at the two higher doses used in this study. Others have not reported an effect of gossypol on FSH (Table 1) with the possible exception of a slight decrease in rabbits [69]. On the basis of the data presently available, it seems reasonable to interpret the influence of gossypol on serum gonadotrophins and testosterone as short-term effects (5 and 7 weeks) and long-term effects (9 and 11 weeks). Thus, although testosterone levels change around the 5th and 7th weeks of treatment at high doses of gossypol, they return to the normal range with time and no overall statistically significant decrease is demonstrated over the long term in either our studies or in those of others [70].

In order to further analyze the effects of gossypol on the steroidogenic pathway, we have studied its effects on steroidogenic enzymes of the Δ_4 and Δ_5 pathway in rats and human testicular microsomes [71]. Two separate rat studies (n = 4) and three separate human studies were conducted. The concentrations of gossypol employed varied from 0–250 μM. The substrate (s) and the product (p) for the enzymes assayed were: 17α-hydroxylase – S, progesterone; P, 17-α-hydroxyprogesterone; 3-β-hydroxysteroid dehydrogenase (3-β-HSD) – S, dehydroepiandrosterone; P, androstenedione; 17-β-hydroxysteroid dehydrogenase (17-β-HSD) – S, androstenedione; P, testosterone. The results are shown in Figs. 19 and 20. The activity of 3-β-HSD in rat testis was strongly inhibited in each of two experiments; by contrast 3-β-HSD was poorly inhibited by gossypol in two of three human testes and moderately inhibited in the third. 17α-hydroxylase activity in rat and two human testes was strongly inhibited by gossypol; in the third human testis, 17α-hydroxylase was weakly inhibited. Finally, 17-β-HSD activity in rat testis was not inhibited by gossypol; in fact, all concentrations of inhibitor tested mildly stimulated this enzyme in the rat. In the human, 17-β-HSD in two of three testes was inhibited only at high concentrations of gossypol while the third was moderately inhibited. These results demonstrate a direct inhibitory effect of various concentrations of gossypol on certain testicular steroidogenic enzymes in vitro in both rats and humans. In vivo, the gossypol level in the testis of the infertile rat is reported to be approximately 8 μg/gm or 16 μM [72, 73, 74]. The slight to moderate stimulation of 17-β-HSD observed in our rat microsomal assays with concentrations varying from 10 μM gossypol (the concentration closest to that present in in vivo in rat testis) to 100 μM gossypol may occur by a mechanism(s) similar to that causing the increase in vivo of serum testosterone in rats treated daily for 7 weeks with 20 or 30 mg/kg of gossypol. This intriguing relationship is under continuing investigation in our laboratory.

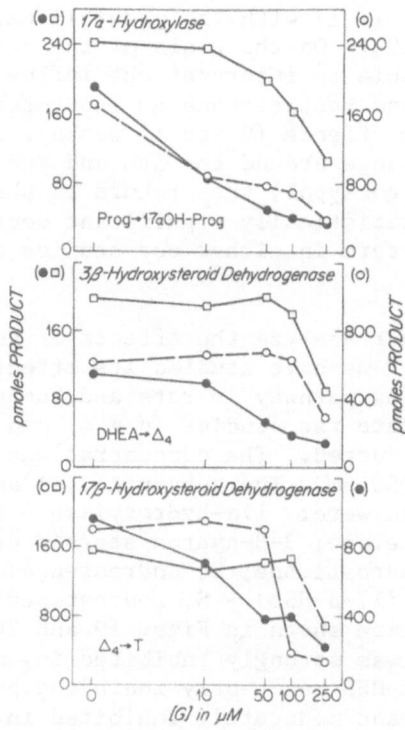

Fig. 20.   In vitro effects of gossypol on steroidogenic enzymes of
           the Δ_4 and Δ_5 pathways for androgen biosynthesis in human
           testicular microsomes.   Inhibition of 17α-hydroxylase,
           3β-hydroxysteroid dehydrogenase and 17β-hydroxysteroid
           dehydrogenase was evaluated at concentrations of gossypol
           varying from 0-250 μM.   Silica gel thin layer chromatog-
           raphy was used to determine conversion of radiolabelled
           substrates to metabolites as shown.   Abbreviations: PROG,
           progesterone; 17α-OH-PROG, 17α-hydroxyprogesterone; DHEA,
           dehydroepiandrosterone; Δ_4, androstenedione; T, testo-
           sterone.   Activity of 17α-hydroxylase was strongly in-
           hibited in two human testes and weakly inhibited in the
           third whereas 3β-hydroxysteroid dehydrogenase was poorly
           inhibited in two of three testes and only moderately in-
           hibited in the third.   High concentrations of gossypol pro-
           duced strong inhibition of 17β-hydroxysteroid dehydro-
           genase in two testes and mild inhibition in the third
           testis.

Specific and Non-Specific Nucleotide Metabolizing Enzymes of the Male Reproductive Tract

LDH-X, a homotetrameric isozyme of LDH, is found in the mature testis and sperm of many species with internal fertilization. One of its most noteworthy characteristics is its cellular specificity. It is contained exclusively in germ cells and is first expressed in the pachytene stage of primary spermatocytes. In mature sperm, isozyme x constitutes more than 80% of the total LDH activity. The exact function of LDH-X is not definitely known but it has been proposed that LDH-X may function as part of an α-keto-hydroxyacid shuttle which transfers reducing equivalents across the sperm mito-chondrial membrane to the respiratory chain [75].

Three years ago, a preliminary report claimed that gossypol produces a selective inhibition of LDH-X in mouse testis in vitro [76]. Gossypol appeared also to inhibit the isozymes LDH-A$_4$ and LDH-B$_4$ but its greatest effect was on testis and sperm-specific LDH-X. The authors concluded that this inhibition is the key to gossypol's mechanism of action as a male contraceptive.

We undertook the analysis of the effects of gossypol on LDH-X in vivo and in vitro in rat testes; for the sake of comparison, the effects of gossypol on LDH-M$_4$ (Sigma), an isozyme from rabbit heart muscle, were also studied [77, 78]. LDH-X was measured according to the method of Lee et al. [79], which exploits the high affinity of LDH-X for α-ketoacids other than pyruvate, a property not shared by the other isozymes; LDH-M$_4$ was measured according to the method of Yoshida and Freese [80]. In vitro, in the rat, we were able to confirm the sensitivity of LDH-X to gossypol at an ED$_{50}$ of 220 μM (Fig. 21A) but we were unable to confirm the report of others that this effect is specific for the X isozyme [81] since LDH-M$_4$ was far more sensitive to gossypol in vitro (ED$_{50}$ = 10 μM) than LDH-X (Fig. 21B). Evaluation of the in vivo effects of gossypol on LDH-X was carried out in rats fed the vehicle (control), 20 or 30 mg/kg/day by gavage for 7 weeks. A 5.6-fold decrease in basal LDH-X activity was observed in the highest treated group over controls (Fig. 22). In order to eliminate the possibility that these differences in ac-tivity are due to exogenous gossypol remaining in the tissues at the time of assay, the dose-dependence of LDH-X from the gossypol-treated rats to additional added gossypol was measured and no significant differences between the ED$_{50}$'s of the control and treated groups was found (data not shown).

We also examined the effects of gossypol on two other key nu-cleotide metabolizing enzymes, adenyl cyclase and phosphodiesterase, in rat testis, cauda epididymidis (sperm-free) and vasal sperm [82, 83]. Adenylate cyclase, a key regulatory enzyme in spermatogenesis, is involved in the production of cyclic AMP. In most mammalian cells, adenylate cyclase is a membrane-bound hormone-sensitive enzyme but in

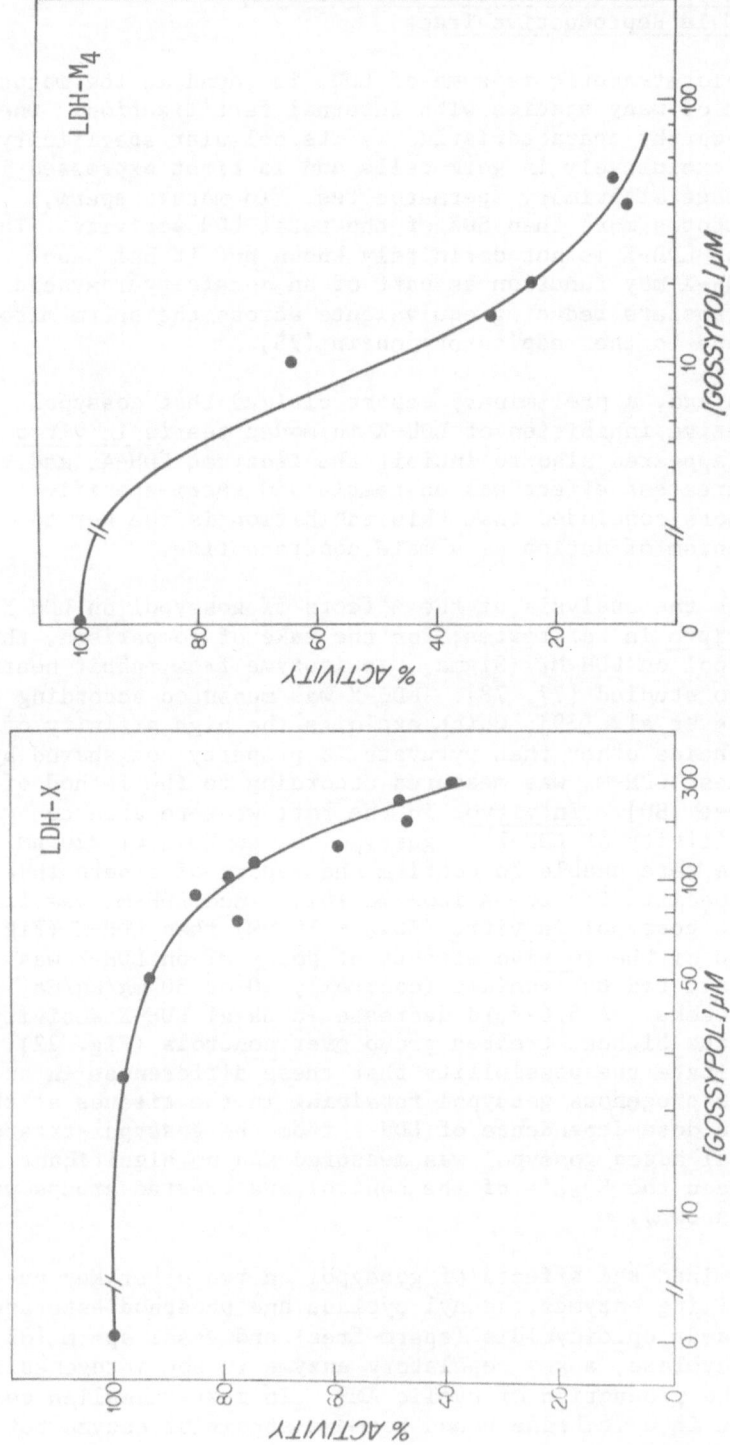

Fig. 21. A) In vitro gossypol inhibition of testicular lactate dehydrogenase-x (LDH-X), an isozyme of LDH localized exclusively in the testis. The ED₅₀ of gossypol inhibition of this enzyme is 220 μM. B) An isozyme of lactate dehydrogenase from rabbit heart muscle. LDH-M₄, is significantly more sensitive to the inhibitor effect of gossypol in vitro than LDH-X; ED₅₀ = 10 μM.

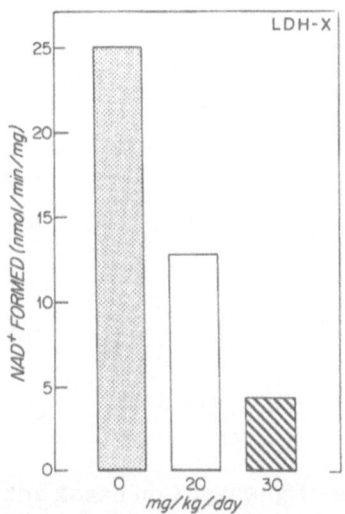

Fig. 22. Gossypol inhibition of LDH-X <u>in vivo</u> in rats fed the
          vehicle (0), 20 or 30 mg/kg/day by gavage for 7 weeks.
          A 5.6-fold decrease in basal LDH-X activity is observed
          in the highest treated group over controls.

rat testis it also occurs in a soluble form and is associated with
late spermatocytes and spermatids [84, 85]. Testicular soluble
adenyl cyclase can be differentiated from the membrane-bound form
by its insensitivity to gonadotropins, its absolute requirement for
Mn^{2+}-ATP as a substrate and its lack of a guanyl nucleotide binding
subunit. The adenylate cyclases in both sperm and the epididymal
epithelium are membrane-bound.

Adenylate cyclase was purified and assayed according to routine
procedures [86, 87] in rats fed vehicle (control), 20 or 30 mg/kg/
day of gossypol for 7 weeks. Administration of these doses of
gossypol produced only slight changes in basal activities of membrane-associated testicular adenyl cyclase (Fig. 23A) whereas soluble testicular adenyl cyclase activity fell to 70% of control levels
in rats treated with 30 mg/kg/day (Fig. 23B). In caudal sperm,
membrane-associated adenyl cyclase showed a 4-fold decrease in basal
activity with increasing dose of the drug (Fig. 23C). Epididymal
adenylate cyclase was not affected under the conditions of our study
(data not shown). The sensitivity of sperm membrane adenylate cyclase to the inhibitory effects of gossypol increased 4-fold (from an
ED_{50} of 200 µM to 50 µM) as the dose of administered gossypol increased (Fig. 24). The ED_{50} values of gossypol inhibition of adenyl
cyclase from other tissues remained unchanged (data not shown).
Basal phosphodiesterase (PDE) activity increased in sperm and
liver, but not in testis, with increasing doses of gossypol.

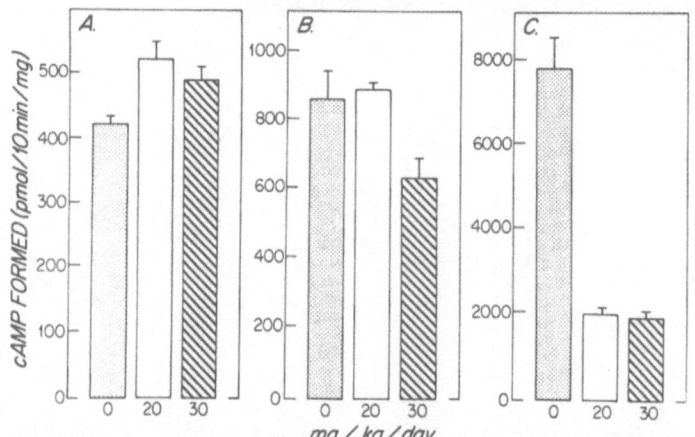

Fig. 23.   In vivo effects of gossypol on basal activities of sperm mem-
           brane adenyl cyclase and on testicular soluble and membrane-
           bound adenyl cyclase. A) Testicular membrane-bound adenyl
           cyclase: administration of 20 or 30 mg/kg/day of gossypol
           for 7 weeks produces slight changes in basal activities of
           the insoluble adenyl cyclase of the rat testis. B) Soluble
           testicular adenyl cyclase: in rats treated orally with 20
           or 30 mg/kg/day of gossypol, enzyme activity fell to 70%
           of control levels in the highest treated group. C)
           Caudal sperm membrane-bound adenyl cyclase: a four-fold
           decrease in enzyme activity over controls was observed in
           both gossypol-treated groups of rats. Epididymal adenyl
           cyclase was not affected under the conditions of the study
           (data not shown).

However, in all cases, addition of 100 μm gossypol inhibited
PDE activity (Fig. 25). The mechanism of gossypol inhibition of
these enzymes is not clear. However, since each of these enzymes
is nucleotide-dependent, it seems likely that gossypol may inhibit
their activity by occupying the nucleotide-binding domain. Further
work is underway to confirm this intriguing possibility and to determine why these nucleotide-binding enzymes in testis and sperm
should be more sensitive to gossypol than their counterparts elsewhere in the body.

ISOMERIC DERIVATIVES OF GOSSYPOL

     Gossypol has been shown to have antibacterial, antiviral, and
antitumor activity in vitro [88, 89, 90, 91], in addition to its
antifertility effect. Moreover, certain derivatives of gossypol are
reported to be less toxic than the parent compound in mammals [92].

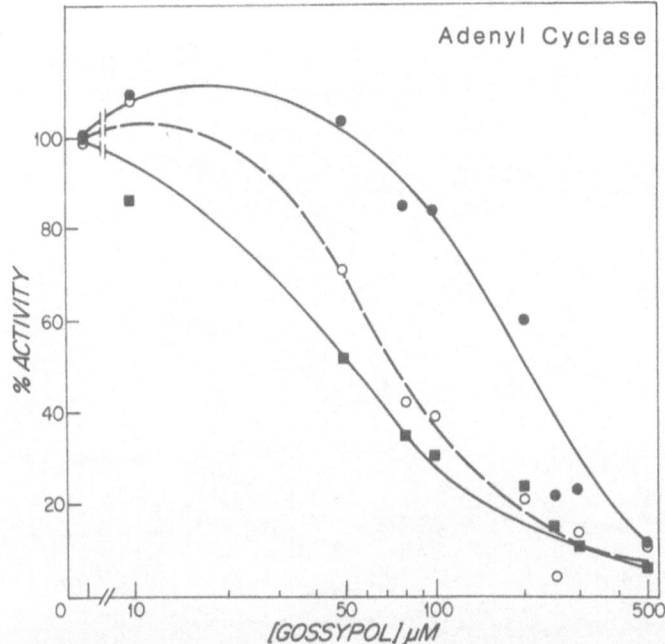

Fig. 24. <u>In vitro</u> inhibitory effects of gossypol on caudal sperm
membrane-bound adenyl cyclase. The ED_{50} of gossypol inhibition of this enzyme from control rats (●) was 200
μM; this shifted to 75 μM in the 20 mg/kg/day group (o),
and to 50 μM in the 30 mg/kg/day group (■).

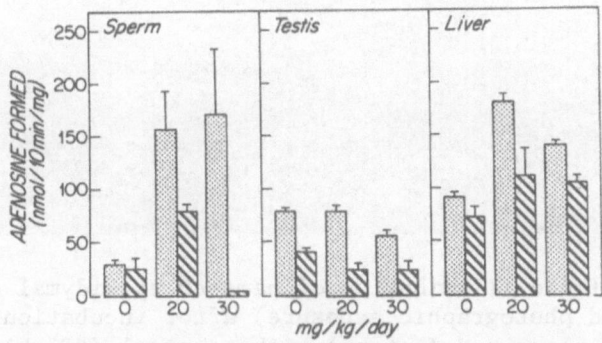

Fig. 25. Effects of gossypol administration on basal phosphodiesterase (PDE) activity. Gossypol administration increased basal PDE activity over controls in sperm and
liver, but not in testis (▨). In all cases, addition of
100 μM gossypol (▨) inhibited PDE activity.

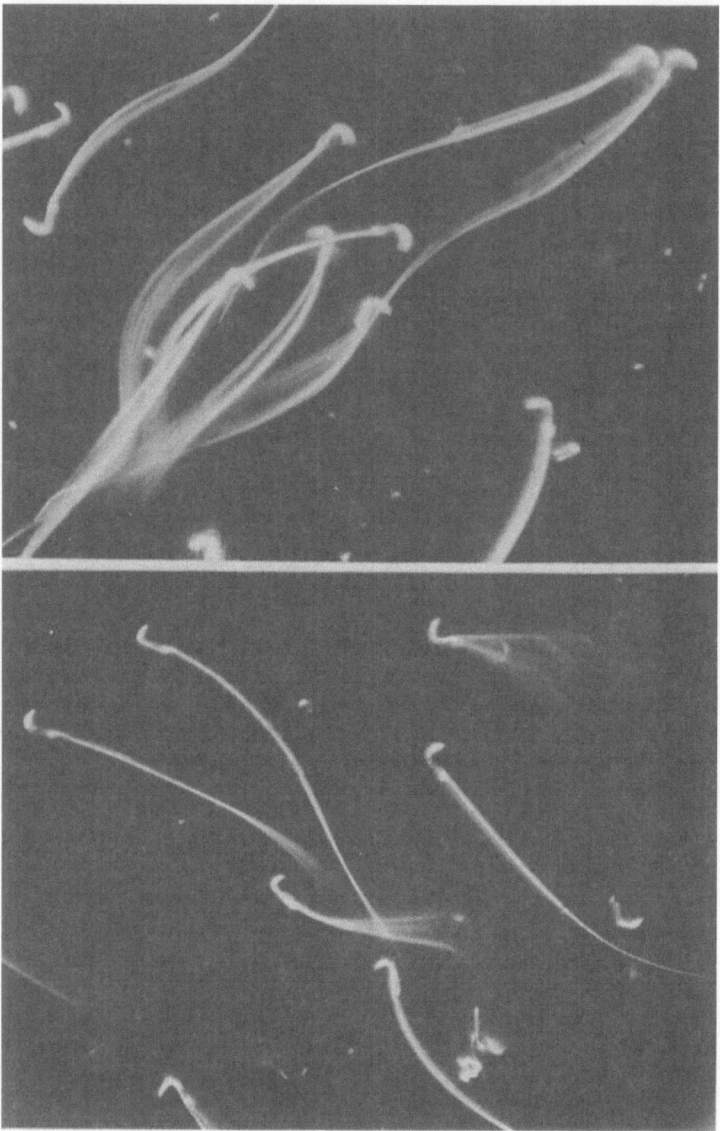

Fig. 26. Dark-field illumination of hamster epididymal sperm (2
          second photographic exposure) after incubation (top) with
          media alone and (bottom) with gossypol (50 μM) for 2 min.
          In the assay, the percent of motile sperm are measured as
          a function of time and the data from the experimental ana-
          logs and derivatives of gossypol are normalized to five
          minutes, the time of complete inhibition of hamster sperm
          by gossypol, the standard.

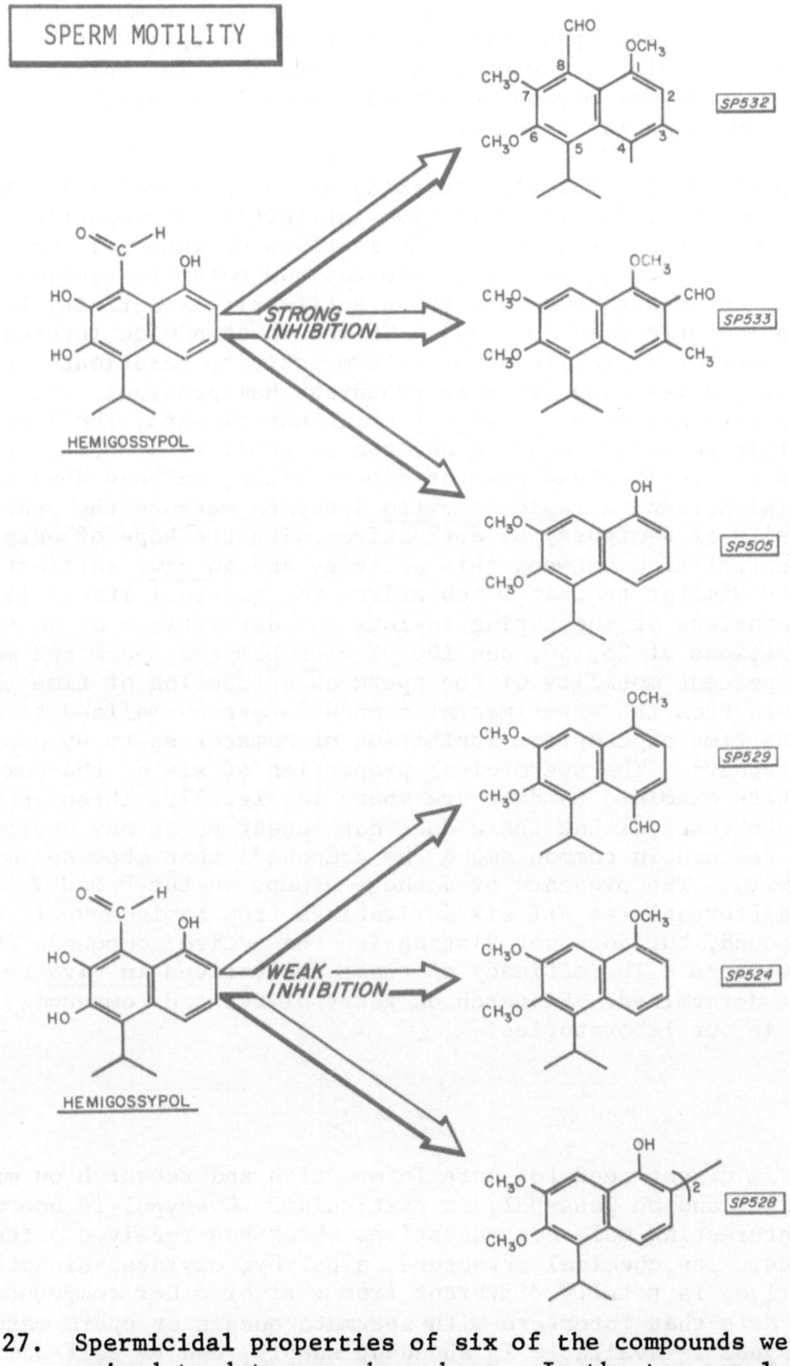

Fig. 27. Spermicidal properties of six of the compounds we have examined to date are shown here. In the top panel, the three
hemigossypol derivatives are equiactive to gossypol in the
in vitro assay; in the bottom panel, the derivatives shown
produce only a weak inhibition of sperm motility in vitro.

One of these, apogossypol, has been shown to retain some of the desirable pharmacological properties of gossypol in spite of the modifications in molecular structure. We believe that the antifertility action of gossypol may be separated from its potentially toxic effects by modifying its structure.

The specific structural features(s) of the gossypol molecule which is responsible for its selective antifertility properties is as yet unknown. A large number of derivatives of gossypol including amino compounds, esters, acetate, formate, and metallic complexes have been prepared but none have shown antifertility activity better than gossypol acetic acid [93, 94]. There has been wide interest in the development of a profile of structure-activity relationships for gossypol and its sesquiterpene precursor hemigossypol. Because of the long-term nature of in vivo feeding experiments, the large amount of test compound required and the instability of hemigossypol and some of its derivatives towards dimerization, we have developed, as an initial screen, a rapid in vitro assay to measure the spermicidal activity of hemigossypol derivatives with the hope of establishing a correlation between this activity and in vivo antifertility activity similar to that which exists for gossypol itself [95]. The assay consists of incubating analogs and derivatives of gossypol at concentrations of 25, 50, and 100 μM with hamster sperm and measuring the percent motility of the sperm as a function of time (Fig. 26); the data from the experimental compounds are normalized to five minutes, the time of complete inhibition of hamster sperm by gossypol, the standard. The spermicidal properties of six of the compounds we have examined to date are shown in Fig. 27. Three appear equiactive to gossypol but there does not appear to be any obvious structural feature in common among the compounds that show spermicidal activity. The presence of methoxy groups in the 6 and 7 positions differentiates all six derivatives from hemigossypol, the parent compound, but does not distinguish the active compounds from the inactive ones. The efficacy of these derivatives in vivo remains to be determined. Research on gossypol-related compounds is continuing in our laboratories.

CONCLUSION

There is urgent need for more information and research on male contraceptives and on gossypol, in particular. Gossypol is one of the most interesting male contraceptives which has received attention to date. Its chemical structure, a polyhydroxylated binapthalene derivative, is totally different from that of other compounds studied to date that interfere with spermatogenesis or sperm maturation. Gossypol is available in abundant supply, can be self-administered and is convenient to use. It has undergone extensive clinical trials in the Peoples Republic of China and also has been evaluated in volunteers in Brazil, Japan, and Austria. Its efficacy is well-documented in man and experimental animals alike and recent studies are demonstrating fewer side effects than initially suspected. At therapeutic doses, gossypol is relatively non-toxic [96, 97] although the acute toxicity in vivo of gossypol at doses >1000-fold those needed to achieve contraception has been well documented [98, 99].

The full reversibility of this contraceptive in man has not been conclusively demonstrated however. The evidence available thus far appears to indicate that the likelihood of recovery is a function of time and is more likely to occur in subjects who have used gossypol for less than two years at a time. Optimal loading and maintenance doses have been determined through years of trial and readjustment [100], but to date, the possibility that lower loading and/or maintenance doses may promote a better rate of recovery in human subjects remains relatively unexplored. The long-term effects of using gossypol as a contraceptive in alternation with other forms of birth control on an annual or biennial basis has also received little investigative attention.

Regardless of the practical outcome of some of these questions about gossypol, the preliminary results to date are exciting. Even if gossypol should ultimately prove unsatisfactory as a human male contraceptive, there is little doubt that chemical modifications of this substance will be developed which may lead to better alternatives.

ACKNOWLEDGMENT

The author would like to thank Dr. Harriet Petersen of the Biostatistics Consulting Laboratory Harvard School of Public Health, for her assistance in statistical evaluation of the radioimmunoassay data on serum FSH, LH, and testosterone in gossypol-treated rats.

REFERENCES

1.   National Coordinating Group on Male Antifertility Agents, Gossypol - A New Antifertility Agent for Males, Chinese Med. J., 4:417 (1978).
2.   Ibid.
3.   F. Coutinho, J. F. Melo, I. Barbosa, and S. J. Segal, Biphasic action of gossypol in men, Fertil. Steril., in press (1984).
4.   W. Bardin, Plasma testosterone in monkeys, in: "Gossypol-A possible male antifertility agent: Report of a Workshop, Vol. 1" (G. Zaruchni and K. Osborne, eds.), Research Frontiers in Fertility Regulation, PARFR, Chicago (1981).
5.   L. Shandilya, T. B. Clarkson, M. R. Adams, and J. C. Lewis, Effects of gossypol on reproductive and endocrine functions of

     male cynomolgus monkeys (Macaca fascicularis), Biol. Reprod.,
     27:241 (1982).

6. National Coordinating Group on Male Antifertility Agents, 1978,
     op. cit. (see Ref. 1).

7. E. Coutinho, et al., 1983, op. cit. (see Ref. 3).

8. M. R. N. Prasad and E. Diczfalusy, Gossypol, in: "Proceedings
     of Second International Congress of Andrology," Int. J. Androl.
     Suppl. 5:53 (1981).

9. Z. Liu, 1981, personal communication.

10. A. McFadzean and R. Yeung, Periodic paralysis complicating
     thyrotoxicosis in Chinese, Brit. Med. J., 1:45 (1967).

11. M. B. Abou-Donia, Physiological effects and metabolism of gossy-
     pol, Residue Rev., 61:125 (1978).

12. L. C. Berardi and L. A. Goldblatt, Gossypol, in: "Toxic Con-
     situents of Plant Foodstuffs" (I. E. Liener, ed.), Academic
     Press, New York (1980).

13. X. S. Pu, Studies on the antifertility effect of gossypol, a
     new contraceptive for males, in: "Recent Advances in Fertility
     Regulation" (C. F. Chang, D. Griffin, and A. Woolman, eds.), Atar
     S.A., Geneva (1980).

14. G. I. Zatuchni and K. Osborne, Gossypol - "A possible male anti-
     fertility agent, Report of a Workshop, Vol. 1," Research
     frontiers in fertility, Chicago (1981).

15. M. R. Prasad and E. Diczfalusy, 1982, op. cit. (see Ref. 8).

16. H. Jackson, "Gossypol. In Progress Towards a Male Contracep-
     tive II, Vol. 8: (S. L. Jeffcoate and M. Sandler, eds.), John
     Wiley and Sons, New York (1982).

17. S. P. Xue, Z. H. Zhou, Y. Liu, Y. W. Wu, and S. D. Zong, The
     pharmacokinetics of ^{14}C-gossypol acetic acid in rats. I. Whole
     body and micro-autoradiographic studies on the distribution and
     fate of ^{14}C-gossypol in the rat body, Doc. 4th Natl. Conf. Male
     Antifertil. Agents, Suzhou (1975), Acta Biol. Exp. Symp., 12:
     179 (1979).

18. S. P. Xue, Y. Zhou, Y. Lin, Y. W. Liu, Y. W. Wu, and S. D. Zong,
     The pharmacokinetics of distribution, excretion and metabolism
     of studies on the kinetics of distribution, excretion and
     metabolism of ^{14}C-gossypol acetic acid in the rat body, Doc.
     4th Natl. Conf. Male Antifertil. Agents, Suzhou (1975), Acta
     Biol. Exp. Sin., 12:275 (1979).

19. H. C. Haspel, Y. F. Ren, K. A. Watanabe, M. Sonenberg, and R. E.
     Corin, Toxicity of gossypol: a cytocidal effect on cultured
     murine erythroleukemia cells is prevented by serum protein, J.
     Pharmacol. Exp. Therap. (in press).

20. P. B. Coulson, R. Snell, and C. Parise, In vitro effects of the
     antifertility agent, gossypol, on the reproductive organs in
     male mice, Int. J. Androl., 3:507 (1980).

21. L. Zhou, C. Chen, N. Wang, and H. Lai, Observations on long-
     term administration of gossypol acetic acid to rats, Doc. 4th
     Natl. Conf. Male Antifertil. Agents, Suzhou (1975), Natl. Med.
     J. Chin., 60:343 (1980).

22. S. A. Bozek, D. R. Jensen, and J. N. Tone, Scanning electron
     microscope study of spermatozoa from gossypol-treated rats,
     Cell Tissue Res., 219:659 (1981).
23. M. A. Hadley and M. H. Burgos, Inhibition of rat epididymal
     sperm by gossypol, paper presented at the New York Academy of
     Sciences meeting on the Cell Biology of the Testis, April,
     1981.
24. H. Jackson, Comparative effects of some antispermatogenic
     chemicals, in: "The Regulation of Mammalian Reproduction"
     (S. Segal, R. Crozier, P. Carfman, and P. Candliffe, eds.),
     Thomas, Sprinfield, Illinois (1973).
25. P. B. Coulson, et al., 1980, op. cit. (see Ref. 20).
26. M. A. Hadley and M. H. Burgos, 1981, op. cit. (see Ref. 23).
27. A. Bozek, et al., 1981, op. cit. (see Ref. 22).
28. A. P. Hoffer, Ultrastructural studies of spermatozoa and the
     epithelial lining of the epididymis and vas deferens in rats
     treated with gossypol, Archives Androl., 8:233 (1982).
29. Z. P. Gu, S. D. Tsong, and C. C. Chang, Effect of gossypol on
     the testis and epididymis of rat and hamster, Contracep. Deliv.
     Systems 3 (3/4):279 abstract (1982).
30. P. Wong, W. Lee, A. Tsang, W. Fu, and Q. Chen, Lack of an
     effect of gossypol on the epididymis of the rat, Contraception,
     27:391 (1983).
31. A. P. Hoffer, 1984, unpublished results.
32. M. C. Chang, Z. Gu, and S. K. Saksena, Effects of gossypol on
     the fertility of male rats, hamsters, and rabbits, Contracep-
     tion, 21 (5):451 (1980).
33. D. W. Hahn, C. Rusticus, A. Probst, R. Homm, and A. N. Johnson,
     Antifertility and endocrine activities of gossypol in rodents,
     Contraception, 24:97 (1981).
34. D. P. Waller, H. H. S. Fong, G. A. Cordel, and D. D. Soejarto,
     Antifertility effects of gossypol and its impurities on male
     hamsters, Contraception, 23:653 (1981).
35. A. P. Hoffer, Effects of gossypol on the seminiferous epithe-
     lium in the rat: A light and electron microscope study, Biol.
     Reprod., 28:1007 (1983).
36. A. P. Hoffer, 1984, unpublished results.
37. R. Oko and F. Hrudka, Segmental aplasia of the mitochondrial
     sheath and sequelae induced by gossypol in rat spermatozoa,
     Biol. Reprod., 26:183 (1982).
38. M. Flores and D. W. Fawcett, Ultrastructural effects of the
     antispermatogenic compound, WIN 18446 (bis dichloroacetyl di-
     amine), Anat. Record., 172:310 (1972).
39. A. H. ElJack and F. Hrudka, Pattern and dynamics of teratospermia
     induced in rams by parental treatment with ethylene dibromide,
     J. Ultrastruct. Res., 67:124 (1979).
40. T. J. Lobl and J. Mathews, Effect of 1-(2,4-dichlorobenzyl)-
     indazole-3-carboxylic acid on sperm tails in rhesus monkeys,
     J. Reprod. Fertil., 52:275 (1978).
41. A. P. Hoffer, 1983, op. cit. (see Ref. 35).

42. I. H. Chen and R. D. Yates, Effects of simulated high altitude on hamster testes (Abstract), Anat. Rec., 178:326 (1974).
43. P. M. Krueger, G. D. Hodgens, and R. J. Sherins, New evidence for the role of the Sertoli cell and spermatogonia in feedback control of FSH secretion in male rats, Endocrin., 95:995 (1974).
44. C. J. Flickinger, Regional differences in synthesis, intracellular transport, and secretion of protein in the mouse epididymis, Biol. Reprod., 25:871 (1981).
45. J. B. Kerr, K. A. Rich, and D. M. deKretser, Effects of expermental cryptorchidism on the ultrastructure and function of the Sertoli cell and peritubular tissue of the rat testis, Biol. Reprod., 21:823 (1979).
46. M. Flores and D. W. Fawcett, 1972, op. cit. (see Ref. 38).
47. D. Waller, N. Bunyapraphatsara, A. Martin, C. Vournazos, M. Ahmed, D. Soejarto, G. Cordell, L. Russell, and J. Malone, Effect of (+)-gossypol on fertility in male hamsters, J. Androl., 4:276 (1983).
48. A. P. Hoffer, 1984, unpublished results.
49. L. Zhuang, D. Phillips, G. Gunsalus, C. W. Bardin, and J. P. Mather, Effects of gossypol on rat Sertoli and Leydig cells in primary culture and established cell lines, J. Androl., 4:336 (1983).
50. A. P. Hoffer and R. Todd, 1984, unpublished results.
51. National Coordinating Group on Male Antifertility Agents, 1978, op. cit. (see Ref. 1).
52. S. P. Xue, Studies on the antifertility effect of gossypol, a new contraceptive for males, in: "Recent Advances in Fertility Regulation" (C. F. Chang, D. Griffin, and A. Woolman, eds.), Atar S.A., Geneva (1981).
53. W. Bardin, 1980, op. cit. (see Ref. 4).
54. Z. Liu, G. Liu, L. Hei, R. Zhang, and C. Yu, Clinical trial of gossypol as a male antifertility agent, in: "Recent Advances in Fertility Regulation" (C. F. Chang, D. Griffin, and A. Woolman, eds.), Atar S.A., Geneva (1981).
55. E. Coutinho, et al., 1983, op. cit. (see Ref. 3).
56. L. Shandilya, et al., 1982, op. cit. (see Ref. 5).
57. M. Hadley, T. Lin, and M. Dym, Effects of gossypol on the reproductive system of male rats, J. Androl., 2:190 (1981).
58. M. C. Chang, et al., 1980, op. cit. (see Ref. 32).
59. A. P. Hoffer, S. J. Klein, S. Weston, and J. A. Canick, Direct effects of gossypol on steroidogenic enzymes in rat and human testis microsomes, Endocrin., 112:104 (1983).
60. A. P. Hoffer and B. Hinton, Morphological evidence for a blood-epididymis barrier and the effects of gossypol on its integrity, Biol. Reprod., 30:991 (1984).
61. L. F. Zhou and H. P. Lei, Recovery of fertility in rats after gossypol treatment, in: "Recent Advances in Fertility Regulation" (C. F. Chang, D. Griffin, and A. Woolman, eds.), Atar S.A., Geneva (1980), pp. 147-151.

62. A. P. Hoffer and S. L. Lisser, Recovery of normal testicular ultrastructure and sperm motility after cessation of gossypol treatment in rats, J. Andol., in press (1984).
63. A. P. Hoffer and R. Todd, 1984, op. cit. (see Ref. 50).
64. S. Wallenstein, C. L. Zucker, and J. L. Fleiss, Some statistical methods useful in circulation research, Circul. Res., 47(1):1 (1980).
65. C. C. Chang, Z. Gu, and Y. Y. Tsong, Studies on gossypol. I. Toxicity, antifertility, and endocrine analyses in male rats, Int. J. Fertil., 27:213 (1982).
66. Ibid.
67. Ibid. Hadley et al. (1981).
68. Ibid. Chang et al. (1982).
69. National Coordinating Group on Male Infertility Agents, 1978, op. cit. (see Ref. 1).
70. C. C. Chang, et al., 1982, op. cit. (see Ref. 65).
71. A. P. Hoffer, 1983, op. cit. (see Ref. 35).
72. Y. B. Ko, X. K. Lin, Y. H. Chang, Y. Z. Mar, S. E. Yu, and Y. Din, Studies on the antifertility effect of gossypol III. The determination of the quantities of gossypol in blood and related internal organs after administration of the drug in rats, Acta. Biol. Exp. Sinica, 12:69 (1979).
73. Y. E. Wang, T. G. Lou, and X. C. Tang, Studies on the antifertility actions of cottonseed meal and gossypol, Acta Pharmacol. Sinic., 14:663 (1979).
74. W. W. Tso and C. S.Lee, Effect of gossypol on boar spermatozoa in vitro, Arch. Androl., 7:85 (1981).
75. A. Blanco, On the functional significance of LDHX, John Hopkins Med. J., 146:231 (1980).
76. Chi-Yu Lee and H. V. Malling, Selective inhibition of sperm-specific lactate dehydrogenase-x by an antifertility agent, gossypol, Fed. Proc., 40(3):718 (1981).
77. K. Olgiati, A. P. Hoffer, and W. A. Toscano, Jr., Gossypol modulation of nucleotide metabolizing enzymes in the male reproductive tract, Biol. Reprod., 28 (Suppl):159 (1983).
78. K. Olgiati, A. P. Hoffer, and W. A. Toscano, Effects of gossypol on nucleotide metabolism in the reproductive system of male rats, submitted.
79. Chi-Yu Lee, Y. S. Moon, J. H. Yan, and A. F. Chen, Enzyme inactivation and inhibition by gossypol, Molec. Cell Biochem., 47:65 (1982).
80. A. Yoshida and E. Freese, Lactate dehydrogenase from Bacillus Subtilis, Meth. Enzymol., 41:304 (1975).
81. C. Y. Lee and H. V. Malling, 1981, op. cit. (see Ref. 76).
82. K. Olgiati, et al., 1983, op. cit. (see Ref. 79).
83. K. Olgiati, et al., 1984, op. cit. (see Ref. 80).
84. T. Braun and R. Dods, Development of a Mn^{2+}-sensitive, "soluble" adenylate cyclase in rat testis, Proc. Natl. Acad. Sci. (USA), 72:1097 (1975).
85. A. R. Kornblihtt, M. M. Flawia, and H. M. Torres, Manganese ion dependent adenylate cyclase activity in rat testis: Purification and properties, Biochem., 20:1262 (1981).

86. Ibid.
87. Y. Salomon, G. Landos, and M. Rodbell, A highly sensitive adenylate cyclase assay, Anal. Biochem., 58:541 (1974).
88. P. Margalith, Inhibitory effect of gossypol on microorganisms, Appl. Microbiol., 15:952 (1967).
89. P. H. Dorsett and E. E. Kerstine, Antiviral activity of gossypol and apogossypol, J. Pharm. Sci., 64:1073 (1975).
90. E. M. Vermel, The search of antitumor substances of plant origin, Acta Uni. Int. Cancrum., 20:211 (1964).
91. K. Wichmann, A. Vaheri, and T. Luukkainen, Inhibiting herpes simplex virus type 2 infection in human epithelial cells by gossypol, a potent spermicidal and contraceptive agent, Am. J. Obstet. Gynecol., 142(5):593 (1982).
92. P. H. Dorsett and E. E. Kerstine, 1975, op. cit. (see Ref. 91).
93. Y. E. Wang, et al., 1979, op. cit. (see Ref. 73).
94. M. R. N. Prasad and E. Diczfalusy, 1981, op. cit. (see Ref. 8).
95. A. Manmade, P. Herlihy, J. Quick, R. P. Duffley, M. Burgos, and A. P. Hoffer, Gossypol: Synthesis and in vitro spermicidal activity of isomeric hemigossypol derivatives, Experientia, 39:1276 (1983).
96. H. Jackson, 1973, op. cit. (see Ref. 24).
97. N. K. Kalla, Gossypol - the male antifertility agent, IRCS-Med. Sci., 10:766 (1982).
98. M. B. Abou-Donia, 1976, op. cit. (see Ref. 11).
99. L. C. Berardi and L. A. Goldblatt, 1980, op. cit. (see Ref. 12).
100. Z. Liu, et al., 1981, op. cit. (see Ref. 54).

A SOLID PHASE RADIOIMMUNOASSAY FOR GOSSYPOL

Y. Y. Tsong and C. C. Chang

Center for Biomedical Research
The Population Council
New York, New York

INTRODUCTION

Gossypol has been shown to uncouple oxidative phosphorylation [1] to inhibit adenosine triphosphatase [2, 3], and lactodehydrogenase-X [4, 5], and to cause degeneration of mitochondria and sperm flagella [6].

Gossypol interacts with free amino groups of amino acids and proteins to form complexes [7], and is also capable of chelating with iron to form metal complexes and decreasing iron absorption from the gut. The absorption of gossypol as well as manifestations of its toxicity were greatly affected by the dietary intake of proteins and iron [8]. Following oral administration of a single dose of radioactive gossypol, labeled compound was eliminated slowly from animals with half life of 60 h for rats and 78 h for swine [9, 10]. Concentrations reached a peak in the rat testis on the ninth day following administration [11].

Since the uptake, elimination and the extent of accumulation of gossypol in the serum and tissues were related to its toxicity, a method to measure low concentration of gossypol is important to the evaluation of its safety. Furthermore, production of antibodies specific to gossypol would facilitate the elucidation of its mechanism of action.

In the present study, we have synthesized gossypol-protein conjugates as antigens. Antibodies against gossypol were produced and a solid phase sandwich radioimmunoassay was developed.

MATERIALS AND METHODS

Reagents

All chemicals were reagent grade. Gossypol acetic acid was obtained from Bejing Institute of Zoology, Bejing, China, Polystyrene tube (10 × 75 mm) and polyethylene tube were from Falcon, Oxnad, Ca. and Sarstedt, W. Germany, respectively. Bovine serum albumin and Freund's complete adjuvant were from Miles Laboratories, Elkhart, Ind. Bovine thyroglobulin and lactoperoxidase were purchased from Sigma Chemical Co., St. Louis, Mo. Sodium cyanoborohydride and ammonium sulfate were obtained from Aldrich Chemical Co., Milwaukee, Wi., and Schwarz/Mann, Inc., Spring Valley, N.Y. DEAE cellulose was from Whatman Co., Clifton, N.J. and Sephadex G-25 from Pharmacia Co., Piscataway, N.J.

Preparation of Gossypol Protein Carrier Conjugates

1) Reaction via Aldehyde Group: Bovine serum albumin (20 mg), gossypol (15.7 mg) and 42.5 mg of sodium cyanoborohydride were dissolved in 20 ml of 0.1 M phosphate buffer in 50% methanol (pH 8.0). The reaction mixture was stirred at room temperature under nitrogen in the dark for 24 h. The solution was evaporated under nitrogen to 10 ml. Ice-cold acetone (50 ml) was added and the precipitate was collected by centrifugation at 5000 g for 20 min. The precipitate was dissolved in 1.5 ml of 50% methanol-water and loaded into a Sephadex G-25 column. Distilled water was used as eluent. The yellow protein peak that came out at the void volume was pooled and lyophilized. The recovery of the conjugates was 22.4 mg.

Conjugation with thyroglobulin was carried out by a reaction mixture containing 20 mg thyroglobulin, 15.7 mg gossypol and 42.5 mg sodium cyanoborohydride. The reaction was allowed to continue for 24 h at room temperature. The reaction mixture was concentrated with nitrogen gas and loaded directly into a Sephadex G-25 column. After the void volume peak was pooled and lyophilized, the recovery of the conjugate was 16.2 mg.

2) Reaction via Hydroxyl Group: Five mg of gossypol, 20 mg of 1-ethyl-3 (3-dimethyl aminopropyl)carbodiimide and 5 mg of either bovine serum albumin or bovine thyroglobulin were dissolved in 6 ml of water containing 70% dimethylformamide. The reaction was carried out at room temperature overnight under nitrogen in the dark. Ethyl alcohol (54 ml) was added to precipitate the conjugate and the precipitate washed twice with 5 ml of alcohol and lyophilized. None of the conjugates was soluble in water. The yield for gossypol-bovine serum albumin and gossypol-thyroglobulin were 4.3 mg and 3.8 mg respectively.

Preparation of Gossypol Carrier Protein Complexes

Gossypol binds to protein to form non-covalently linked complexes. We prepared such complexes and used them as antigens. Twenty mg of either bovine serum albumin or thyroglobulin and 15.7 mg of gossypol were dissolved in 7.5 ml of 0.1 M phosphate buffer (pH 8.0) in 50% methanol. The mixture was incubated at 37° for 3 h under nitrogen. The complexes were purified by Sephadex G-25 chromatography after concentrated down to 1 ml under a stream of nitrogen. The yellow protein peak at the void volume was collected and lyophoilized. The recovery of gossypol-bovine serum albumin and gossypol-thyroglobulin complex were 19 mg and 21 mg, respectively.

Immuniziation of Rabbits

New Zealand albino rabbits weighing approximately 3 kg were used for immunization. Five mg of gossypol conjugate in 2 ml of an emulsion made up of equal volume of saline and Freund's complete adjuvant were injected intradermally into rabbits at two sites. Five rabbits per group were used for each gossypol conjugate. Three initial immunizations were given one month apart. Booster injection was followed 6 months after the third injection. Animals were bled at two week intervals after immunization. Sera were collected and stored at -20°C.

Double Diffusion Studies

Ouchterlongy discs consisting of a circle of six wells around a single 6 mm well were used. Bovine serum albumin and bovine thyroglobulin were dissolved in saline for introduction into the wells. Gossypol and gossypol-protein conjugate were dissolved in saline containing 10% methanol and 20 mM phosphate buffer, pH 8.0. Antiserum was used without dilution. Wells were filled with sera or test solution as designated in the Results section. Discs were placed in a humid chamber and developed at room temperature for three days.

Purification of Immunoglobulin (IgG)

Purification of γ-immunoglobulin was performed according to the method of Campbell [12], with some modifications. The serum from immunized rabbit was precipitated with ammonium sulfate at a final concentration of 40%. The precipitate was collected by centrifugation and chromatographed successively through Sephadex G100 and DEAE cellulose. After extensive dialysis, the IgG was lyophilized. The final yield was 87 mg from 20 ml of serum.

Iodination of Immunoglobulin

Immunoglobulin was iodinated with lactoperoxidase according to the method of Marchalonis [13]. The iodinated product was purified through a Sephadex G-25 column which was eluted with 1% bovine serum albumin in phosphate buffer-saline. The specific activity of ^{125}I-IgG was 25 μC/μg.

Treatment of Rats with Gossypol

Adult male rats of the Sprague-Dawley strain weighing 280-300 g was obtained from Charles River Breeding Laboratories (Waltham, MA). Animals were housed in a temperature-(24.5-26.5°C) and illumination-(14 h light, 10 h dark) controlled room and maintained on Purina laboratory chow and tap water ad libitum. Ten animals were used for each group. Rats were fed orally with 15 mg gossypol per kg body weight, six days a week. Animals were sacrificed by decapitation at the third, fourth, and fifth weeks. Sera collected and epididymal sperm counts and sperm motility were examined with a hematocytometer under a microscope as described elsewhere [14].

Extraction of Gossypol from Serum Samples

Tubes containing 0.1 ml serum and 0.3 ml of 0.1 M acetate buffer (pH 4.0) were extracted three times with 2 ml of ethyl acetate saturated with water. Three extracts were pooled and organic solvent was removed to dryness by a stream of nitrogen gas. The sample tubes were individually sealed under nitrogen and stored in a freezer for next day assay.

Procedure for Solid Phase Sandwich Radioimmunoassay

Twenty five μg of purified anti-gossypol immunoglobulin (IgG) in 1 ml of 0.05 M bicarbonate buffer, pH 9.6 was incubated in a polystyrene tube at 37°C for 4 h, then overnight at 4°C. On the second day, the tube was washed twice with 1 ml of phosphate buffer-saline (PBS) by decantation to remove uncoated IgG. Either a standard solution of gossypol or an unknown sample in 1 ml PBS containing 30 μl of 50% methanol, 0.1 M phosphate buffer (pH 8.0) was added to the IgG coated tube and incubated at 37°C for 4 h then at 4°C overnight. On the third day, the contents of tube were decanted and the tube washed twice with 1 ml of 0.05% Tween 20-PBS and once with 1 ml of PBS. One ml of ^{125}I labeled IgG (100,000 cpm) in PBS was added to the tube and incubated at 37°C for 4 h then at 4°C overnight. After the incubation, the tube was washed 3 times with 1 ml of 0.05% Tween 20-PBS, dried and counted directly in an automatic gamma counter (LKB 1270 Rackgamma counter).

RESULTS

Gossypol-Protein Carrier Conjugates

Two functional groups, aldehyde and phenolic hydroxyl, of gossypol were readily available for conjugation to amino and carboxyl

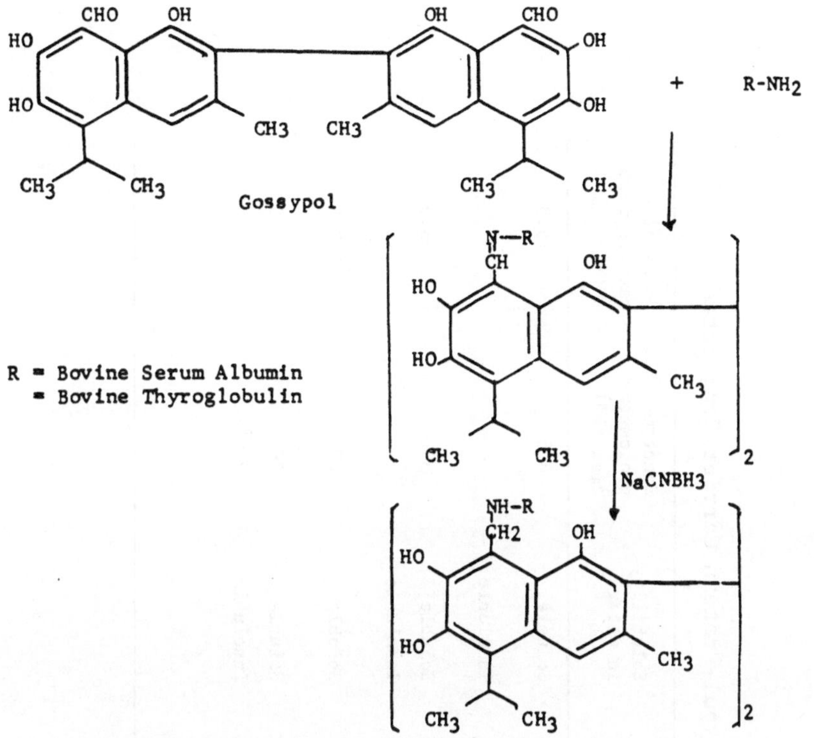

Fig. 1. Scheme of conjugation of gossypol with protein carrier via aldehyde group.

groups of proteins. Bovine serum albumin (BSA) and bovine thyro-globulin (Thy) were used as protein carriers. Covalent linkages between gossypol and protein carrier were achieved by either forma-tion-reduction of Schiff base linkage (via aldehyde) or by formation of an ester linkage (via hydroxyl) as shown in Figs. 1 and 2. So-dium cyanoborohydride and 1-ethyl-3(3-dimethylaminopropyl) carbo-diimide were employed as reducing agent and condensation agent.

Table 1 summarizes the characteristics of seven gossypol-protein carrier conjugate/complexes. Gossypol conjugated via alde-hyde functions with BSA or thyroglobulin (G-BSA-1 or G-Thy) were water soluble. However, when purification by alcohol precipitation was substituted for Sephadex G-25 chromatography, it became in-soluble(G-BSA-2). The formation of covalent linkages between gossy-pol and proteins was evidenced by a shift in gossypol absorption maximum from 390 to 405 nm. The comigration of the coomasie blue stained protein band with the yellow band in 10% SDS polyacrylamide gel electrophoresis was also an indication of covalent linkage. The weight ratio of gossypol to carrier protein was calculated on the basis of spectrophotometric analysis of weighed samples. The molar

TABLE 1.   Properties of Gossypol–Protein Carrier Conjugates

Conjugate	Chemical linkage	Solubility in water	Spectro-photometry λ_{max} (nm)	Gossypol: carrier ratio (w/w)
G-BSA 1	Covalent, via aldehyde	Soluble	405	1:5.8
G-GSA-2	Covalent, via aldehyde	Insoluble	–	–
G-BSA C	Noncovalent	Soluble	390	1:6.0
G-BSA CDI	Covalent, via hydroxyl	Insoluble	–	–
G-Thy	Covalent, via aldehyde	Soluble	405	1:7.5
G-Thy C	Noncovalent	Soluble	390	1:8.9
G-Thy CDI	Covalent, via hydroxyl	Insoluble	380[a]	–

[a]Soluble in DMF–water (7:3).

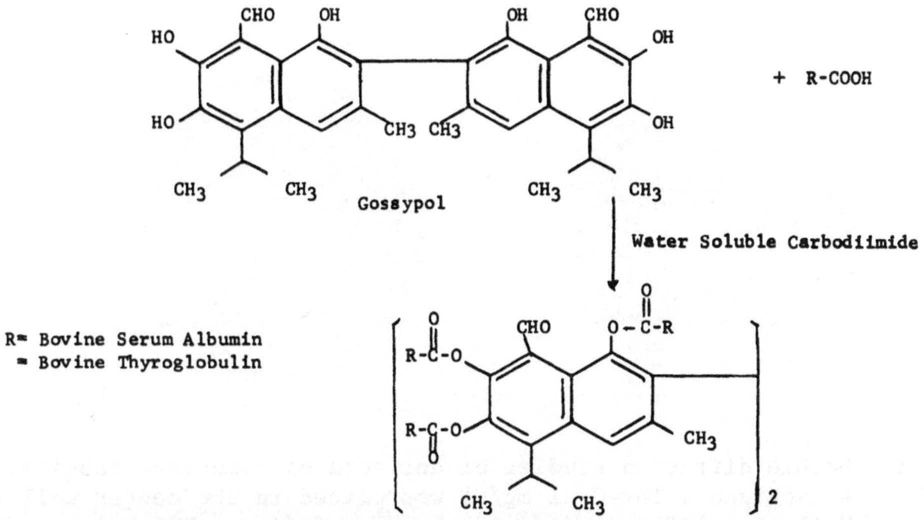

Fig. 2. Scheme of conjugation of gossypol with protein carrier via phenolic hydroxy group.

ratio of gossypol to BSA in G-BSA-1 was 22:1. Since the thyroglobulin used was heterogeneous in SDS-polyacrylamide gel electrophoresis, no attempt was made to calculate its molar ratio with gossypol.

Non-covalently linked gossypol-carrier protein complexes, namely G-BSA-C and G-Thy-C were water soluble. It is interesting to note that the complexes showed an identical spectrophotometric absorption curve in the visible region to gossypol (λ_{max} = 390 nm). G-BSA-C contained 21 moles of gossypol per mole of BSA.

The carbodiimide condensed products of gossypol, G-BSA-CDI and G-Thy-CDI were water insoluble. G-Thy-CDI was soluble in a mixture of dimethylformamide-water (7:3) and showed an absorption maximum at 380 nm. Since they were soluble only with the aid of dimethylformamide and dimethylformamide is not desirable for injection, none of the carbodiimide conjugates were used for immunization.

Double Diffusion Studies

The formation of antibody against gossypol was initially qualitatively examined with Ouchterlony plates. Sera from all immunized rabbits produced a distinctive precipitation line against antigen used for immunization. Typical results were shown in Fig. 3A. G-Thy (1 mg/ml) in the center well produced precipitation lines which coalesced when antisera of five individual rabbits immunized with G-Thy were placed in the outer wells. Although bovine thyroglobulin

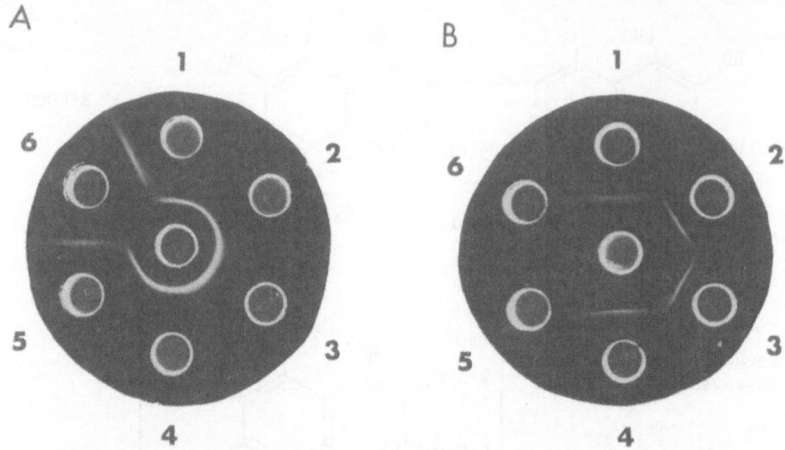

Fig. 3.   Double diffusion studies of antisera of immunized rabbits.
A) Antigen G-Thy-C, 1 mg/ml was placed in the center well.
Wells No. 1-5 were individual sera of five rabbits immunized with G-Thy-C.   Well No. 6 was thyroglobulin, 1
mg/ml.   B) Antiserum of rabbit immunized with G-Thy-C was
in the center well.   Well No. 1: thyroglobulin, 1 mg/ml.
Well No. 2: G-Thy-C, 1 mg/ml.   Well No. 3: G-Thy-C, 0.5
mg/ml.   Well No. 4: thyroglobulin, 0.5 mg/ml.   Well No. 5:
gossypol, 1 mg/ml.   Well No. 6: gossypol, 0.5 mg/ml.   All
test samples were dissolved in saline containing 10% methanol 20 mM phosphate buffer, pH 8.0.   The Ouchterlony plates
were developed in a humid chamber at room temperature for
3 days.

itself (well No. 6) also formed precipitation lines with antisera
of immunized rabbits (well No. 1 and well No. 5), the failure of
these lines to fuse at their intercepts indicated that different
antibodies were involved.

     The results demonstrated that at least two different antibodies
were produced in the immunized rabbits, one was specific to the conjugated antigen and the other was specific to the protein carrier,
thyroglobulin.

     An individual rabbit serum in the center well (Fig. 3B) pro-
duced precipitation lines with thyroglobulin (well No. 1, 4) and
G-Thy (well No. 2, 3).   Similarly, precipitation lines produced between antiserum and thyroglobulin did not fuse with those formed between antiserum and G-Thy.   There was no precipitation line formation between antiserum and gossypol (well No. 5, 6).   Since gossypol
is a small molecule, it is possible that soluble forms of antigen-
antibody complexes were produced.

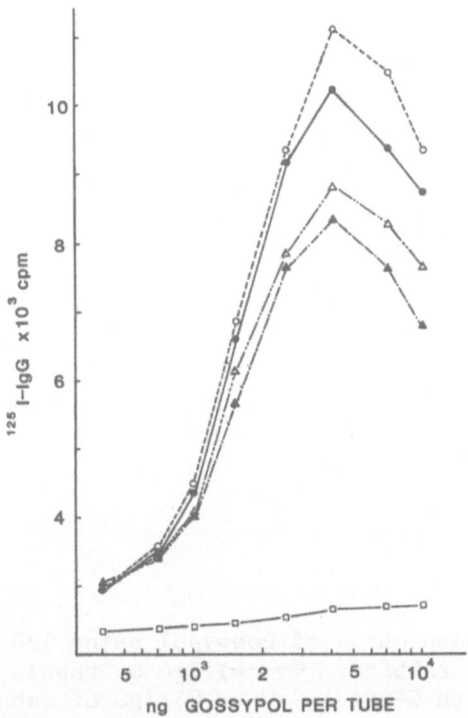

Fig. 4.   Dose response curve of gossypol in solid phase sandwich
          radioimmunoassay.   ○----○) 100 μg IgG per tube was coated
          in polystyrene tubes; ●——●) 25 μg IgG per tube was coated
          in polystyrene tubes; △-·--△) 100 μg IgG per tube was coated
          in polyethylene tubes; ▲-·-▲) 25 μg IgG per tube was coated
          in polyethylene tubes; □——□) polystyrene tubes without
          coating of IgG.   The assay method was described in the
          Method section.

Effect of Polystyrene Tube vs. Polyethylene Tube

     In the solid phase sandwich radioimmunoassay, the most impor-
tant factor was the nature of the solid support. Since we in-
tended to use ^{125}I labeled IgG as tracer and wished to count the
solid phase directly in the gamma counter, test tubes were chosen as
solid supports. The effectiveness of the coating of IgG on tubes
made of different polymers, polystyrene and polyethylene, was examined. Under identical assay conditions, as shown in Fig. 4, polystyrene tubes gave higher counts of ^{125}I-IgG than polyethylene tubes
in the gossypol dose response curve. This was true whether 25 μg or
100 μg of IgG was used for coating the tubes. Thus we chose polystyrene tubes for the assay system.

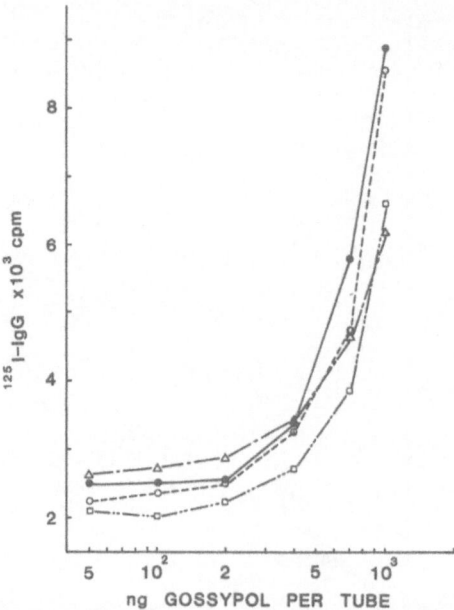

Fig. 5. Dose response curve of gossypol using IgG purified from
        individual rabbits. ●——●) IgG of rabbit (R#943) im-
        munized with G-BSA-1; ○----○) IgG of rabbit (R#944) im-
        munized with G-BSA-1; □-·--□) IgG of rabbit immunized
        with G-Thy-C. △-·-△) IgG of rabbit immunized with G-BSA-C.
        IgG was purified and iodinated individually for each rab-
        bit. The assay was carried out as descrived in the method.

Selection of the Amount of IgG for Coating of Solid Phase

As shown in Fig. 4, coating tubes with 100 μg of IgG resulted
in only slightly higher counts of ^{125}I-IgG than coating with 25 μg.
The coating of 5 μg IgG or 100 μl antiserum gave inferior binding
of ^{125}I-IgG. Since higher binding of ^{125}I-IgG represents higher
sensitivity of the assay, 25 μg of IgG was selected as the optimal
amount for the assay tubes.

In Fig. 4, ^{125}I-IgG binding to the assay tubes increased steadily
as the amount of gossypol increased and reached a peak at 4 μg per
tube, it inhibited the binding of ^{125}I-IgG. This phenomenon is be-
lieved to result from steric hinderance in which the high density of
bound gossypol in the assay tube obstructed the binding of ^{125}I-IgG
to neighboring gossypol moieties.

The assay gave evidence of specificity. In the absence of an
IgG coating on the tube, gossypol in concentration up to 10 μg/tube
did not significantly increase ^{125}I-IgG binding (Fig. 4).

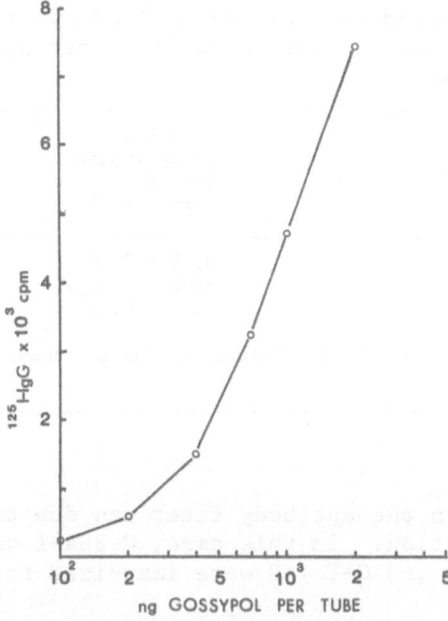

Fig. 6. Standard curve of gossypol for assay of rat serum.

Gossypol Dose Response Curve Produced by IgG
of Individual Rabbits

     Based on the double diffusion studies, all immunized rabbits
produced specific antibody against the antigen used for immunization. In order to examine the characteristics of antiserum produced by individual rabbits receiving the same antigen and individual rabbits receiving different antigens and to examine effects
of these characteristics on the assay, sera from four rabbits were
selected for purification of IgG. Two were immunized with G-BSA-1
and one each immunized with G-Thy-C or G-BSA-C. The sera were individually purified and the purified IgG were individually iodinated
with lactoperoxidase. The specific activities of ^{125}I-IgG were similar (between 20 μCi/μg to 27 μCi/μg). In the assay, IgG for coating
the tube and ^{125}I labeled tracer were from the same rabbit. As
demonstrated in Fig. 5, IgG from different rabbits gave good dose
response curves. The two rabbits immunized with G-BSA-1 showed
higher binding of ^{125}I-IgG (Fig. 5) than the rabbits immunized with
G-BSA-C or G-Thy-C. In the assay, IgG of G-BSA-1-immunized rabbits
gave sensitivity of 50-100 ng gossypol, whereas IgG of rabbits immunized with G-BSA-C or G-Thy-C had inferior sensitivity. Although
it was possible that G-BSA-1 could be a better antigen than G-BSA-C
or G-Thy-C and so give higher antibody titers, it was more likely

TABLE 2.   Rat Serum Concentration of Gossypol After
           Oral Administration of 15 mg per kg Body
           Weight

Length of treatment (weeks)	No. of rats	Gossypol concentration (μg/ml, mean ± SEM)	Fertility[a]
3	7	5.21 ± 0.40	Yes
4	8	5.96 ± 0.46	Yes
5	8	5.38 ± 0.37	No

[a]Fertility was based on the examination of sperms (count and motility from epididymis.

that the difference in the antibody titer was due to the different durations of immunization. In this case, G-BSA-1 was immunized for 12 months and G-BSA-C and G-Thy-C were immunized for eight months.

Assay of Gossypol in Treated Rat Serum

A typical standard curve of solid phase sandwich radioimmuno-assay of gossypol is illustrated in Fig. 6. In the assay, coating of 25 μg IgG on the polystyrene tube was used as solid phase, and extraction of gossypol from serum was carried out with ethyl acetate as described in the method. The recovery of thé exogenously added gossypol by ethyl acetate was about 85%. The results in Table 2 were corrected for background of control rat sera and extraction recovery. Table 2 shows concentrations of gossypol found in rat sera after 3, 4, and 5 weeks of oral administration of 15 mg/kg of gossypol. There were no significant differences in gossypol concentration during this period of treatment. It is of interest that the appearance of infertility as evidenced by low sperm counts and no motility in the treated animals (5 weeks) was not associated with an increment in circulating gossypol concentration.

DISCUSSION

Many methods have been developed for analysis of gossypol. Spectrophotometric measurement of colored derivatives of gossypol such as para-anisidine or anidine derivatives has been widely used [15]. The method is relatively insensitive. In addition, colored materials which might derive from biological samples would interfere with its accuracy. A paper chromatographic method has also been studied [16]. Although the sensitivity was improved over that of colorimetric methods, the visual comparison of the phloroglucinal sprayed spot with standards is subjedt to many uncontrollable errors.

A gas liquid chromatographic method has also been reported [17]. Gossypol was converted to its volatile trimethylsilyl ether derivative prior to analysis. Due to its tautometric forms, three component peaks were observed for gossypol in the analysis. The increased sensitivity of gas liquid chromatography was undermined by its complexicity in the analysis of three tautomeric peaks. More recently, high performance liquid chromatography using reverse phase column was also developed.

Gossypol (2,2'-bis(8-formyl-1,6,7-trihydroxy-5-isopropyl-3 methyl(naphthyl)) has a symmetrical structure with naphthyl nucleus on each side of the molecule. The symmetrical structure could serve as two identical binding sites for antibodies. On this basis, we have developed successfully the solid state sandwich radioimmunoassay of gossypol. In the process, antigen containing gossypol as heptan was synthesized and antibody was produced in rabbits. In the assay system, IgG was purified and used to coat a polystyrene tube which served as a solid support. Gossypol was introduced into the tube. During the antigen-antibody binding process, one end of the gossypol molecule bound to the coated IgG. Finally, the ^{125}I labeled IgG was added to the system to bind the other end of gossypol molecule. The formation of IgG-gossypol-^{125}I IgG complexes on the test tube was proportional to the concentration of gossypol in the sample. This method is the most sensitive method that has yet been developed for the analysis of gossypol. The lowest detection limit was 50-100 ng of gossypol.

Among seven antigens prepared (Table 1), three were water insoluble. Preliminary double diffusion and binding studies of antiserum produced by G-BSA-2, a water insoluble antigen showed that it gave little or no antibody titer against gossypol. Therefore, our studies were countered on water soluble antigens. We have also synthesized gossypol-(^{3}H)-tyramine and gossypol-(^{14}C)-methylamine as tracers. Unfortunately, the tracers had very low specific activities (less than 0.1 μCi/μg). They showed very poor specific binding to antisera.

Our assay method in the present form requires four days to complate. Studies are under way to examine the feasibility of shortening the assay time as well as increasing its sensitivity.

We have used the solid phase sandwich radioimmunoassay to measure the serum concentration of gossypol of rats administered gossypol orally. Based on the definition of Clark [18] and Lyman [19] and of Smith [20], the organic solvent extractable gossypol was termed "free gossypol." Gossypol remaining in the extracted residues was termed "bound gossypol." Since we assayed ethyl acetate extracts of samples, the results in Table 2 represent free gossypol concentrations.

Other researchers, using the anidine spectrophotometric method, measured gossypol concentrations in the serum and liver of rats treated with 5 mg gossypol 5 days a week for one month [21]. Their report did not specify whether the amount measured was free, bound or otal gossypol. The gossypol concentration in the liver increased, reached plateau at 7 days and remained at the same level for one month. The concentration of gossypol in serum increased to reach a plateau in 3 days (2 µg/ml). It remained at this level until 14th day, then increased to reach 5 µg/ml at 30th day of treatment. Our results (Table 2) showed that the free gossypol concentrations in rat serum stayed at the same level from the third to the fifth week of gossypol treatment. These were somewhat different from those of the researchers just referred to. Perhaps, the discrepancy was due to method used for analysis of gossypol.

Our results indicated that the appearance of infertility after five weeks of treatment was not associated with the increment of free gossypol concentration in the sera. This may suggest that gossypol act on an early stage of spermatogenesis and only the cumulative effect of such intervention resulted in the damage of spermatids and sperms leading to infertility. Further analysis of gossypol in sperm and various tissues of treated rats may give some clue to the mechanism of action of gossypol.

The solid phase sandwich radioimmunoassay has several advantages. The method is simple and is the most sensitive method for analysis of gossypol yet reported. It can be easily adapted to enzyme immunoassay procedures thus eliminating handling of radio-isotopes. The conjugation of enzymes such as β-galactosidase, phosphatase, etc., to IgG has been well studied. The method has a wide range of application in clinical studies for monitoring the concentration of gossypol.

RFFERENCES

1. M. B. Abou-Donia and J. W. Diekert, Gossypol: Uncoupling of respiratory chain and oxidative phosphorylation, Life Science, 14:1955 (1974).
2. O. Adeyemo, C. Y. Chang, S. J. Segal, and S. S. Koide, Gossypol action on theproduction of ATP in sea urchin spermatozoa, Arch. Androl., 9:343 (1982).
3. W. W. Tso, C. S. Lee, and M.-Y. W. Tso, Effect of gossypol on boar spermatozoal adenosine triphosphate metabolism, Arch. Androl., 9:319 (1982).
4. W. W. Tso and C. S. Lee, Lactate dehydrogenase-X an isozyme particularly sensitive to gossypol inhibition, Int. J. Androl., 5:205 (1982).
5. R. Eliasson and N. Virji, Effects of gossypol acetic acid on the activity of LDH-C$_4$ from human and rabbit spermatozoa, Int. J. Androl., 6:109 (1983).

6. A. P. Hoffer, Ultrastructural studies of spermatozoa and the epithelial lining of the epididymis and vas deferens in rat treated with gossypol, Arch. Androl., 8:233 (1982).

7. C. M. Lyman, B. P. Baliga, and M. W. Saly, Reaction of proteins with gossypol, Arch. Biochem. Biophys., 84:486 (1959).

8. M. B. Abou-Donia and J. W. Dieckert, Metabolic fate of gossypol: The metabolism of ^{14}C-gossypol in rats, Lipids, 5:938 (1970).

9. National Coordinating Group on Male Antifertility Agents, Gossypol - a new antifertility agent for male, Chinese Med. J., 4:417 (1978).

10. M. B. Abou-Donia and J. W. Diekert, Metabolic fate of gossypol: The metabolism of ^{14}C-gossypol in swine, Toxicol. Appl. Pharmacol., 31:32 (1975).

11. National Coordinating Group on Male Antifertility Agents, 1978, op. cit. (see Ref. 9).

12. D. H. Campbell, J. S. Gravey, N. E. Cremer, and D. H. Sussdorf, Isolation of rabbit antibodies and their subunits, in: "Methods in Immunology," 2nd ed _D. H. Campbell, J. S. Gravey, N. E. Cremer, and D. H. Sussdorf, eds.), Benjamin, New York, p. 189 (1970).

13. J. J. Marchalonis, An enzymic method for trace iodination of Immunoglobulins and other proteins, Biochem. J., 113:299 (1969).

14. C. C. Chang, Z.-P. Gu, and Y. Y. Tsong, Studies on gossypol I: Toxicity, antifertility, and endocrine analyses in male rats, Intl. J. Fertil., 27:213 (1982).

15. W. A. Pons, Jr., C. L. Hoffpauir, and R. T. O'Conner, Determination of total gossypol pigments in cotton seed materials, J. Amer. Oil Chemist Soc., 27:390 (1950).

16. G. Schramm and J. H. Bendict, Quantitative determination of traces of free gossypol in fats, oils, and fatty acids, by paper chromatography, J. Amer. Oil Chemist Soc., 35:371 (1958).

17. P. K. Raju and C. M. Carter, Gas liquid chromatographic determination of gossypol as the trimethysilyl ether derivative, J. Amer. Oil Chemist Soc., 44:465 (1967).

18. E. P. Clark, Studies on gossypol II, Concerning the nature of Carruth's gossypol, J. Biol. Chem., 76:229 (1928).

19. C. M. Lyman, et al., 1959, op. cit. (see Ref. 7).

20. F. H. Smith, Determination of free and bound gossypol in swine tissues, J. Amer. Oil Chemist Soc., 42:145 (1965).

21. Y.-B. Ko, X.-K. Lin, X.-Y. Lin, Y.-H. Chang, Y.-Z. Mar, S.-E. Yu, and Y. Din, Studies on the antifertility effect of gossypol III: The determination of the quantities of gossypol in blood and related internal organs after administration of the drugs in rats, Acta Biol. Expt. Sinica, 12:69 (1979).

EVALUATION OF GOSSYPOL'S EFFECT

ON BULL SPERMATOZOA IN VITRO

Erwin Rovan,* Natwar R. Kalla,†
Julian Frick,‡ and H. Adam*

*Institute of Zoology
 University of Salzburg
 Salzburg, Austria

†Visting Scientist
 Department of Biophysics
 Panjab University
 Chandigarh, India

‡Urological Department
 General Hospital
 Salzburg, Austria

INTRODUCTION

It has been reported over the past several years that gossypol inhibits the motility of spermatozoa in vitro [1, 2, 3]. Although the precise mechanism causing this inhibition is not known, it is clear that gossypol inhibits the activities of certain enzymes involved in the metabolic regulation of spermatozoa. The major enzymes reported to be affected by gossypol treatment are ATPase [4], lactic dehydrogenase and LDH-X [5, 6]. These enzymes are associated with specific morphological compartments of the spermatozoa. The purpose of the present investigation was to examine, by electron-microscopy, the morphological changes in these compartments of bull spermatozoa after gossypol treatment.

MATERIAL AND METHODS

Gossypol acetic acid (GAA) was obtained from the Institute Materia Medica, Beijing, China through the courtesy of the Rockefeller Foundation in New York City. Fresh bull semen, collected by means of an artificial vagina, was obtained from the Agricultural Station for Artificial Insemination, Klessheim, Salzburg.

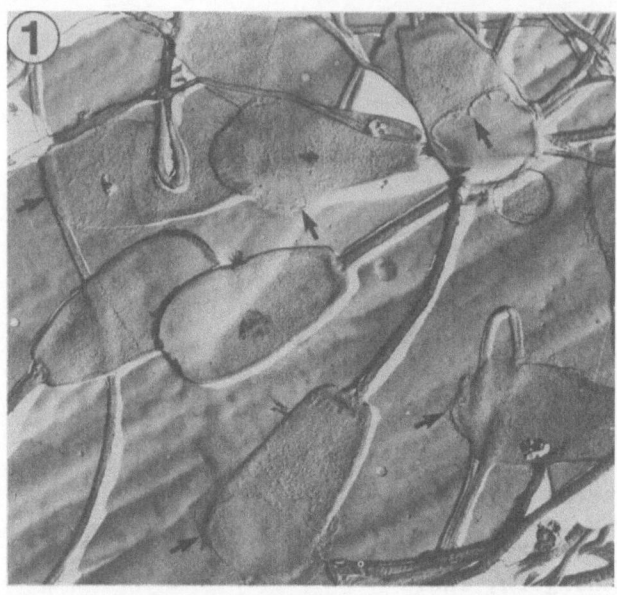

Fig. 1.   One ml of native bull semen was incubated, with no dilut-
          ing media, as an untreated control (A); 1 ml of native
          bull semen was incubated with 1 ml of 1% glycerol (B) and
          with 1 ml 1% Tween 80 buffered solution (C) as treated
          controls.   One ml of native semen was mixed with 1 ml of
          1% glycerol made in tyrode-buffer containing 1000 μg GAA
          (D), and 1 ml of the native semen was diluted in 1 ml 1%
          Tween 80 made in isotonic tyrode-buffer (pH 7.2) contain-
          ing 1000 μg GAA (E).

     Samples of proven motility (progressive motility not less than
80%, and sperm counts of not less than 800 million/ml) were used in
these investigations.   One ml of native bull semen (1 ml having a
spermatozoa concentration of 8.5×10^8/ml and a progressive motility of 87.4%) was diluted in 1 ml of 1% Tween 80 made in isotonic
tyrode-buffer (pH 7.2) containing 1000 μg GAA.   In another set of
experiments, 1 ml of native semen was mixed with 1 ml of 1% glycerol
made in tyrode-buffer, containing 1000 μg GAA.   For controls, 1 ml
of 1% Tween 80 buffered solution or 1 ml of 1% glycerol buffered
suspendant was mixed with equivalent volumes of native semen.   One
ml of native semen was incubated as an untreated control with no
diluting media.

     All the samples were incubated at 37°C in a water bath, and
semen analyses were done at intervals of 5 minutes.   After 30 minutes of incubation, parts of each group were prepared for electron

microscopical investigations. After fixation in 2% glutaraldehyde
(buffered in 300 mOsmol cacodylate-Na; pH = 7.2) and 2% osmium
tetroxide (buffered in cacodylate-Na), the samples were subdivided
into two groups. One group was prepared for fine structure analysis
on ultrathin sections. The samples were placed in small agar tubes
and subjected to the preparatory steps described by Rovan and Simonsberger [7]. In the second group, the cell suspensions were de-
hydrated in ethanol and small volumes of each were mounted on form-
varcoated grids. After air drying, the grids were brought into a
high vacuum device (Balzers 201). The samples were coated with
platinum-carbon (evaporation angle: 35°) and carbon alone (evaporation angle: 90°) under high vacuum conditions (air pressure: less
than 10^{-6} Torr). The thickness of coated metal and carbon layers
was standardized by a Quartz Crystal Film Monitor (QSC 201, Balzers).
After this procedure the grids were transferred into chromic acid
(40% aqueous solution) for 2 hours so as to remove the organic sperm
material and to obtain a purified replica. The metal replicas were
washed several times in distilled water, mounted on coated grids and
examined with a TEM Phillips 300.

Preparation as described above and examination on a TEM guaran-
tee a ten times higher resolution of the cell surface fine structure
than is possible with a scanning EM.

RESULT

The data of native examination (evaluation of motility) are
summarized in Fig. 1. The motility rate of control samples did not,
over a period of 30 minutes, differ significantly from untreated
controls (Fig. 8A-C). In contrast, the GAA-treated sperm suspensions show a marked motility decrease within 20 minutes of incubation (Fig. 8D, E), and no motile sperms were found after 30 minutes.
It is evident that GAA in this concentration produces a toxic effect
on the vitality of bull spermatozoa.

In electron microscopical evaluation, 250 single sperm or sperm
fractions were observed in all groups, both on surface replicas and
ultrathin sections. In the untreated (native) group, the morphological analysis indicated 87.6% of counted cells to be normal and 12.4%
to be damaged in membrane compartment arrangement and organell archi-
tecture. The percentage relation of unaffected and damaged cells
was equivalent to untreated sperms (75.6% normal; 24.4% damaged).

These data correspond to those found in native spermiogram
analysis over the incubation period (Fig. 8A-C).

In GAA-treated groups (1000 μg GAA/ml-diluting media), a high
percentage of analyzed sperm show marked abnormalities in fine
structure (92.1% damaged; 7.9% normal).

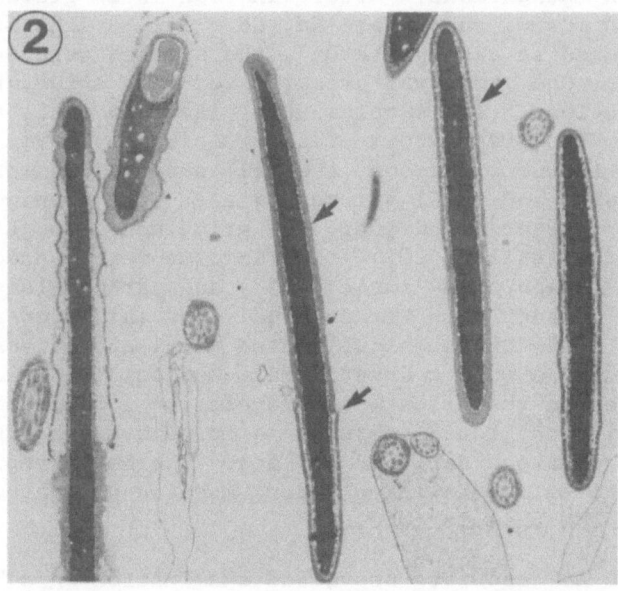

Fig. 2.   A large number of GAA-treated sperm show severe damage to
         the membrane compartment and to the acrosomal complex
         (arrows) (Magnification: 2300:1)

Figures 1 and 4 show that a large number of GAA-treated sperm
demonstrate severe damage to membrane compartment and to the
acrosomal complex.

In GAA-treated groups (1000 μg GAA/ml diluting media), a high
percentage of analyzed sperm show marked abnormalities in the fine
structure (92.1% damaged, 7.9% normal). In cross sections of different sperm head regions, there is, after GAA incubation, a dis-
ruption of the cytoplasmic membrane mainly in the region of the
acrosome. The post-acrosomal cap and its microfibrillar content
appear less affected (Fig. 2).

Figure 3 demonstrates the unaltered head morphology of control
sperms incubated only in the solvents (1% glycerol buffered in
Tyrode-solution or 1% Tween 80 buffered in Tyrode-solution).

In fine structure analysis of different GAA-incubated sperm
tail regions, there was found, in a distinct number, a separation
of microtubules in the end piece (Fig. 5). This defect was never
present in untreated or control sperm. Head-tail separations were
not observed.

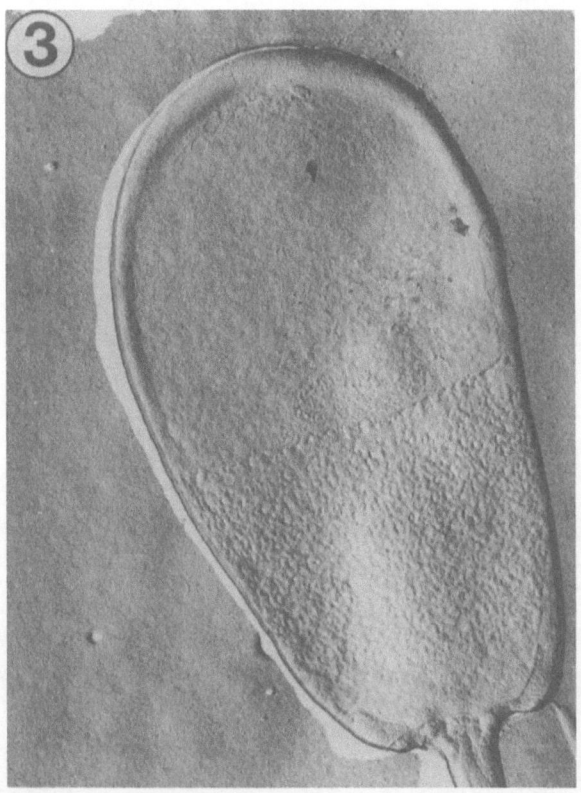

Fig. 3.   Morphological damages to sperm heads after GAA-treatment
          (Magnification: 8700:1.)

The cytoplasmic membrane and the acrosomal cap were markedly
affected by GAA incubation. The acrosomal material seems to be
extracted or coagulated to spheric granules (Fig. 6). The post-
acrosomal cap, however, with its typical microfibrillar pattern,
did not show obvious morphological alterations in GAA-incubated
sperm (Fig. 7).

DISCUSSION

The data confirm the assumption that GAA in a biogenic concentration of 1000 µg/ml solvent has a strong immobilizing effect
on spermatozoa in vitro.

The results show that GAA induces strong defects on the cellular membrane system. This can be related to the reaction of GAA
with membrane compounds or to inactivation of metabolic enzymes.

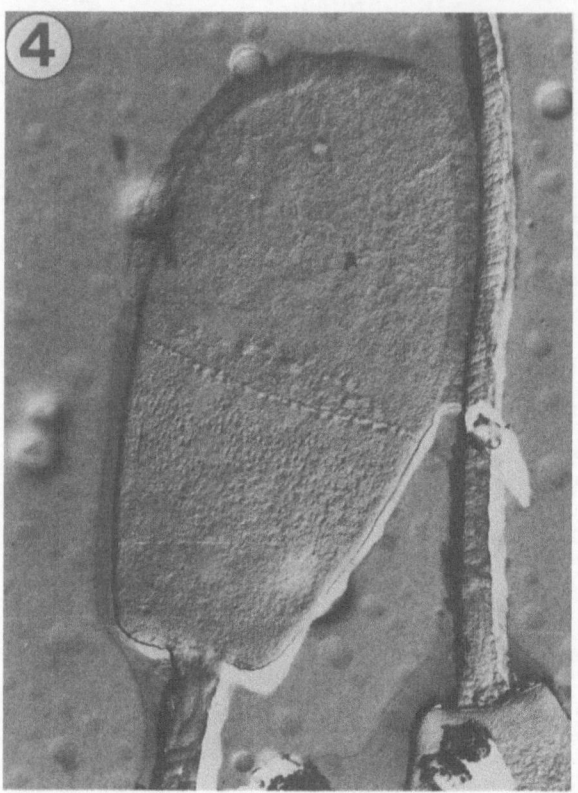

Fig. 4.   Cross sections of different sperm head regions after GAA
          incubation. The cytoplasmic membrane is disrupted prefer-
          entially in the region of the acrosome; the postacrosomal
          cap and its microfibrillar content appear less affected
          (arrows). (Magnification: 23000:1.)

Essential kinetic enzymes such as ATPase and LDH, are reported to
be partially inactivated by this drug [8, 9, 10].

        Furthermore, if the cytoplasmic membrane system is altered,
the membrane transport and the membrane electric potential must
also be affected and the cells must perish. The extent of cellular necrosis can be related to the incubation times of drug media.
Therefore, it is very difficult to compare sperm cell morphological changes during long-term _in vivo_ experiments with brief _in_

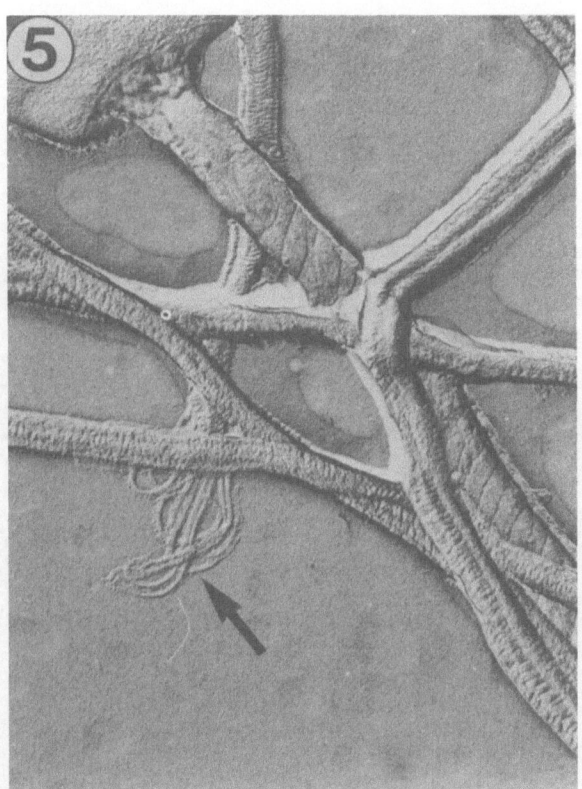

Fig. 5.   The unaltered head morphology of control semen incubated in
          the solvents (1% glycerol buffered in Tyrode-solution or
          1% Tween 80 buffered in Tyrode-solution). (Magnification:
          8700:1.)

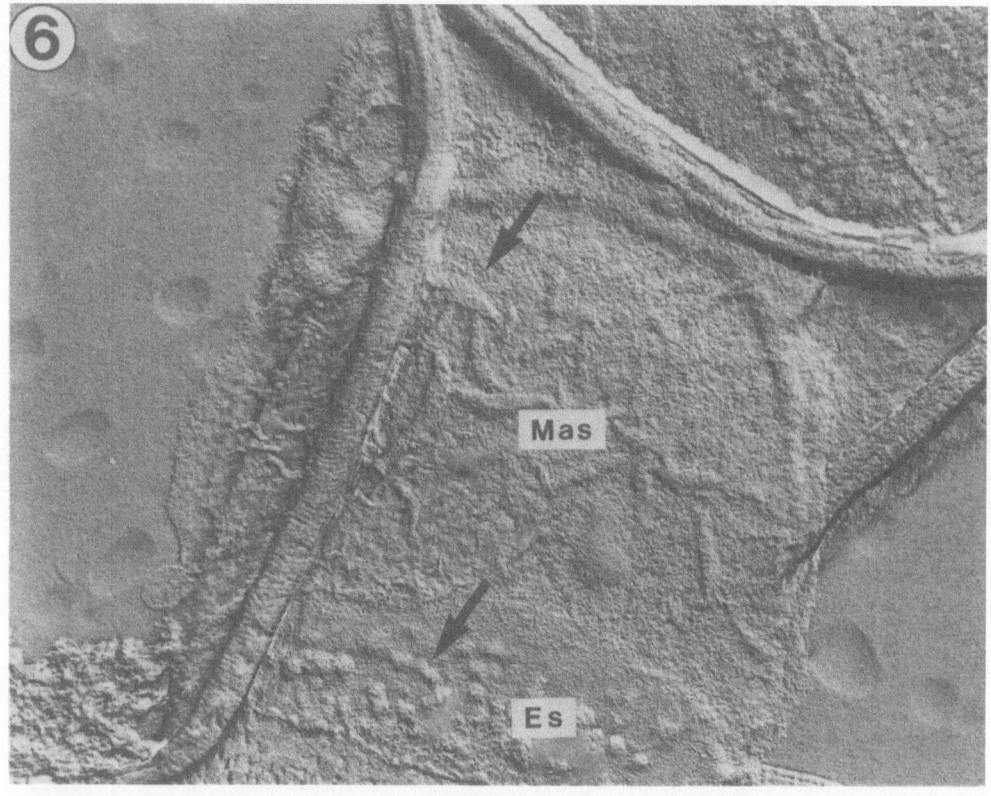

Fig. 6. The fine structure of different sperm tail regions after
        GAA-incubation. Note the sepration of microtubules in the
        end piece (arrow).

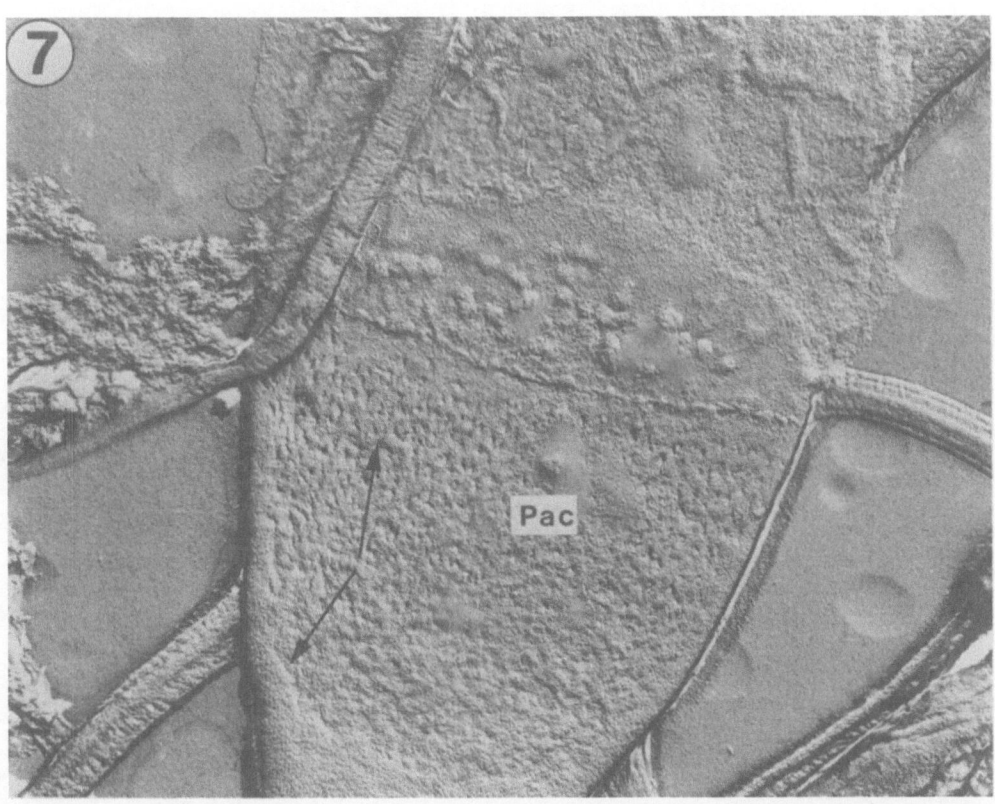

Fig. 7. The acrosomal cap (Mas) and the cytoplasmic membrane ap-
         pear hardly affected by GAA-treatment. The acrosomal mate-
         rial seems to be extracted or coagulated to spheric granules
         (arrow) (Es = equatorial segment). (Magnification:
         35000:1.)

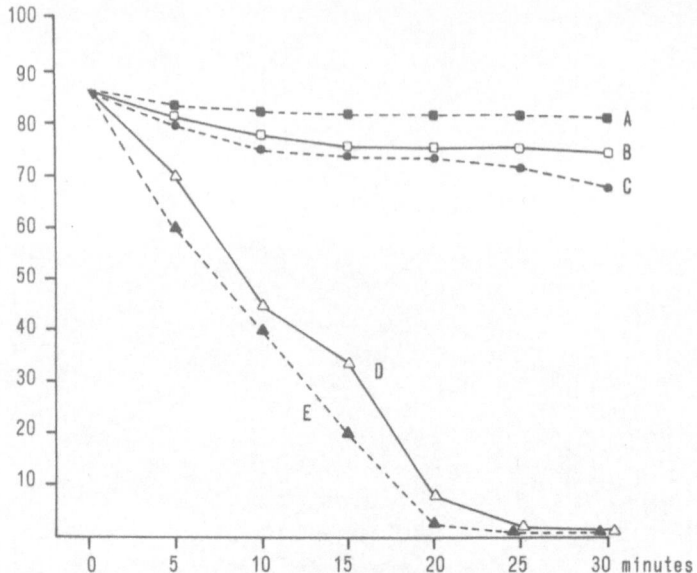

Fig. 8.   In contrast to the acrosomal complex, the postacrosomal
          cap (Pac) with its typical microfibrillar pattern did not
          obvious morphological alterations after GAA-incubation
          (arrow).   (Magnification: 35000:1.)

vitro studies [11, 12, 13].   The aim of a future experiment would
be to show the working mechanism of GAA on enzymes which are preferentially involved in the kinetic mechanism of mature sperms.

ACKNOWLEDGMENT

        This investigation was supported by The Rockefeller Founda-
tion, New York.

REFERENCES

1.   N. R. Kalla and M. Vasudev, Studies on the male antifertility
      agent, gossypol acetic acid: II.   Effect of gossypol acetic
      acid on the motility and ATP-ase activity of human sperma-
      tozoa, Andrologia, 13(20):95 (1981).
2.   J. Pösö, K. Wichmann, J. Jänne, and T. Luukkainen, Gossypol,
      a powerfull inhibitor of human spermatozoa metabolism, Lancet,
      19:885 (1980).
3.   D. P. Waller, L. J. Zaneveld, and H. H. S. Fong, In vitro
      spermacidal activity of gossypol, Contraception, 22(20):183
      (1980).

4. N. R. Kalla and M. Vasudeo, 1981, op. cit. (see Ref. 1).

5. C. Y. Lee and H. Y. Malling, Selective inhibition of sperm specific lactate dehydrogenase X by an antifertility agent, gossypol, Fed. Proc., 40:718 (1981).

6. W. Tso and C. S. Lee, Effect of Gossypol on Boar Spermatozoa in vitro, Arch. Andrology, 7:85 (1981).

7. E. Rovan and P. Simonsberger, Die Agarröhrchenmethode fur elektronmikroskopische Präparation von Zellsuspensionen und kleinen Gewebestuckchen, Mikroskopie, 30:129 (1974).

8. N. R. Kalla and M. Vasudeo, 1981, op. cit. (see Ref. 1).

9. C. Y. Lee and H. Y. Malling, 1981, op. cit. (see Ref. 7).

10. W. W. Tso and C. S. Lee, 1981, op. cit. (see Ref. 6).

11. A. Bozek, D. R. Jensen, and J. N. Tone, Scanning electron microscopic study of spermatozoa from gossypol-treated rats, Cell Tissue Res., 219:659 (1981).

12. M. J. Nadakavukaren, R. H. Sorensen, and J. N. Tone, Effect of gossypol on the ultrastructure of rat spermatozoa, Cell Tissue Res., 204:293 (1979).

13. D. P. Waller, et al., 1980, op. cit. (see Ref. 3).

INFLUENCE OF GOSSYPOL ON THE MOTILITY AND DYNEIN

ATPase ACTIVITY OF SEA URCHIN SPERM

Hideo Mohri,* Sheldon J. Segal,†
and Samuel S. Koide‡

*Department of Biology
 University of Tokyo
 Tokyo, Japan

†Rockefeller Foundation
 New York, U.S.A.

‡Center for Biomedical Research
 The Population Council
 New York, U.S.A.
 and
 Marine Biological Laboratory
 Woods Hole, Massachusetts, U.S.A.

INTRODUCTION

That gossypol affects spermatogenesis and sperm maturation in
the epididymis [1, 2, 3], testicular steroidogenesis [4] and metabolism of male accessory organs [5], resulting in a reduction of
sperm count, have all been demonstrated, as has its capacity to inhibit in vitro the motility of spermatozoa of various species, including that of human beings [6, 7], other mammals [8], and even sea
urchins [9, 10]. Gossypol interacts with various macromolecules
such as acrosin [11]. The motility arrest may result from a reduction in energy supply through inhibition of lactate dehydrogenase-X [12], pyruvate dehydrogenase [13], and the succinate to
cytochrome c segment of the electron transport chain [14]. Oxidative phosphorylation and mitochondrial Mg^{2+}-ATPase are also suppressed by gossypol [15, 16]. However, the influence of this compound on the motile machinery of sperm flagella, i.e., the tubulin-
dynein system that converts the chemical energy of ATP to mechanical
energy to be used for flagellar movement [17], has not been reported
although it has been claimed that the flagellar ATPase activity of
boar spermatozoa is probably not inhibited by gossypol [18].

215

The present study was undertaken to examine whether or not gossypol directly influences the motility apparatus of sea urchin spermatozoa. The effect of this compound on sperm models demembranated with Triton X-100 and dynein ATPase preparations isolated from sperm flagella were investigated. A preliminary account of this work was reported elsewhere [19].

MATERIALS AND METHODS

Sperm from the sea urchins, <u>Arbacia punctulata</u> and <u>Hemicentrotus pulcherimus</u>, were studied. Semen was obtained by injecting 0.5 M KCl into the coelomic cavity. Gossypol was obtained from the Institute of Zoology, Chinese Academy of Sciences, Beijing, China. he powder was dissolved in 95% ethanol to make a 10 mM stock solution. The solution was stored in the dark until use. The stock solution was diluted with either filtered sea water or other assay media to the appropriate concentration.

To examine intact spermatozoa, semen was diluted 500–1000 times with filtered sea water containing various concentrations gossypol. Demembranated sperm models were prepared according to Okuno [20], namely 10 μl of semen was mixed with 200 μl of an extraction medium containing 0.15 M KCl, 1 mM dithiothreitol, 0.1 mM $CaCl_2$, 2 mM Tris-HCl, pH 8.2, and 0.04% (v/v) Triton X-100. After 30 sec, 10 μl of the mixture was added to 500 μl of a reactivation medium consisting of 0.2 M KCl, 2 mM dithiothreitol, 0.5 mM $CaCl_2$, 1.8 mM $MgCl_2$, 1.8 mM EGTA, 2% polyethyleneglycol, 20 mM Tris-HCl, pH 8.2, and 1 mM ATP. Gossypol was added to the reactivation medium at varying concentrations. Spermatozoa were preincubated with gossypol, demembranated and reactivated with ATP. The procedure consisted of diluting 10 μl of semen with 500 μl of filtered sea water containing gossypol. The tubes were left standing at room temperature for 10 min and centrifuged in an Eppendorf centrifuge model 5412 for 1 min. Then, 100 μl of filtered sea water was added to the sedimented spermatozoa. The sperm suspension was treated with 10 vol. of the extraction medium and diluted with 10 vol. of the reactivation medium.

Sperm motility was assessed by visual examination under a phase contrast microscope and scored as ++++, very vigorous; +++, vigorous; ++, moderate; +, weak; -, inactive; and ±, indicating that a few spermatozoa showed head oscillation.

Separation of spermatozoa into head-plus-midpiece and flagellar fractions and preparation of axonemes, crude dynein extract and purified 21S dynein were performed with slight modification according to the methods described by Mohri [21] and by Gibbons and Fronk [22]. Semen was suspended in 10 vol. of Ca^{2+}, Mg^{2+}-free artificial sea water and homogenized in a Teflon homogenizer. The homogenate

was centrifuged at 900 × g for 15 min. The head–plus–midpieces
were located in the sediment. The supernatant was centrifuged again
at 900 × g for 15 min to remove any contaminating head–plus–midpieces.
The flagella were collected from the second supernatant by centrifugation at 10,000 × g for 10 min. The flagellar fraction was suspended in a demembranating medium containing 0.1 mM phenazine metho-
sulfate (PMSF), 10 mM Tris-HCl, pH 8.2, and 0.4% Triton X-100, and
centrifuged at 10,000 × g for 10 min. The precipitate was washed
with the same medium containing no Triton X-100, and the final pellet obtained was used as the axoneme fraction. The axonemes were
extracted with 0.5 M NaCl, 1 mM $CaCl_2$, 4 mM $MgCl_2$, 0.1 mM dithiothreitol, 0.1 mM PMSF and 10 mM Tris-HCl, pH 8.2, for 20 min. The
mixture was centrifuged at 10,000 × g for 30 min. The supernatant
contained the crude dynein. The crude dynein extract was concentrated using Acquacide II or Diaflo PM30. The concentrated extract
was layered onto a 5–20% sucrose density gradient cushioned with a
small volume of 40% sucrose at the bottom of the centrifuge tube.
The tubes were centrifuged at 24,000 rpm for 23 h using a RPS 25-2
rotor, in a Hitachi 55P-3 ultracentrifuge.

ATPase activity was measured in a system consisting of 0.1 M
KCl, 0.1 mM dithiothreitol, 1 mM $CaCl_2$, 4 mM $MgCl_2$, 0.5 mM EDTA,
10 mM Tris-HCl, pH 8.0, 1 mM ATP and enzyme preparation in a final
volume of 1 ml. After appropriate incubation at 25°C, the reaction
was stopped by adding 0.1 vol. of 55% trichloroacetic acid. The reaction mixture was centrifuged in an Eppendorf centrifuge for 1 min.
For the kinetic studies, an ATP-regenerating system consisting of
1 mM phosphoenolpyruvate and pyruvate kinase was included in the
above assay system. The liberated inorganic phosphate was determined by the method of Taussky and Schorr [23].

Protein content was estimated by the method of Lowry with modification [24] using bovine serum albumin as the standard. Fractions
obtained from the sucrose density gradient centrifugation were monitored by measuring absorption at 280 nm.

RESULTS

Effect of Gossypol on the Motility of Intact Spermatozoa

The effect of gossypol on the motility of intact Arbacia spermatozoa was observed under the microscope. In the control experiment,
ethanol up to 0.1 vol. of filtered sea water was tested on sea
urchin motility and found to have no effect. As summarized in Table
1, spermatozoa movements stopped immediately when exposed to 300 μM
gossypol. Motility was arrested within 5 min at 100 μM and within
20 min at 10 μM. At a final concentration of 1 μM, gossypol had no
effect on sperm motility. This result is comparable to previous reports showing that gossypol in vitro at concentrations from 10-100
μM stopped sperm motility within 12 min [25].

TABLE 1. Effect of Gossypol on Motility of Intact Arbacia Spermatozoa

Gossypol μM	Sperm motility (min after dilution)						
	0	5	10	15	20	25	30
0	++++	+++	+++	+++	+++	+++	+++
1	++++	+++	+++	+++	+++	+++	+++
3	++++	+++	+++	+++	+++	+++	+++
10	++++	+++	++	++	+	±	±
30	+++	+	-	-	±	-	-
100	+	-	-	-	-	-	-
300	-	-	-	-	-	-	-

Note: ++++, very vigorous; +++, vigorous; ++, moderate; +, weak; -, inactive, and ±, a few spermatozoa showed head oscillation.

TABLE 2. Effect of Gossypol on Motility of Demembranated *Arbacia* Spermatozoa

Gossypol μM	Sperm motility (min after ATP addition)						
	0	5	10	15	20	25	30
0	+++	+++	+++	+++	+++	++	±
1	+++	++++	+++	++	++	±	-
3	+++	++++	+++	++	++	±	-
10	+++	++++	++	++	+	±	-
30	+++	+++	++	++	+	±	-
100	+++	+++	+++	±	±	±	-
300	-	-	++	-	-	-	-
1000			-		-	-	-

Note: See Table 1.

Effect of Gossypol on ATP-Induced Motility
of Demembranated Spermatozoa

When Arbacia spermatozoa were demembranated with Triton X-100 and reactivated with ATP, they exhibited vigorous progressive movement similar to that of intact sperm. For gossypol to arrest completely ATP-induced motility, concentrations as high as 1 mM were required (Table 2). Even at 300 μM of gossypol which caused an immediate cessation of sperm motility, the demembranated spermatozoa were as vigorous as those of untreated control sperm up to 15 min providing ATP is made available. These sperm models were also more resistant to lower concentrations of gossypol in comparison to intact spermatozoa, except that motility was somewhat reduced after 10-15 min exposure to this compound even at 1 μM.

ATP-Induced Motility of Demembranated Spermatozoa
Models After Pretreatment with Gossypol

When spermatozoa were exposed to 300 μM gossypol for varying durations, centrifuged, washed and suspended in filtered sea water, some sperm regained motility with variable activity providing the pretreatment time with gossypol was less than 5 min. However, beyond 10 min of treatment, motility did not resume even after extensive washing. Spermatozoa were pretreated with 300 μM gossypol for 10 min and subsequently extracted with Triton X-100. The resulting demembranated sperm moved as vigorously as the controls when ATP was added to the medium. However, when spermatozoa were pretreated with 1 mM gossypol for 10 min, demembranated and reactivated, the sperm models remained immobile in spite of being supplied with exogenous ATP.

Effect of Gossypol on Mg^{2+}-ATPase Activity
of Sperm Fractions

The above results suggest that gossypol inhibits the energy-generating system of the mitochondria to a greater degree than it does the sperm's motility apparatus. To determine whether gossypol has a direct effect on the flagellar ATPase or dynein, Arbacia spermatozoa were separated into head-plus-midpiece and flagellar fractions. The latter was further demembranated with Triton X-100 to obtain the axonemes. As shown in Fig. 1, Mg^{2+}-ATPase activities of all fractions were suppressed by gossypol. At about 500 μM the compound induced a 50% inhibition. The flagellar and axoneme fractions were slightly more sensitive to the inhibitory effect of gossypol than to the head-plus-midpiece fraction in spite of the fact that mitochondria are located in the midpiece.

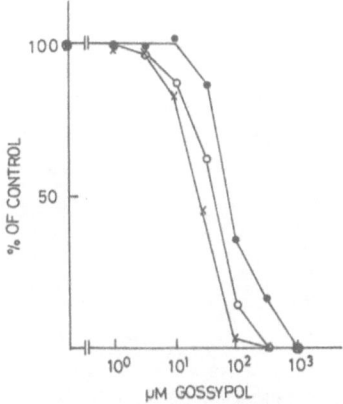

Fig. 1.   Effect of gossypol on Mg^{2+}-ATPase activities of sperm fractions (<u>Arbacia punctulata</u>). ●) Head-plus-midpiece fraction; ○) axoneme fraction; X) flagellar fraction

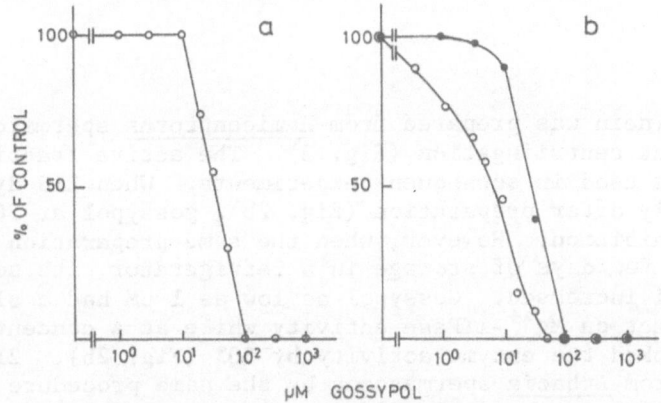

Fig. 2.   Effect of gossypol on Mg^{2+}-ATPase activities of crude
dynein and purified 21S dynein from <u>Hemicentrotus pul-
cherrimus</u> spermatozoa. a) Crude dynein extract; b) 21S
dynein (●, fresh preparation; ○, stored preparation).

Effect of Gossypol on Mg^{2+}-ATPase Activity of Crude Dynein Extract and Purified 21S Dynein

The crude dynein extracts, i.e., axonemes in 0.5 M NaCl, were
prepared from both <u>Arbacia</u> and <u>Hemicentrotus</u> spermatozoa. The degree of inhibition of the Mg^{2+}-ATPase activities in the crude extracts and in the axoneme fraction was similar (Fig. 2). At concentrations of 30 to 50 µM, gossypol induced a 50% inhibition (Fig. 2a).

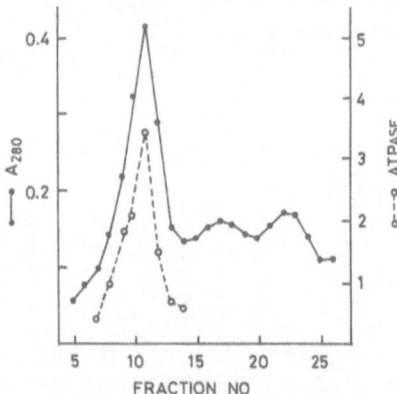

Fig. 3.   Sucrose density gradient centrifugation of crude dynein
          extract from Hemicentrotus spermatozoa. ATPase activity
          is expressed as μg Pi liberated/10 min/10 μl.

Purified 21S dynein was prepared from Hemicentrotus spermatozoa by
sucrose gradient centrifugation (Fig. 3).   The active fraction (No.
11, Fig. 3) was used in subsequent experiments. When 21S dynein was
used immediately after preparation (Fig. 2b), gossypol at 30 μM induced a 50% inhibition. However, when the same preparation was examined after a few days of storage in a refrigerator, its sensitivity to gossypol increased. Gossypol as low as 1 μM had a slight
inhibitory effect on Mg^{2+}-ATPase activity while at a concentration
of 5 μM it blocked the enzyme activity by 50% (Fig. 2b).   21S dynein
was prepared from Arbacia spermatozoa by the same procedure and the
effect of gossypol on the Mg^{2+}-ATPase activity was examined. Inhibition of the Arbacia and stored Hemicentrotus 21S dynein by gossypol was similar [26]. However, the dynein peak obtained from Arbacia
appears to have a smaller S value than that of Hemicentrotus. The
present results suggest the possibility that dynein may be more accessible to gossypol on purification since the purified product
tends to dissociate into subunits.

    Finally, the effect of ATP concentrations on the reaction
velocity of 21S dynein ATPase activity was examined in the presence
and absence of gossypol. Figure 4 shows the Lineweaver-Burk plots
drawn from the data obtained. The Km value for the 21S dynein in
the absence of the inhibitor was about 25 μM. The inhibition is of
the competitive type in spite of the considerable difference in
chemical structure between the substrate and the inhibitor. Gossypol may act by reducing the affinity of dynein ATPase for ATP.

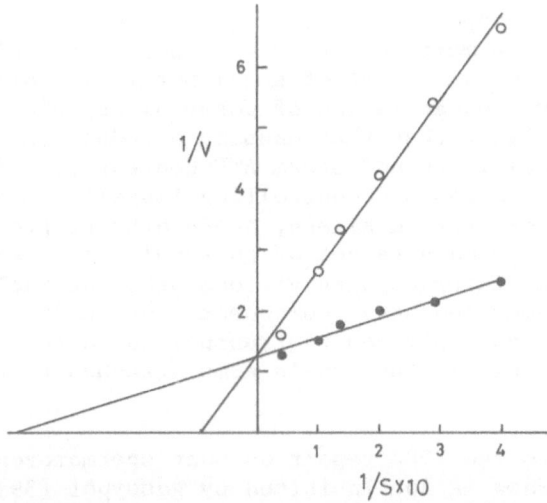

Fig. 4. Lineweaver-Burk plots for 21S dynein ATPase from Hemi-
         centrotus spermatozoa. ●) Control; ○) in the presence of
         30 μM gossypol. V is given as μmole Pi/min/mg protein and
         S as 10^{-1} mM. Lines were obtained by the method of least
         squares.

DISCUSSION

     The present study confirms the reports that gossypol has a di-
rect suppressing effect on the motility of mature sea urchin spermatozoa [27]. The motility of intact spermatozoa was more sensitive
to gossypol than the ATP-induced motility of the demembranated sperm
models. Furthermore, when intact sperm are pretreated with gossypol
at a specified concentration sufficient to cause complete arrest of
their movement, demembranated with Triton X-100 and reactivated with
ATP, the derived demembranated sperm models exhibited vigorous motility. This reactivation of sea urchin spermatozoa suppressed with
gossypol and subsequently demembranated was also observed and recorded by using a video system [28]. These findings indicate that
gossypol may act primarily on site(s) other than the sperm's motility apparatus which consist mainly of the doublet microtubules and
the dynein arms.

     It has been demonstrated that gossypol inhibits enzymes of the
glycolytic pathway and of the respiratory chain [29, 30, 31] and uncouples oxidative phosphorylation [32, 33]. The net result is a reduction in ATP synthesis [34]. ATP utilization may also be affected since Mg^{2+}-ATPase activity of sperm mitochondria is inhibited
by this compound as other investigators have reported [35, 36] and
as can be seen in Fig. 1. Although dynein ATPase and other enzymes

are inhibited by gossypol, the energy-generating system in mitochondria might be the main target of gossypol. This will result in
a shortage of ATP and an arrest of sperm motility. Alternatively,
since the effective concentration of gossypol capable of inhibiting
sperm motility is lower than that causing a reduction in mitochondrial enzymatic activities and sperm ATP content [37, 38], it is con-
ceivable that some components controlling flagellar movement, such
as adenyl cyclase or protein kinase, among others, present in the
membrane might be the main target of gossypol. In intact spermatozoa, gossypol may interact with various proteins including the
mitochondrial enzymes and other components surrounding the flagellar axoneme before gossypol can be transported to the sperm's motile elements, especially the dynein arms attached to the doublet
microtubules.

In contrast to the 1982 report on boar spermatozoa which found
that flagellar ATPase is not inhibited by gossypol [39], our present
study shows that purified 21S dynein ATPase and Mg^{2+}-ATPase activities of flagellar and axoneme fractions of sea urchin spermatozoa
are inhibited by gossypol. In the boar spermatozoa study, ATPase
activity present in sonicated sperm fraction that can be stimulated
with ouabain and oligomycin was considered as flagellar ATPase.
Hence, the flagellar ATPase complex is composed of dynein and other
ATPases. Furthermore, the structure of the flagellum of mammalian
spermatozoon is more complex than that of sea urchin spermatozoon.
The mammalian sperm contain additional structures such as outer
coarse fibers and fibrous sheaths. It is possible that gossypol
binds preferentially to these structural proteins rather than to the
dynein arms which are situated at a considerable distance from the
flagellar membrane. The finding that the inhibition of dynein ATP-
ase by gossypol was of the competitive type is unusual because of
the marked difference in chemical structure between ATP and gossypol.
It is possibly that gossypol binds to the dynein molecule and blocks
the active site(s) of dynein so that the substrate is less accessible
in an all-or-none fashion.

In the present study, we observed that the 21S dynein ATPase
of Hemicentrotus spermatozoa becomes more sensitive to gossypol on
storage. It is known that the 21S dynein consists of at least two
subunits [40] and tends to dissociate on storage. Moreover, Arbacia
21S dynein tends to disperse into smaller subunits during its preparation. This dissociation of dynein into subunits might be the
basis for the observed susceptibility to gossypol. At any event,
gossypol does affect flagellar dynein and the sperm energy-generating system. Our present results suggest that it is unlikely that
this compound acts as a specific inhibitor of dynein ATPase and that
the inhibition of this enzyme system is not the primary cause of the
observed arrest in sperm motility.

ACKNOWLEDGMENTS

    This work was supported by The Rockefeller Foundation 8208;
NICHD, NIH, ROI HD13184; and the Ministry of Education, Science,
and Culture of Japan. We thank Miss Kyoko Matsuda and Mrs. Toshiko
Mohri for their skillful technical assistance. We also thank
Miss Yoko Yano-Toyoshima and Dr. Mary Porter for some dynein prepa-
rations. Hideo Mohri was the Rand Lecturer at the Marine Biological
Laboratory, Woods Hole, in 1982.

REFERENCES

1. R. Adam, T. A. Geissman, and F. D. Edwards, Gossypol - a pig-
    ment of cottonseed, Chem. Rev., 60:555 (1960).
2. S. A. Bozek, D. R. Jensen, and J. N. Tone, Scanning electron
    microscopic study of spermatozoa from gossypol-treated rats,
    Cell Tissue Res., 219:659 (1981).
3. R. Oko and F. Hrudka, Segmental aplasia of the mitochondrial
    sheath and sequelae induced by gossypol in rat spermatozoa,
    Biol. Reprod., 26:183 (1982).
4. T. Lin, E. P. Murono, J. Osterman, H. R. Nankin, and P. B.
    Coulson, Gossypol inhibits testicular steroidogenesis, Fertil.
    Steril., 35:563 (1979).
5. P. B. Coulson, R. L. Snell, and C. Parise, Short term metabolic
    effects of the antifertility agent, gossypol, on various re-
    productive organs of male mice, Int. J. Androl., 3:507 (1980).
6. N. R. Kalla and M. Vasudev, Studies on the male antifertility
    agent gossypol acetic acid: in vitro studies on the effect of
    gossypol acetic acid on human spermatozoa, IRCS Medical Sci-
    ence, 8:375 (1980).
7. A. J. Ridley and L. Blasco, Testosterone and gossypol effects
    on human sperm motility, Fertil Steril., 36:632 (1981).
8. W.-W. Tso and C.-S. Lee, Effect of gossypol on boar spermatozoa
    in vitro, Arch. Androl., 7:85 (1981).
9. M. H. Burgos, C. Y. Chang, L. Nelson, and S. J. Segal, Gossypol
    inhibits motility of Arbacia sperm, Biol. Bull., 159 (1980).
10. M. H. Burgos, J. L. Fridovich, G. Weissman, and S. J. Segal,
    Delivery of gossypol by liposome: inhibition of sperm motil-
    ity, Biol. Bull., 161 (1981).
11. W.-W. Tso and C.-S. Lee, Gossypol: an effective acrosin
    locker, Arch. Androl., 8:143 (1982).
12. T. H. Maugh, Male 'pill' blocks sperm enzyme, Science, 212
    (1981).
13. O. Adeyemo, C. Y. Chang, S. S. Koide, and S. J. Segal, Gossypol
    action on the production and utilization of ATP by sea urchin
    spermatozoa, Arch. Androl., 9:343 (1982).
14. W.-W. Tso and C.-S. Lee, Variations of gossypol sensitivity in
    boar spermatozoal electron transport chain segments, Contra-
    ception, 24:569 (1981).

15. O. Adeyemo, et al., 1982, op. cit. (see Ref. 13).
16. W.-W. Tso, C.-S. Lee, and M.-Y. W. Tso, Effect of gossypol on
     boar spermatozoal adenosine triphosphate metabolism, Arch.
     Androl., 9:319 (1982).
17. H. Mohri, The function of tubulin in motile systems, Biochem.
     Biophys. Acta, 456:85 (1976).
18. W.-W. Tso, et al., 1982, op. cit. (see Ref. 16).
19. H. Mohri, K. Matsuda, S. S. Koide, and S. J. Segal, Effect of
     gossypol on Arbacia sperm ATPase, Biol. Bull., 163 (1982).
20. M. Okuno, Inhibition and relaxation of sea urchin sperm flagella
     by vanadate, J. Cell Biol., 85:712 (1980).
21. H. Mohri, Adenosinetriphosphatases of sea urchin spermatozoa,
     J. Fac. Sci. Univ. Tokyo, IV, 8:307 (1958).
22. I. R. Gibbons and E. Fronk, A latent adenosine triphosphatase
     form of dynein 1 from sea urchin sperm flagella, J. Biol. Chem.,
     254:187 (1979).
23. H. H. Taussky and E. Schorr, A microcolorimetric method for the
     determination of inorganic phosphorus, J. Biol. Chem., 202:675
     (1953).
24. G. R. Schacterle and R. L. Pollack, A simplified method for the
     quantitative assay of small amounts of protein in biological
     material, Anal. Biochem., 51:654 (1973).
25. M. H. Burgos, et al., 1980, op. cit. (see Ref. 9).
26. H. Mohri, 1976, op. cit. (see Ref. 17).
27. M. H. Burgos, et al., 1980, op. cit. (see Ref. 9).
28. S. Inoue, personal communication.
29. T. H. Maugh, 1981, op. cit. (see Ref. 12).
30. O. Adeyemo, et al., 1982, op. cit. (see Ref. 13).
31. W.-W. Tso and C.-S. Lee, 1981, op, cit. (see Ref. 14).
32. Ibid.
33. W.-W. Tso, et al., 1982, op. cit. (see Ref. 16).
34. Ibid.
35. O. Adeyemo, et al., 1982, op. cit. (see Ref. 13).
36. W.-W. Tso and C.-S. Lee, 1981, op. cit. (see Ref. 14).
37. Ibid.
38. W.-W. Tso, et al., 1982, op. cit. (see Ref. 16).
39. Ibid.
40. Y. Yano, H. Mohri, C. Toyoshima, and T. Wakabayashi, Molecular
     composition and structure of dynein arms, in: "Biological
     Functions of Microtubules and Related Structures" (H. Sakai,
     H. Mohri, and G. G. Borisy, eds.), Academic Press, Inc., New
     York (1982), pp. 125-135.

BINDING OF [¹⁴C]GOSSYPOL BY Arbacia SPERM

Eimei Sato,* Sheldon J. Segal,†
and Samuel S. Koide‡

*Center for Biomedical Research
The Population Council
New York, New York, U.S.A.

†The Rockefeller Foundation
New York, New York, U.S.A.

‡Marine Biological Laboratory
Woods Hole, Massachusetts, U.S.A.

INTRODUCTION

At concentrations of 10 to 100 μM, gossypol blocks the motility of Arbacia sperm, in vitro. The cessation of sperm motility is attributed to an inhibition of mitochondrial enzymes, Mg^{2+} and Na^+, K^+-dependent ATPases and pyruvate dehydrogenase [2], to a suppression in the transport of ATP to the sperm's motility apparatus [3] and to an inhibition of dynein ATPase [4].

In the present study, the uptake of [¹⁴C]gossypol by Arbacia sperm, and the nature of the physico-chemical binding were determined.

MATERIALS AND METHODS

The investigation was conducted at the Marine Biological Laboratory, in Woods Hole, during July and August of 1983. Specimens of Arbacia punctulata were obtained from the Department of Marine Resources. All experiments, unless otherwise specified, were performed at 22°C.

Chemicals

Gossypol acetic acid was provided by the Institute of Zoology, Chinese Academy of Sciences, China. The sample was analyzed by high performance liquid chromatography by Dr. H. Ueno, of The Rockefeller University, in New York City, and its purity was estimated to be better than 99%. [^{14}C]gossypol radiolabeled on the aldehyde group with specific activity of 3.33×10^5 dpm per micromole, was prepared by Drs. K. Watanabe and Y. F. Fen of Memorial Sloan-Kettering Cancer Center, in New York City. It was dissolved in 95% ethanol, and diluted a 100-fold with artificial sea water (ASW). Because of its photosensitivity [5], the gossypol solution was stored in a brown bottle and kept in a refrigerator. Other chemicals were purchased from the Sigma Chemical Co. ASW and Ca^{2+}, Mg^{2+}-free ASW were obtained from the Chemical Department of the Marine Biological Laboratory.

Preparation of Sperm and Eggs

Sperm and eggs were obtained from Arbacia by electrical stimulation. The oozing semen were collected and diluted with ASW. The eggs suspended in ASW were allowed to settle by gravity and the suspending medium was siphoned off. The washing process was repeated at least three times. Suspensions of sperm and eggs prepared in this manner were used within 1 h after collection. Sperm motility was determined by visual examination under the light microscope at a magnification of 150 ×.

Assay for [^{14}C]gossypol Binding to Sperm and Eggs

Sperm and washed eggs were suspended in ASW to the appropriate final concentration. Aliquots (0.9 ml) of the cell suspension were pipetted into 12 × 100 mm test tubes containing 0.1 ml of 100 μM of [^{14}C]gossypol. The mixtures were incubated at 22°C for varying durations according to the design of the experiment. The mixture was centrifuged at 2500 × g for 10 min. Aliquots of 0.5 ml of the supernatant were transferred to a vial containing 15 ml of the scintillator fluid (Dioxane cocktail, New England Nuclear, U.S.A.). The radioactivity of the supernatant was measured in an automatic scintillation counter (Hitachi 3300). The counting efficiency was 93.1%. The amount of [^{14}C]gossypol bound to sperm and eggs was determined by measuring the reduction in radioactive counts of the suspending medium. Values were expressed as percentage of the original amount of gossypol added. The number of moles of gossypol bound was calculated and corrected for the non-specific binding of [^{14}C]gossypol to the surface of the glass tubes.

The amount of [^{14}C]gossypol bound to sperm and eggs was determined by measuring the radioactivity in the suspending medium before and after the incubation with the cells. The reason for using

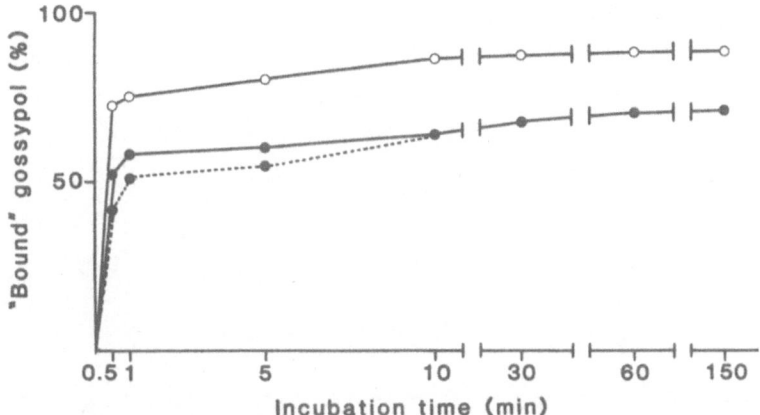

Fig. 1.   Time course of gossypol binding to <u>Arbacia</u> sperm. ●,
          7×10^7 sperm/ml; (O), 7×10^8 sperm/ml; temperature of
          incubation: 4°C (O——O) and 22°C (●---●). Final concen-
          tration of [^{14}C]gossypol 10 µM.

this indirect method of measuring the bound radioactivity is that the
direct determination of the amount incorporated into the cells requires several washing steps and complete solubilization of the
samples. Difficulty was encountered in avoiding loss of cells when
aspirating off the supernatant that marked variations in counting
values resulted. Also, solubilization of sperm was incomplete, e.g.,
only about 50% of the [^{14}C]gossypol was released on heating at 60°C
for 1 h in 1 M hyamine hydroxide. To validate that that the values
obtained by the indirect measurement paralleled the quantities bound
by sperm and eggs, the following controls were carried out. First,
the amount of [^{14}C]gossypol bound to the surface of the test tubes
was determined and used in the calculation to obtain the corrected
value of bound gossypol. Second, after washing the sperm and egg
several times with ASW, only 0.1% of the bound radioactivity could
be extracted. This finding indicates that the difference in the
amounts of radioactivity in the medium before and after incubation
with the cells corresponded to the amount bound or incorporated by
the eggs or sperm. Since the amount of extractable radioactivity
was less than 0.1%, this small value was neglected in the calculation. The radioactivity values obtained by indirect measurement
were consistent and reproducible.

RESULTS

Binding of Gossypol to Motile and Immotile Sperm

     Approximately 90% of the sperm in the semen collected from
specimens of <u>Arbacia</u> showed vigorous motility. To obtain prepara-

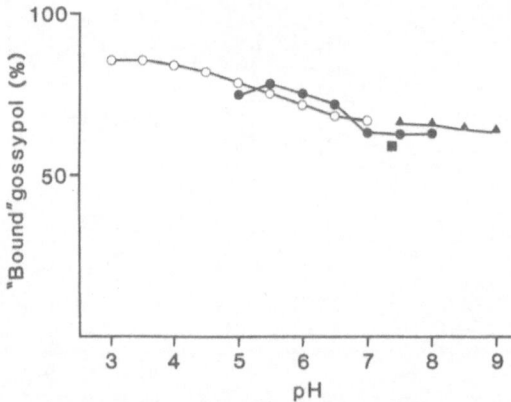

Fig. 2.   Effect of pH on the binding of gossypol to sperm. The re-
          action mixture containing 7×10^7 sperm/ml and 10 µM
          [^{14}C]gossypol was incubated for 2 h at 22°C. The incuba-
          tion media containing 145 mM NaCl was adjusted to the proper
          pH with 10 mM citric acid and 20 mM Na_2HPO_4 (O); 6.7 mM
          KH_2PO_4 and 6.7 mM Na_2HPO_4 (●); 20 mM Tris and 10 mM HCl
          (Δ), artificial sea water (ASW) (□).

tions of immotile sperm they were suspended in Ca^{2+}, Mg^{2+}-free ASW
for 20 min. Both motile and immotile preparations of sperm were incubated with 10 µM of [^{14}C]gossypol at 22°C for 10 min. Both preparations showed similar binding capacities (data not shown).

Time Course of Gossypol Binding to Sperm

     The degree of binding was dependent upon sperm density and tem-
perature. It was higher at 22°C compared to 4°C, as Fig. 1 shows.
The uptake of gossypol was rapid and occurred within a min after
exposure. At one minute of exposure, the amount of gossypol bound
to sperm was 58% and 74% at sperm densities of 7×10^7 and 7×10^8,
per ml, respectively. Subsequently, the binding increased gradually
and reached a steady state at 60 min.

Effect of pH on the Binding of Gossypol to Sperm

     Three different buffer systems were used with pHs ranging from
3 to 9. Figure 2 indicates that binding was slightly greater under
acidic condition (pH 3-4) compared to basic buffer, (pH 7-9). As
can be seen in the figure, similar results were obtained with different buffer systems at the same pH.

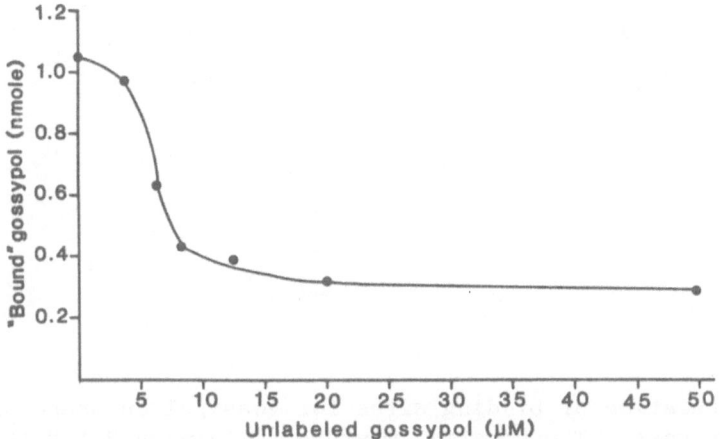

Fig. 3. Competitive binding of radiolabeled and unlabeled gossypol
         to sperm. The reaction mixture containing 2.5×10^6/ml
         sperm, 5 μM of [^{14}C]gossypol and varying concentrations of
         unlabeled gossypol. Incubation time of 2 min at 22°C.

Competitive Binding of Radiolabeled and Unlabeled Gossypol

Sperm (2.5×10^6/ml) was incubated in ASW containing 5 μM
radiolabeled gossypol and varying concentrations of unlabeled gossypol (Fig. 3). After 2 min of incubation, the amount of bound radiolabeled gossypol was determined. In the presence of unlabeled gossypol, the binding of labeled gossypol was competitively inhibited
(Fig. 3). Unlabeled gossypol at a concentration of 7 μM affected a
50% inhibition.

Specific Binding Sites for Gossypol
on Sperm and Egg Surfaces

Specific binding sites became saturated at a concentration of
25 μM of gossypol with sperm density of 2.5×10^6/ml and eggs density
of 5×10^2/ml, as Fig. 4 shows. Non-specific binding occurred when
the concentration of unlabeled gossypol exceeded 50 μM. The amount
of gossypol bound was 3.2 nmoles/2.5×10^6 of sperm and 0.5 nmole/
5×10^2 oocytes. Based on these values, the specific binding sites
per cell was calculated to be about 8×10^8 per spermatozoa and
6×10^{11} per oocyte. Thus, the oocyte possesses about 1000 times
more specific binding sites than spermatozoa. The amount of [^{14}C]-
gossypol bound per mg of dry weight of cells was calculated to be
about 28.2 and 16.3 nmoles per mg of sperm (ca 2.2×10^7) and eggs
(ca 1.6×10^4), respectively. The ratio of gossypol bound to sperm
and egg was about 1.8 based on the dry weight of the cells.

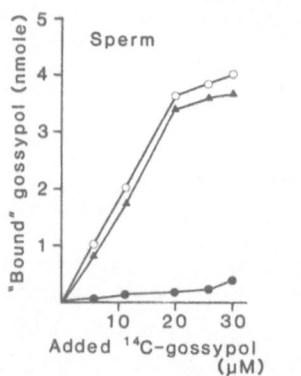 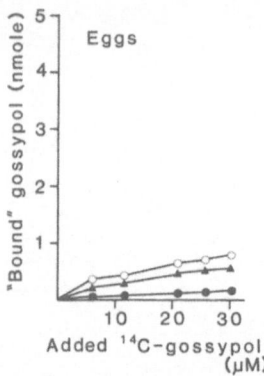

Fig. 4.   Saturation of binding sites for gossypol on sperm and egg
          surfaces.   The reaction mixture containing 2.5×10^6 sperm/
          ml or 5×10^2 eggs/ml and varying concentrations of [^{14}C]-
          gossypol.   Incubation time of 2 h.   (O), total binding;
          (●) non-specific binding.   Non-specific binding values,
          were determined in the presence of 50 μM of unlabeled
          gossypol.   (Δ), specific binding values, difference be-
          tween the amount of total and non-specific binding.

DISCUSSION

The present finding that the binding of gossypol was the same
with motile and immotile sperm suggests that motility is not a prerequisite for binding.   The binding of gossypol by sperm is rapid
and complete within 1 min after exposure (Fig. 1) while cessation
of motility occurs after 10 min of exposure [6].   Thus, during the
latent period following the binding a cascade of events may occur,
resulting in the loss of motility.

Although peptide hormones and gossypol interact with cell surface components, their binding characteristics are quire different.
Peptide hormones bind to surface receptors of target cells over a
prolonged period and the binding reaches a steady state after an
hour [7].   In contrast, the binding of gossypol to sperm surface
components is rapid and occurs principally at the midpiece followed
by internalization [8].   Also, the binding of polypeptides varies
with the temperature, while that of gossypol remains relatively constant to temperature changes.

Although the number of binding sites on spermatozoa is about
8×10^8 per cell, this value far exceeded the number of surface receptors on target cells for polypeptide hormones, e.g., the number
of binding sites for human chorionic gonadotropin on the plasma
membrane of granulosa cells is estimated to be about 10^2 per cell

[9]. The present finding of numerous binding sites for gossypol
suggest that the membrane-gossypol interaction is by chemical bonding probably via covalent linkage. It has been reported that gossypol interacts rapidly and tenaciously with serum albumin [10, 11].
The bonding is postulated to be between the aldehyde group of gossypol and the primary amines of proteins by the formation of a Schiff
base [12]. Moreover, bonding may occur by other mechanisms such as
oxidation of phenolic groups forming reactive quinones, hydrogen
bonding, Van der Waals interaction, and charge transfer complex
formation [13]. Hence, gossypol may interact with a variety of
determinants on surface molecules, manifested by a large number of
binding sites.

     The solubility of gossypol may also influence its binding since
it is relatively insoluble at neutral condition [14]. ASW, and
buffers of phosphate, citrate and Tris were used in the present
study as the incubation media and the solubility of gossypol in
these media did not pose a problem. Although we found that gossypol binding was slightly greater under acidic condition than under
basic conditions and comparatively less in ASW (Fig. 2), nonetheless, ASW was used as the incubation medium in several experiments
because the motility of Arbacia sperm was maximal in ASW.

     The binding of [^{14}C]gossypol was higher with Arbacia eggs than
with sperm, i.e., the number of gossypol binding sites per egg was
greater than that of the sperm. This finding can be attributed to
the larger size of the egg. It should be pointed out, however, that
gossypol at concentrations that totally inhibit sperm motility did
not influence fertilizability, maturation or development of fer-
tilized Arbacia eggs [15]. This inability to demonstrate any biological or morphological alteration in the structure or function of
the egg by gossypol suggest that the egg plasma membrane is im-
permeable to the compound in spite of the binding to the surface.

     Whole body autoradiographic studies after administration of
[^{14}C]gossypol showed that the drug is incorporated into the liver,
lung, kidney, heart, ·fat, and testes [16, 17]. However, the testis
is the only organ to show discernible damage at low dosages of
gossypol, indicating a selective uptake by the testes [18, 19]. In
rats, the seminiferous spermatids and spermatocytes show pathological alterations, while the morphological structures of Sertoli cells,
Leydig cells, epithelial cells and spermatogonia appear unaffected
[20, 21]. Most, if not all, of the spermatozoa found in the epididymis of gossypol-treated animals are immotile. Their mitochondrial sheath and cristae are disorganized. The inner and outer
tail fibres are disrupted and the cell membrane of the head region
are detached [22, 23].

     The inhibitory effects of gossypol on sperm motility may re-
sult from its interaction with the sperm motility apparatus and/or

with the associated proteins that regulater motility [24, 25, 26] or with the enzymes involved in ATP production and utilization [27, 28, 29]. Thus, the mechanism of the selective uptake of gossypol and the sensitivity of sperm to gossypol and especially its inter-action with the mitochondria and plasma membrane need to be clari-fied.

ACKNOWLEDGMENTS

Dr. E. Sato is a Rockefeller Foundation fellow. This study was supported in part by Grant GA PS 8210 from The Rockefeller Foundation and Grant R01-HD13184 from NICHD, NIH.

REFERENCES

1. M. H. Burgos, C. Y. Chang, L. Nelson, and S. J. Segal, Gossypol inhibits motility of Arbacia sperm, Biol. Bull., 159:467 (1980).
2. O. Adeyemo, C. Y. Chang, S. J. Segal, and S. S. Koide, Gossypol action on the production and utilization of ATP in sea urchin psermatozoa, Arch. Androl., 9:343 (1982).
3. H. Mohri, S. Matsuda, S. S. Koide, and S. J. Segal, Effect of gossypol on Arbacia sperm ATPase, Biol. Biol., 163:374 (1982).
4. Ibid. Chapter 15, this volume.
5. R. Adams, T. A. Geissmann, and J. D. Edwards, Gossypol, a pig-ment of cottonseed, Chem. Rev., 60:555 (1960).
6. M. H. Burgos, et al., 1980, op. cit. (see Ref. 1).
7. C. P. Channing and S. Kammerman, Characteristics of gonadotropin receptors of porcine granulosa cells during follicle maturation, Endocrinology, 92:531 (1973).
8. M. H. Burgos, et al., 1980, op. cit. (see Ref. 1).
9. S. Kammerman, R. E. Canfield, J. Kolena, and C. P. Channing, The binding of iodinated hCG to porcine granulosa cells, Endo-crinology, 91:65 (1972).
10. C. M. Lyman, B. P. Baliga, and M. W. Slay, Reactions of proteins with gossypol, Arch. Biochem. Biophys., 84:486 (1959).
11. R. Adams, et al., 1960, op. cit. (see Ref. 5).
12. C. M. Lyman, et al., 1959, op. cit. (see Ref. 10).
13. M. B. Abou-Donia, Physiological effects and metabolism of gossypol, Residue Rev., 61:125 (1976).
14. C. M. Lyman, J. T. Cronin, M. M. Trant, and G. V. Odell, Metab-olism of gossypol in the chick, J. Amer. Oil Chem. Soc., 46: 100 (1969).
15. M. H. Burgos, et al., 1980, op. cit. (see Ref. 1).
16. M. B. Abou-Donia, C. M. Lyman, and J. W. Dieckert, Metabolic fate of gossypol: the metabolism of [^{14}C]gossypol in rats, Lipids, 5:938 (1969).

17. C. M. Lyman, et al., 1969, op. cit. (see Ref. 14).
18. R. X. Dai, S. N. Pang, and Z. L. Liu, Studies on antifertility
     effect of gossypol. II. A morphological analysis of anti-
     fertility effect of gossypol, Acta Biol. Exp. Sinica, 11:27
     (1978).
19. S. Xue, S. Zong, S. Su, Y. Lin, Z. Zhou, and X. Ma, Anti-
     spermatogenic effect of gossypol on the germinal epithelium
     of the rat testis, Sci. Sin., 22:642 (1980).
20. R. X. Dai, et al., 1978, op. cit. (see Ref. 18).
21. S. Xue, et al., 1980, op. cit. (see Ref. 19).
22. A. P. Hoffer, Ultrastructural studies of spermatozoa and the
     epithelial lining of the epididymis and vas deferens in rats
     treated with gossypol, Arch. Andol., 8:233 (1982).
23. A. P. Hoffer, Effects of gossypol on the seminiferous epi-
     thelium in the rat: a light and electron microscope study,
     Biol. Reprod., 28:1007 (1983).
24. W. W. Tso and C. S. Lee, Lactate dehydrogenase-X: an isozyme
     particularly sensitive to gossypol inhibition, Int. J. Androl.,
     5:205 (1982).
25. H. Mohri, et al., 1982, op. cit. (see Ref. 3).
26. K. L. Olgiati and W. A. Toscano, Jr., Kinetics of gossypol in-
     hibition of bovine lactate dehydrogenase-X, Biochem. Biophys.
     Res. Commun., 115:180 (1983).
27. W. W. Tso and C. S. Lee, Effect of gossypol on boar sperma-
     tozoa in vitro, Arch. Androl., 7:85 (1981).
28. O. Adeyemo, et al., 1982, op. cit. (see Ref. 2).
29. M. B. Abou-Donia and J. W. Dieckert, Gossypol uncoupling of
     respiratory chain and oxidative phosphorylation, Life Sci.,
     14:1955 (1963).

BIOCHEMICAL STUDIES OF GOSSYPOL

Chi-Yu Gregory Lee, Young S. Moon,
Anthony Duleba, Albert F. Chen, James H. Yuan,
and Victor Gomel

Department of Obstetrics and Gynaecology
The University of British Columbia
Vancouver, Canada

INTRODUCTION

Gossypol does indeed prove to be a simple, safe, economical, and reversible method of male contraception, an understanding of its biochemical mechanism of action will be essential, since such elucidation may lead to the development of synthetic compounds exhibiting the desired antifertility effect without the toxicity so far noted in animals and in humans.

Extensive research has been under way in the last several decades regarding the toxicology of gossypol so as to ensure the safe consumption of cotton seed oil and meal by humans and domestic animals. However, the mechanisms by which gossypol cause tissue damage are as yet poorly understood. Research suggests that the toxicity may be associated with its binding to specific enzymes or proteins, or with its interference with amino acid, protein or ion metabolism.

Recently, we initiated biochemical studies of gossypol in an attempt to elucidate its possible mechanism of action as a male antifertility agent [1, 2].

GOSSYPOL INACTIVATION OF LDH-X AND STABILITY OF GOSSYPOL

We proposed three working hypotheses regarding gossypol's antifertility mechanisms. First, spermatogenesis is a well-programmed

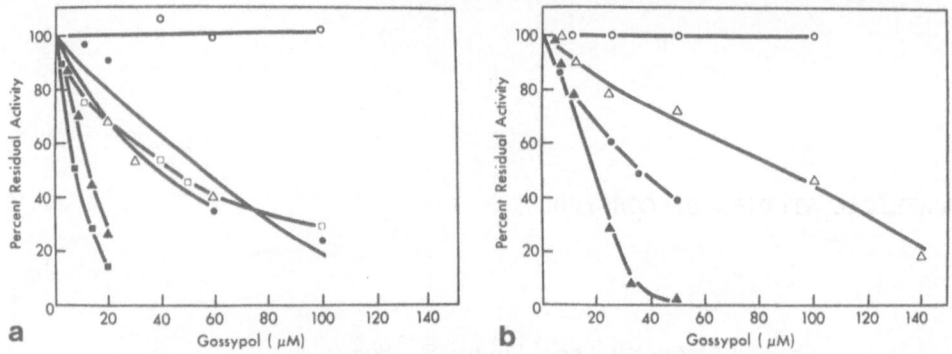

Fig. 1.   a) Activity of mouse lactate dehydrogenase isozymes in a mix-
           ture of NADH, pyruvate and gossypol [open symbol; O) LDH-1,
           Δ) LDH-5, and □) LDH-X] and activity of mouse lactate de-
           hydrogenase isozymes, when the enzyme was mixed with gossy-
           pol prior to the addition of NADH and pyruvate within 10
           seconds before assay [closed symbol; ●) LDH-1, ▲) LDH-5,
           and ■) LDH-X].   b) Activity of human LDH-1 (O) and LDH-X
           (Δ) in a mixture of NADH, pyruvate and gossypol; and ac-
           tivity of human LDH-1 (●) and LDH-X (▲), when the enzyme
           was mixed with gossypol prio to the addition of NADH and
           pyruvate within 10 seconds before assay.   Initial enzyme
           activity in each assay was about 0.01 unit/ml.

event during which specific isozymes of certain enzymes are expressed to fulfill metabolic functions of certain spermatogenic
cells [3].   If any of the sperm- or testis-specific enzymes are
selectively inhibited or inactivated by gossypol, its presence may
lead to metabolic disturbance of some spermatogenic cells, but not
other types of cells or tissues.   Second, spermatogenic cells may
have specific receptors to gossypol.   The binding of gossypol to
these cells may result in cytotoxicity.   Third, since spermatogenic
cells divide rapidly, gossypol may have a specific inhibitory effect
on DNA/RNA or protein synthesis during the active mitosis or meiosis
of spermatogenesis.

MATERIALS AND METHODS

     To test the first of these hypotheses, an initial biochemical
study was conducted regarding the effect of gossypol on the activity of about 20 enzymes from mouse testis in vitro [4].   Among the
enzymes examined, isozymes of lactate dehydrogenase and malate dehydrogenase as well as glutathione S-transferase were shown to be
significantly inactivated or inhibited by low concentrations of
gossypol in neutral aqueous solution [5, 6].

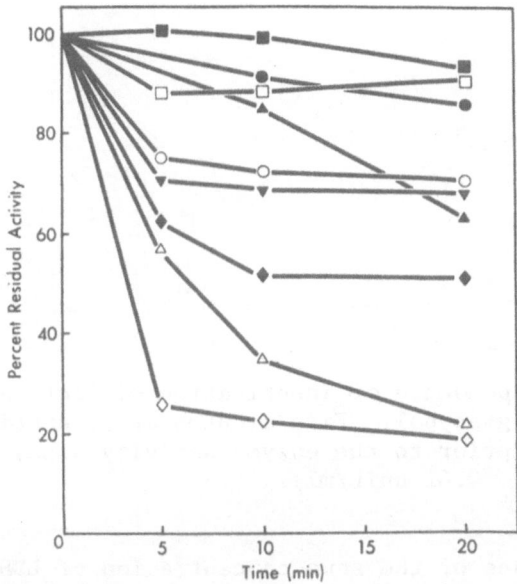

Fig. 2.   Time-dependent inactivation of mouse LDH-X under different conditions of incubation: ■) 0.01 unit/ml LDH-X in
50 mM potassium phosphate, pH 7.0 (control); □) 0.01 unit/
ml LDH-X + 1 µM gossypol; ○) 0.01 unit/ml LDH-X + 5 µM
gossypol; △) 0.01 unit/ml LDH-X + 10 µM gossypol; ●) 0.01
unit/ml LDH-X + 5 µM gossypol + 100 µM NADH; ▲) 0.01 unit/
ml LDH-X + 10 µM gossypol + 100 µM NADH; ▼) 0.4 unit/ml
LDH-X + 10 µM gossypol; ♦) 0.4 unit/ml LDH-X + 50 µM
gossypol; ◇) 0.4 unit/ml LDH-X + 100 µM gossypol.

As shown in Fig. 1, among the isozymes of lactate dehydrogenase, lactate dehydrogenase-X(LDH-X) from the mouse and humans was
selectively inactivated by gossypol. The degree of enzyme inactivation or inhibition depends on time, concentration of gossypol and
enzyme as well as the order of additions of assay components. If
LDH was first mixed with gossypol, a significantly higher degree of
inactivation or inhibition of enzyme activity was observed compared
to the assay in which the enzyme was added to the assay solution
containing pre-mixed NADH, pyruvate and gossypol. By either procedure, LDH-X and LDH-5 were consistently inactivated faster than
LDH-1.

Inactivation of LDH isozymes by gossypol is time-dependent.
When 0.01 unit/ml of LDH-X was incubated with 10 µM gossypol at
room temperature in 50 mM potassium phosphate, pH 7.0, 50, 35, and
20% of the initial enzyme activity was observed, respectively, after
5, 10, and 20 min of incubation.

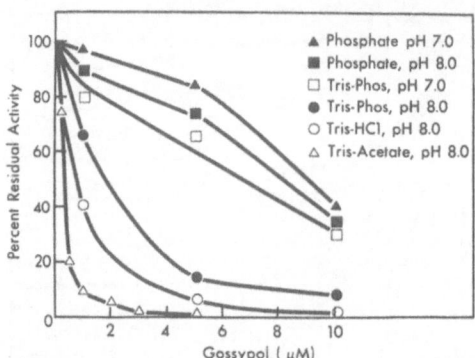

Fig. 3. Buffer dependence of inactivation of lactate dehydrogen-
         ase-X by gossypol. Five minutes of incubation of gossypol
         was made prior to the enzyme activity assay (initial enzyme
         activity: 0.01 unit/ml).

        In the presence of the same concentration of LDH-X, the extent
and the degree of time-dependent inactivation by gossypol is gossy-
pol-concentration dependent. After 20 min of incubation of gossypol
with 0.01 unit/ml LDH-X, the percent residual enzyme activity observed is 95, 70, and 21%, respectively, in the presence of 1, 5,
and 10 µM gossypol. The results of this study are presented in
Fig. 2.

        The degree of enzyme inactivation by gossypol is also enzyme-
concentration dependent. In the case of LDH-X, when 0.4 unit/ml
enzyme was incubated with 10 µM gossypol, greater than 70% of the
enzyme activity remained after 20 min of incubation. In contrast,
upon incubation of 0.01 unit/ml of LDH-X with the same concentration
of gossypol, only 20% of the original activity remained after the
same incubation time as Fig. 2 shows.

        Inactivation of LDH-X by gossypol was found to be irreversible.
Upon inactivation by gossypol, a further incubation with coenzyme
or substrate failed to restore the original enzyme activity. On the
other hand, the presence of NADH appeared to partially protect LDH-X
from inactivation by gossypol. For example, in the absence of NADH,
greater than 80% of LDH-X activity was inactivated by 10 µM gossypol
after 20 min of incubation. However, in the presence of 100 µM NADH
and 10 µM gossypol, only 40% inactivation of LDH-X activity was observed after the same incubation time (Fig. 2).

        Recently, we also found that the degree of LDH-X inactivation
by gossypol is pH- and buffer-dependent. As shown in Fig. 3, at a
given pH, the relative potency of enzyme inactivation by gossypol
varied more than 10-fold depending on the counter-anions of the

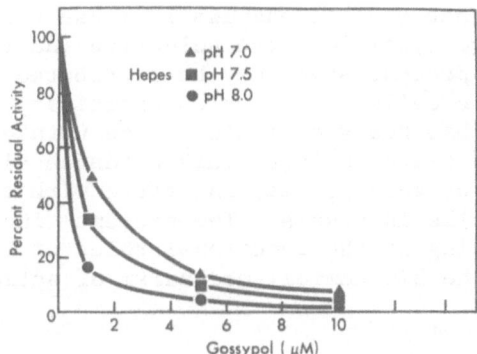

Fig. 4.   pH-dependence of inactivation of lactate dehydrogenase-X
          by gossypol in HEPES buffer. The enzyme assay was per-
          formed after 5 min incubation of enzyme with gossypol
          (initial activity: 0.01 unit/ml).

Tris buffer according to the following order: Acetate > Cl⁻ > gly-
cine > phosphate.

     To a given buffer solution, the degree of enzyme inactivation
increases with increasing pH from 7.0 to 8.0 as clearly demonstrated
in the case of HEPES buffer (Fig. 4).

     The rsults of this biochemical study seem to indicate that
gossypol is a selective inactivator of sperm-specific LDH-X from
mouse and human. The degree of LDH-X inactivation by gossypol was
found to depend on gossypol concentration, even though its apparent
concentration is always in great excess compared to that of LDH-X.
This observation strongly suggests that the presence of minor active
components in gossypol (which is a limiting factor) may be responsible for LDH-X inactivation in neutral aqueous solution. Based on
the study of enzyme- and gossypol-dependent inactivation of LDH-X,
it is estimated that the minor active components may amount to only
0.1 to 0.5% of the total gossypol in solution.

     The fact that the enzyme inactivation by gossypol is partially
blocked by NADH indicates that the inactivation processes may be
coenzyme binding site-directed. The irreversible inactivation of
LDH-X by gossypol could result from the covalent interaction between the active components of gossypol and the enzyme. To elucidate this point, we are currently employing C^{14}-labeled gossypol
for further analysis.

     It has been reported that LDH-X is not expressed until the male
germ cells have reached their pachytene stage, and is found only in
spermatocytes, spermatids, and spermatozoa [7]. Although it has

been demonstrated that several enzymes in mouse testis are inhibited or inactivated by gossypol [8], the selective inactivation of LDH-X by gossypol in the present study may be attributed to its cytotoxicity on spermatogenic cells and to male infertility. Recently, it has been reported that gossypol inhibits the uptake of sugar and lactate by human spermatozoa [9]. This evidence also suggests that LDH-X inactivation by gossypol may interfere with the metabolism of spermatogenic cells in testis. The present finding may lead to a better understanding of the functional roles of LDH-X in spermatogenic cells and the biochemical mechanism of action of gossypol on male infertility.

STABILITY OF GOSSYPOL

Since gossypol is a polyphenolic compound, we would expect a high degree of instability in aqueous solution. The decomposition of gossypol may occur via air oxidation, alcohol-aldehyde dismutation or chelation/oxidation by metal ions such as Fe^{3+} [10].

The minor active components of gossypol that irreversibly inactivate LDH-X may arise from either the impurities present in the original gossypol sample, or in the decomposition products or minor tautomeric forms of gossypol. In view of the instability of gossypol, it is likely that the minor decomposition products of gossypol are responsible for the inactivation of LDH-X in aqueous solution. Therefore, the decomposition or the metabolic fate of gossypol may play a key role in its physiological actions. Based on this assumption, the stability of gossypol in aqueous solution was investigated in our laboratory in an attempt to search for the minor gossypol components that inactivate LDH-X. Factors which affect the stability of gossypol in solutions were elucidated by thin-layer chromatography, high pressure liquid chromatography and by uv/visible spectrophotometry.

In absolute ethanol, gossypol exhibits high solubility, but undergoes gradual spectral changes with time either in the presence of, or in the absence of, oxygen. By thin-layer chromatography (on polyamide plates using a solvent system: benzene/acetic acid/H_2O of 57/28/15), one can clearly demonstrate the appearance of two additional uv-positive spots on thin-layer plates with Rf values of 0.6 and 0.4, respectively instead of 0.75 for the parent compound, gossypol, after 96 h incubation in absolute ethanol. The gradual decomposition or transformation of gossypol in ethanol is not oxygen-dependent and is accompanied by a shift in uv λ_{max} from 238 to 259 nm and a decrease in absorbance at 370 nm.

pH- and time-dependent stability of gossypol in aqueous solution was also studied by high pressure liquid chromatography (C18-reverse phase column, 2.3 × 250 mm, 10 μ particle size, Altex). At

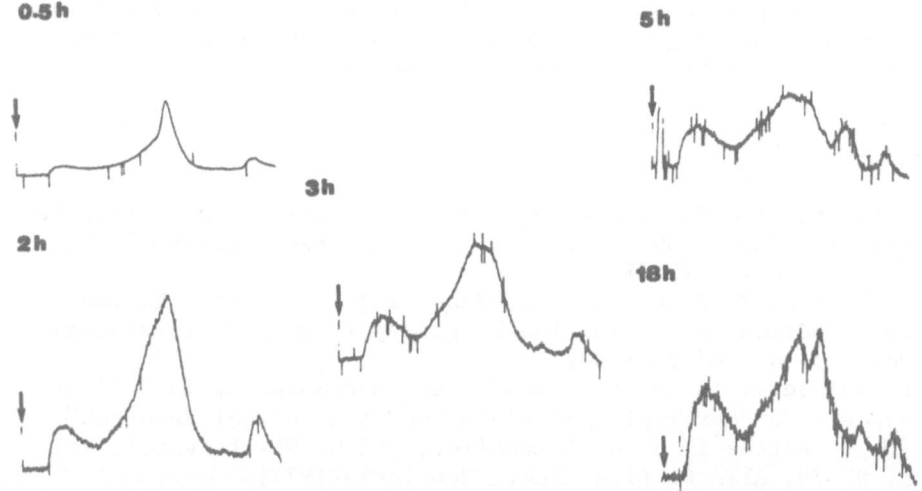

Fig. 5. Decomposition of gossypol in 0.05 M sodium bicarbonate, pH
         8.5 as a function of time, when analyzed by high pressure
         liquid chromatography. Solvent system used and conditions:
         40% CH_3CN in 0.01% acetic acid for 1 min, 70% CH_3CN in
         0.01% acetic acid for 4 min linear gradient, 100% CH_3CN in
         0.01% acetic acid for 3 min linear gradient, and 100% CH_3CN
         in 0.01% acetic acid for 3 isocratic conditions.

pH 4.5 in 0.05 M citrate buffer, gossypol is stable indefinitely as
judged from tracings by high pressure liquid chromatography. At pH
7.0 in 50 mM phosphate, gossypol is slowly decomposed with time.
A faster decomposition of gossypol was observed at higher pH. Typical tracings of HPL chromatogram are presented in Fig. 5 to demonstrate the time-dependent decomposition of gossypol in aqueous solution.

     The instability of gossypol in aqueous solution is also con-
firmed by thin-layer chromatography and uv/visible spectrophotometry. Generally speaking, in the oxygenated neutral aqueous solution, gossypol exhibits a marked decrease in absorbance at uv λ_{max}
of 238 and 370 nm and a concomittant increase in absorbance at λ_{max}
of 315 nm. In the absence of oxygen, no apparent changes in uv
spectra of gossypol were observed with time. Similarly, by thin-
layer chromatography, one can show the appearance of three additional uv-positive spots on thin-layer plates with Rf values of 0.1,
0.2, and 0.65, respectively, upon incubation in oxygenated phosphate buffer at pH 7.0 and 96 h. It was noted that the Rf values
of these three uv-positive spots are not identical to those observed
for gossypol in absolute ethanol. This indicates the difference in
pathways of decomposition between that in ethanol and in aqueous

solution, gossypol remains stable without apparent decomposition. On the other hand, light may not be an important factor that catalyzes the decomposition of gossypol in solution.

REFERENCES

1. C. Y. Lee and H. V. Malling, Selective inhibition of lactate dehydrogenase-X by a male antifertility agent-gossypol, Fed. Proc., 40:2790 (1981).
2. C. Y. Lee, Y. S. Moon, J. H. Yuan, and A. F. Chen, Enzyme inactibation and inhibition by gossypol, Mol. Cell. Biochem., Vol. 47, pp. 65-70 (1982).
3. E. Goldberg, Isozymes in testes and spermatozoa, in: "Isozymes: Current Topics in Biological and Medical Research" (M. C. Rattazzi, J. G. Scandalios, and G. Whitt, eds.), Vol. 1, p. 79, Alan R. Liss, Inc., New York (1977).
4. C.Y. Lee and H. V. Malling, 1981, op. cit. (see Ref. 1).
5. Ibid.
6. C. Y. Lee, et al., 1982, op. cit. (see Ref. 2).
7. E. Goldberg, 1977, op. cit. (see Ref. 3).
8. C. Y. Lee, et al., 1982, op. cit. (see Ref. 2).
9. H. Pöso, K. Wichmann, J. Jänne, and T. Luukkainen, Gossypol, a powerful inhibitor of human spermatozoal metabolism, Lancet 1:885 (1980).
10. M. B. Abou-Donia, Physiological effect and metabolism of gossypol, Residual Reviews, Vol. 61, p. 126, Springer-Verlag, New York (1976).

DEACTIVATION OF SPERMATOZOAL FERTILIZING

CAPABILITY BY GOSSYPOL

Wung-Wai Tso

Department of Biochemistry
The Chinese University of Hong Kong
Shatin, N.T., Hong Kong

INTRODUCTION

Although the toxicology of gossypol has been studied extensively in countries where cottonseed was used as a source of dietary protein for the livestock industry, a renewed interest in this compound was prompted by the recent Chinese discovery of its remarkably anti-fertility effect on males of a variety of mammalian species including humans [1, 2, 3, 4]. Studies have shown that the compound causes a reduction of epididymal spermatozoal motility and a gradual suppression of spermatogenesis [5, 6]. While the relationship of these two effects is not understood, the suppression of spermatogenesis appears to be reversible in most cases. The male gonad is not the main depot of gossypol, and its antifertility action does not stem from its effect on the endocrine system [7, 8, 9, 10]. Many animal studies have focused on adverse gossypol effects on spermatozoal morphology and enzyme activities [11, 12]. The results of most of these studies, though insufficient to establish the precise mechanism of gossypol's antifertility effect, have sketched a simple picture suggesting that an interruption of energy metabolicm might be a vital part of its mode of action.

Our group has demonstrated that the forward progress motility of boar ejaculated spermatozoa can be effectively reduced by gossypol in vitro at a threshold concentration of 10^{-5} M [13]. As sperm immobilization is one aspect of gossypol's action in antifertility treatment, this paper summarizes our present understanding of its effect on mature spermatozoa.

TABLE 1.   Changes of Rat Spermatozoal Motility and ATP Content by Gossypol[a]

Number of weeks forced-fed gossypol	Number of weeks after gossypol cessation	Motility[b] %	ATP content (fg/sperm)[c,d]	ATP %
0		100	52.95 ± 14.06 (6)[e]	100
1		100	53.78 ± 7.79 (3)	102
2		91	53.19 ± 16.24 (4)	100
3		60	36.00 ± 17.50 (5)	67
4		0	5.32 ± 1.70 (4)	10
	1	0	4.89 ± 2.27 (5)	9
	2	10	5.85 ± 3.09 (5)	11
	3	10	10.12 ± 2.51 (5)	21
	4	33	29.62 ± 10.90 (3)	56
	6	94	46.74 ± 3.92 (4)	94

[a]Adapted from Y.-B. Ye and W.-W. Tso, see Reference 16.
[b]Motility was expressed in motility index.
[c]1 femtogram = 10^{-15} g.
[d]Spermatozoa were collected from caudal epididymis.
[e]The number of rats tested is indicated in parenthesis.

Insufficient Energy to Support Spermatozogenesis

Adenosine triphosphate is required both for spermatogenesis and sperm motility. Based on some early enzyme inhibition studies, it has been suggested that lactate dehydrogenase-X (LDH-X), a gonad-specific enzyme, is the target of gossypol action [14]. As a consequence of such inhibition, the process of spermatogenesis is impeded due to a lack of ATP support. Indeed, with boar semen, we have demonstrated that the LDH-X was particularly sensitive to gossypol inhibition [15]. In order to clarify the relationship between the antifertility effect and energy economy, we have tested both the motility and the ATP content of spermatozoa collected from the caudal epididymal region of rats treated with gossypol for different periods of time according to the established method for inducing infertility [16]. After two weeks of gossypol treatment, the rats began to show a proportional decrease in spermatozoal ATP content and motility (Table 1). Recovering from gossypol-induced ATP decrease also developed at two weeks following the cessation of gossypol administration. The results document a close relationship between spermatozoal motility and its intrinsic ATP content.

The delay in the gossypol antifertility action might have stemmed from the time required either for the specific inhibition to develop along with spermatogenesis or for the sufficient accumulation of gossypol in situ to cause an effect. Since the developmental process of spermatogenesis depends heavily on a continuous supply of energy, it should be severely damaged when energy is lacking.

As described in the introduction, gossypol's antifertility action consists of immobilization of sperm motility and suppression of spermatogenesis. It is quite likely that a deterioration in the cell's energy economy might be a common denominator of both phenomena. It is unclear, however, whether the sperm immobilization is due to a simple depletion of available energy or a group of deactivation reactions including energy depletion. Recently, it has been shown that the introduction of gossypol into the rat epididymal fat pad inhibited epididymal sperm motility within 24 h of administration [17]. This addresses the problem of the nature of the susceptibility of intact mature spermatozoa to gossypol inhibition.

Gossypol's Uncoupling Effects

In addition to its instability in air when dissolved in alkaline solution, gossypol readily reacts with many proteinous molecules because of its reactive aldehyde group [18, 19]. Biochemically, gossypol has been shown to be an uncoupler of oxidative phosphorylation and the electron transport system in rat liver mitochondria [20]. This uncoupling property transcends animal and tissue origin [21]. In boar ejaculated spermatozoa, the addition

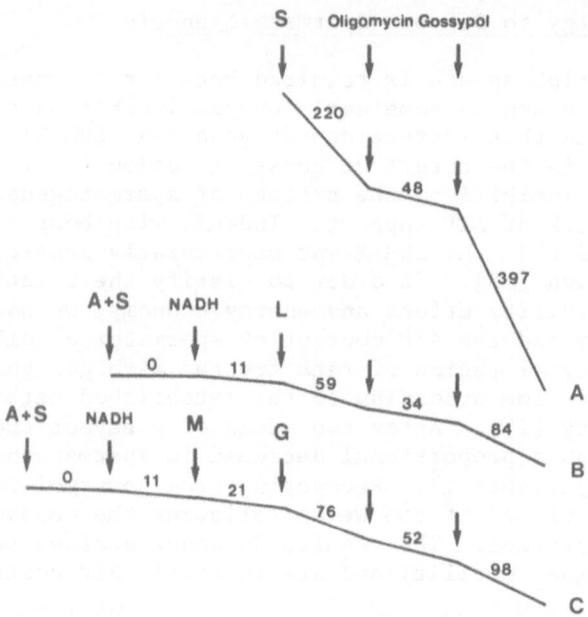

Fig. 1. Effect of gossypol on spermatozoal respiration in the
presence of oligomycin. The values against the slope represent the rate of respiration in nmole O_2/hr/10^8 sperms.
a) Unwashed spermatozoa were diluted with isotonic Tris-HCl
buffer, pH 7.0, containing 10% (v/v) seminal plasma.
Spermatozoa (S), oligomycin, and gossypol, each to a final
concentration of 80 × 10^6 cell/ml, 1 µg/ml, and 3.2 × 10^{-}
M, correspondingly, were added in the designated sequence.
b and c) Hypotonically-treated spermatozoa, 180 × 10^6
sperm.ml, were used. Assay conditions were identical to
that described in a except lactate (L), 1 mM; malate (M),
1 mM; glutamate (G), 5 mM and arsenite (A), 2 mM were added
accordingly. [Adapted from W.-W. Tso and C.-S. Lee, 1982,
op. cit. (see Ref. 22).]

of gossypol relieved the oligomycin-inhibited respiration in both
the unwashed sample and hypotonically-treated ones (Fig. 1). This
uncoupling effect, when taken together with that specific inhibition on the electron transport chain itself, particularly on the
succinate to cytochrome C segment, will create a very rapid depletion of spermatozoal intrinsic ATP [22, 23]. The mechanism of the
gossypol uncoupling action is unknown. As a polyphenolic compound,
gossypol is structurally similar to the classical uncoupler 2,4-
dinitrophenol and may act similarly.

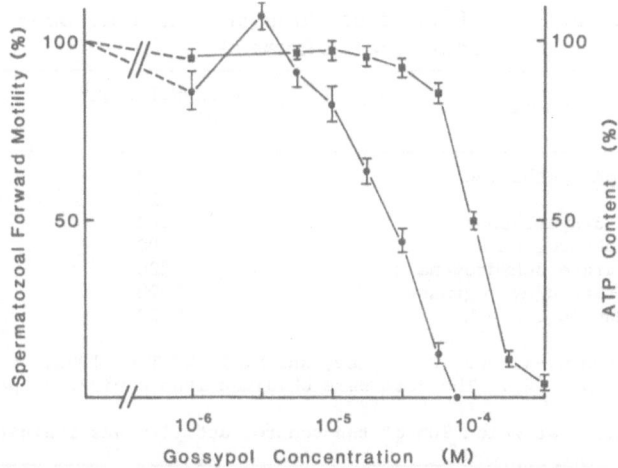

Fig. 2. Effect of gossypol on the spermatozoal forward motility
and spermatozoal ATP content. The effect of gossypol on
the spermatozoal forward motility was assayed by a photographic method [39]. The motility assay medium contained
seminal plasma, 10% (v/v) and the modified Krebs-bicarbon-
ate solution. Unwashed spermatozoa at a final concentration of 1.5×10^6 sperm ml was used. The measured motility
represents an average motility of the motile spermatozoa
(●). At the 5 sec exposure period, usually about 20% of
the spermatozoal population was caught in motion. Each
value at one concentration denotes as an average ± s.d.
For ATP assay, unwashed spermatozoa were suspended in pH
7.4 Krebs-Ringer phosphate solution, supplemented with 10%
(v/v) seminal plasma and 2 mg/ml glucose. The ATP contents
were assayed at 15 min correspondingly after the addition
of gossypol (■). The assay temperature for both experiments was 25°C. [Adapted from W.-W. Tso and C.-S. Lee,
1981, op. cit. (see Ref. 13) and W.-W. Tso, C.-S. Lee,
and M.-Y. W. Tso, 1982, op. cit. (see Ref. 38).]

Energy Depletion and Sperm Immobilization

Our previous studies have established a close relationship between sperm motility and its energy economy. The results reported
by other investigators with spermatozoa collected from various animals have also confirmed this [24, 25, 26]. In spite of the general agreement among investigators that gossypol at a low concentration brings about sperm immobilization, and that this immobilization appeared concomitantly with a depletion of the energy pool,
the main cause of energy depletion has never been clarified. As
noted, uncoupling effect is one of the causes [28]. The inhibition

TABLE 2. The Effect of Gossypol on Some Boar
          Spermatozoal Enzymes[a]

Enzyme	Gossypol IC_{20}[b] (μM)
Succinyl-CoA synthetase	20
Aconitase	20
NAD-malate dehydrogenase	100
Succinyl dehydrogenase	200
α-Ketoglutarate dehydrogenase	200
NAD-isocitrate dehydrogenase	20
Lactate dehydrogenase-X	20

[a]Adapted from W.-W. Tso, C. S. Lee, and M.-T. W. Tso, 1982, op. cit.
   (see Reference 46). The data were obtained from sonicated spermatozoa.
[b]Concentration at which 20% of the control activity was inhibited.

of the electron transport chain is another [29, 30]. And there are
further activity [31, 32, 33, 34, 35]. At the same time, the inhibition of ATPase as a factor in depleting the cell's energy has
also been investigated [36, 37, 38, 39, 40, 41, 42]. Although several investigators accepted the significance of the inhibition of
ATPase in the immobilization phenomenon, other results showed that
gossypol had no effect on renal ATPase or that the effect was slight
at a gossypol concentration that has already exhibited motility
arrest [43, 44]. Moreover, a general inhibitory effect of gossypol
on many enzymes has also been reported [45, 46, 47]. In the list
of enzymes studied, some enzymes are less reactive and some even
inert to gossypol interaction [48]. But of those reactive enzymes,
many are involved in energy generating steps. It is noteworthy to
point out that at a high concentration, at about 10^{-4} M, gossypol
essentially reduces the activities of many enzymes and cellular functions. This emphasizes the importance of having the quantity of
gossypol carefully monitored when it is taken orally. Because of
the wide spectrum of enzymes affected by gossypol, it is plausible
that one of these inhibitions is not responsible for the depletion
of spermatozoal intrinsic ATP, but a combination of many, if not
all, gives rise to the energy reduction. It is natural that the
energy depletion will result in sperm immobilization. An in vitro
study of the spermatozoal motility with respect to its cellular ATP
content (see Fig. 2), however, that the immobilization phenomenon
is by far more sensitive to gossypol inhibition than it is to the
reduction of ATP content. This suggests that apart from ATP depletion, other factors may be involved in sperm immobilization.
Whether the possibility that gossypol interferes with the incorpora-
tion of the sperm forward motility protein onto the maturing sperm
or that a component in the motile machinery has been impaired, cannot be eliminated [49, 50]. This remains to be elucidated.

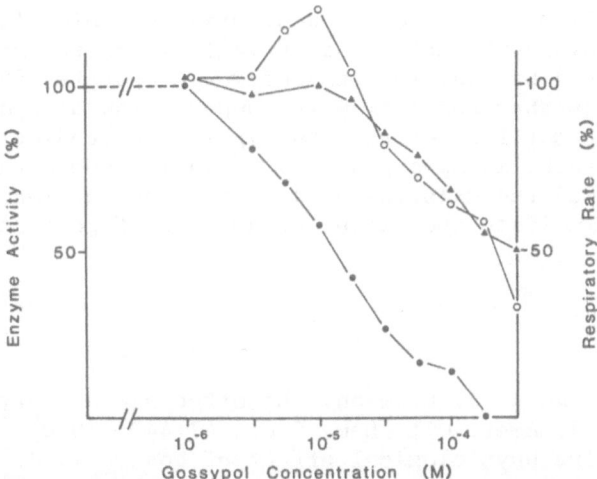

Fig. 3.   Effect of gossypol on spermatozoal enzyme activities and
hypotonically-treated spermatozoal respiration. LDH-X
activity was obtained with α-ketovalerate as substrate (▲).
A 100% activity is equal to 28.5 nmole/min/10^8 sperms.
Boar spermatozoal head proacrosin was fully activated at
0°C for 30 min. Acrosin activity was assayed at 25°C employing p-toluenesulfonylarginine methyl ester (TAME) as
artificial substrate (●). One hundred percent activity is
7.7 μmole TAME hydrolyzed/min/10^8 sperms. For respiration
studies, hypotonically-treated spermatozoa were employed.
Sodium succinate at 10 μM was used as substrate. The control respiratory rate was 100.7 nmole O_2/hr/10^8 sperms (○).
[Adapted from W.-W. Tso and C.-S. Lee, 1982, op. cit. (see
Ref. 15), W.-W. Tso and C.-S. Lee, 1982, op. cit. (see Ref.
51), and W.-W. Tso and C.-S. Lee, 1981, op. cit. (see Ref.
23).]

Acrosin is Highly Susceptible to Gossypol Inhibition

In many mammalian systems, the male gametes have to travel a
long distance to meet the female one and the fertilization process
can only be achieved after a successive completion of a train of
biochemical events starting with a hydrolytic step that requires a
proper functioning of the spermatozoal acrosin activity. We have
compared the gossypol effect on this enzyme activity with respect to
that on the respiration process and that on the LDH-X activity (Fig.
3). Acrosin is about 10- to 30-fold more sensitive. This finding
has led to the suggestion that gossyol or even cottonseed oil be
used as an active ingredient in the manufacture of vaginal contraceptives [51, 52, 53]. The inhibitory effect of gossypol on acrosin

activity was confirmed by a modified autoradiographic plate method
[54]. Its possible applicability as a vaginal contraceptive has
also been suggested by many independent investigators [55, 56]. It
thus seems obvious that apart from its suppression of spermatogenesis and its antimotility effect, gossypol is exceedingly specific
in reducing the fertilizing capability of motile spermatozoa. This
report has analyzed the existing data on gossypol action on mature
spermatozoa to elucidate the different aspects of gossypol inhibition.

REFERENCES

1. F. H. Smith and A. J. Clawson, The effects of dietary gossypol
   on animals, J. Amer. Oil Chem. Soc., 47:443 (1970).
2. P. Menaul, The physiological effect of gossypol, J. Agr. Res.,
   26:233 (1923).
3. E. W. Schwartze, Pharmacology of gossypol, J. Agr. Res., 28:
   191 (1924).
4. B. S. Liu, Suggestions of feeding crude cottonseed oil for
   contraception, Shanghai Acad. Med., 6:43 (1957).
5. National Coordinating Group on Male Antifertility Agents,
   Gossypol - A new antifertility agent for males, Chin. Med. J.
   (Engl. Edn.), 6:417 (1978).
6. R. X. Dai, S. N. Pang, X. K. Lin, Y. B. Ke, Z. L. Lui, and
   R. H. Dong, A study of antifertility of cottonseed, Acta Biol.
   Exp. Sinica, 11:1 (1978).
7. Y. B. Ke, X. K. Lin, X. Y. Lin, Y. H. Chang, Y. Z. Mar, S. E.
   Yu, and Y. Din, Studies on the antifertility effect of gossypol,
   III. The determination of the quantities of gossypol in blood
   and related internal organs after administration of the drug
   in rats, Acta Biol. Exp. Sinica, 12:69 (1979).
8. N. Wang, G. Li, Q. Chen, and H. Lei, The metabolism of gossypol
   in vivo, Zhonghua Yixue Zashi (Natl. Med. J. of China), 59:
   596 (1979).
9. C. C. Chang, Z. Gu, and Y. Y. Tsong, Studies on gossypol. I.
   Toxicity, antifertility and endocrine analyses in male rats,
   Int. J. Fertil., 27:213 (1982).
10. D. W. Halm, C. Rusticus, A. Probst, R. Homm, and A. N. Johnson,
    Antifertility and endocrine activities of gossypol in rodents,
    Contraception, 24:97 (1981).
11. A. P. Hoffer, Ultrastructural studies of spermatozoa and the
    epithelial lining of the epididymus and vas deferens in rats
    treated with gossypol, Arch. Androl., 8:233 (1982).
12. S. Su, Y. Liu, Z. Zhou, S.-P. Shieh, X. Zhao, M. Xu, and Y.
    Zhuang, Studies of the relationship between the gossypol ad-
    ministration and the activity of Na-Ka-ATPase in animals,
    Acta Anat. Sinica, 13:85 (1982).
13. W.-W. Tso and C.-S. Lee, Effect of gossypol on boar sperma-
    tozoa in vitro, Arch. Androl., 7:85 (1981).

14. C. Y. Lee and H. V. Malling, Selective inhibition of sperm-
     specific lactate dehydrogenase-X by an antifertility agent,
     gossypol, Fed. Proc., 40:718 (1981).
15. W.-W. Tso and C.-S. Lee, Lactate dehydrogenase-X: an isozyme
     particularly sensitive to gossypol inhibition, J. Androl., 5:
     205 (1982).
16. Y. B. Ye and W.-W. Tso, Variations of gossypol susceptibility
     in rat spermatozoa during spermatogenesis, Int. J. Fert., 27:
     42 (1982).
17. M. A. Hadley and M. H. Burgos, Inhibition of rat epididymal
     sperm motility by gossypol, Proceedings of the fifth NIH spon-
     sored testis workshop, Abstract, pp. 458-9 (1981).
18. C. Y. Lee, Y. S. Moon, A. Duleba, and A. F. Chan, The instabil-
     ity of gossypol, Arch. Androl, 9:33 (1982).
19. B. P. Baliga and C. M. Lyman, The nutritional significance of
     bound gossypol in cottonseed meal, J. Amer. Oil Chemists' Soc.,
     34:21 (1957).
20. M. B. Abou-Donia and J. W. Dieckert, Gossypol: uncoupling of
     respiratory chain and oxidative phosphorylation, Life Sci., 14:
     1955 (1962).
21. B. D. Myers and G. O. Throneberry, Effect of gossypol on some
     oxidative respiratory enzymes, Plant Physiol., 47:787 (1966).
22. W.-W. Tso and C.-S. Lee, Gossypol uncoupling of respiratory
     chain and oxidative phosphorylation in ejaculated boar sperma-
     tozoa, Contraception, 25:649 (1982).
23. W.-W. Tso and C.-S. Lee, Variations of gossypol sensitivity in
     boar spermatozoal electron transport chain segments, Contra-
     ception, 24:569 (1981).
24. M. Burgos, J. L. Fridovich, G. Weissman, and S. J. Segal,
     Delivery of gossypol by liposomes: inhibition of sperm mo-
     tility, Biol. Bull., 161:334 (1981).
25. N. R. Kalla and M. Vasuder, Studies on the male antifertility
     agent-gossypol acetic acid II. Effect of gossypol acetic acid
     on the motility and the ATPase activity of human spermatozoa,
     Andrologia, 13:95 (1981).
26. R. Oko and F. Hrudka, Effect of gossypol on spermatozoa, Arch.
     Androl., 9:39 (1982).
27. K. Wichmann, K. Kapyacho, R. Sinervirta, and J. Janne, Effect
     of gossypol on the motility and metabolism of human spermatozoa,
     J. Re. Fert., 69:259 (1983).
28. W.-W. Tso and C.-S. Lee, 1982, op. cit. (see Ref. 22).
29. W.-W. Tso and C.-S. Lee, 1981, op. cit. (see Ref. 23).
30. N. R. Kalla and J. F. T. Wei, Effect of gossypol acetic acid
     on respiratory enzymes in vitro, IRCS Med. Sci., 9:792 (1981).
31. C. Y. Lee and H. V. Malling, 1981, op. cit. (see Ref. 14).
32. W.-W. Tso and C.-S. Lee, 1982, op. cit. (see Ref. 15).
33. N. Giridharan, M. S. Bamji, and A. V. B. Sankaram, Inhibition
     of rat testis LDH-X activity of gossypol, Contraception, 26:
     607 (1982).

34. R. Eliasson and N. Virji, Effects of gossypol acetic acid on
     the activity of LDH-C₄ from human and rabbit spermatozoa, Int.
     J. Androl., 6:109 (1983).
35. K. L. Olgiati and W. A. Toscano, Kinetics of gossypol inhibi-
     tion of bovine lactate dehydrogenase X, Biochem. Biophys. Res.,
     Commun., 115:180 (1983).
36. S. Su, Y. Liu, Z. Zhou, S.-P. Shieh, X. Zhao, M. Xu, and Y.
     Zhuang, 1982, op. cit. (see Ref. 12).
37. N. R. Kalla and M. Vasuder, 1981, op. cit. (see Ref. 25).
38. W.-W. Tso, C.-S. Lee, and M.-Y. W. Tso, Effect of gossypol on
     boar spermatozoal adneosine triphosphate metabolism, Arch.
     Androl., 9:319 (1982).
39. X. Bi, Y. Zheng, H. Yang, and Z. Zhang, The effect of gossypol
     on ATPase activity of the kidney, Sci. Sin., 24:573 (1981).
40. Y. Fai, D. Liang, Y. Gou, Y. Liu, X. Gor, C. Chow, and S.-P.
     Xue, Gossypol effect on the activity of renal cell membrane
     Na-Ka-ATPase of rats and guinea pigs, Reprod. and Contracept.,
     2:42 (1982).
41. O. Adeyemo, C. Y. Chang, S. J. Segal, and S. S. Koide, Gossypol
     action on the production and utilization of ATP in sea urchin
     spermatozoa, Arch. Androl., 9:343 (1982).
42. H. Mohri, K. Matsuda, S. S. Koide, and S. J. Segal, Effect of
     gossypol on Arbacia sperm ATPase, Biol. Bull., 163:374 (1982).
43. S. Su, Y. Liu, Z. Zhou, S.-P. Shieh, X. Zhao, M. Xu, and Y.
     Zhuang, 1982, op. cit. (see Ref. 12).
44. W.-W. Tso, C.-S. Lee, and M.-Y. W. Tso, 1982, op. cit. (see
     Ref. 32).
45. N. R. Kalla and J. F. T. Wei, 1981, op. cit. (see Ref. 28).
46. W.-W. Tso, C.-S. Lee, and M.-Y. W. Tso, Sensitivity of various
     spermatozoal enzymes to gossypol inhibition, Contraceptive
     Delivery Syst., 3:280 (1982).
47. E. E. Montamat, C. Burgos, N. M. G. Burgos, L. E. Bovai, and
     A. Blanco, Inhibition action of gossypol on enzymes and growth
     of trypanosoma cruzi, Sci., 218:288 (1982).
48. W.-W. Tso, C.-S. Lee, and M.-Y. W. Tso, 1982, op. cit. (see
     Ref. 46).
49. T. S. Acott and D. D. Hoskins, Bovine sperm forward motility
     protein, J. Biol. Chem., 253:6774 (1978).
50. W.-W. Tso and W.-M. Lee, Seminal plasma and progressive mo-
     tility of boar spermatozoa, Int. J. Androl., 3:243 (1980).
51. W.-W. Tso and C.-S. Lee, Gossypol: an effective acrosin
     blocker, Arch. Androl., 8:143 (1982).
52. W.-W. Tso and C.-S. Lee, Cottonseed oil as a vaginal contra-
     ceptive, Arch. Androl., 8:11 (1982).
53. W.-W. Tso and C.-S. Lee, Cottonseed - a source of vaginal con-
     traceptive, Contraception Fertilite Sexualite, 10:465 (1982).
54. O. Johnsen, J. M. Diaz, and R. Eliasson, Gossypol: a potent
     inhibitor of human sperm acrosomal proteinase, Int. J. Androl.,
     5:636 (1982).

55. L. W. William, New antifertility agents active in the rabbit
     vaginal contraception method, Contraception, 22:659 (1980).
56. D. P. Waller, L. J. D. Zaneveld, and H. H. S. Fong, In vitro
     spermicidal activity of gossypol, Contraception, 22:183 (1980).
57. D. P. Waller, H. H. S. Fong, G. A. Cordell, and D. D. Soejarto,
     Antifertility effects of gossypol and its impurities on male
     hamsters, Contraception, 23:653 (1981).

UPTAKE OF ^{14}C-GOSSYPOL BY MURINE ERYTHROLEUKEMIA CELLS:
A MODEL OF UNMEDIATED DIFFUSION FOR GOSSYPOL UPTAKE
BY A NONTESTICULAR CELL

Robert E. Corin, Howard C. Haspel,
Andrew Peretz, Yun-Feng Ren,
Kyoichi A. Watanabe, and Martin Sonenberg

Laboratories of Membrane Regulation
and Organic Chemistry
Memorial Sloan-Kettering Cancer Center and the
Cornell University
Graduate School of Medical Sciences
New York, N. Y., U.S.A.

INTRODUCTION

Gossypol (G) has been shown to be a highly efficacious oral
male contraceptive [1, 2, 3]. G has potential for wide use as a
contraceptive agent. Additionally, the study of G may provide a
useful model for the development of new male oral contraceptives.
The mechanism of contraceptive action and the pharmocokinetics of
G are not well defined. At therapeutic (contraceptive) doses G is
relatively non-toxic [2, 3]. Acutely toxic doses of G, in vivo, are
∿1000 fold greater than contraceptive doses of the drug [4, 5].
Thus, the in vivo pharmacology of G may be viewed as having two important facets. One involves the basis for selective toxicity to
testicular tissues, i.e., what is the nature of the uptake system
or target for drug action that accounts for testicular sensitivity
to G? A second consideration is that contraceptive doses of G are
not acutely toxic to most body tissues. We have approached the
latter issues by studying the toxicity of G, in vitro, to an established cell line. Murine erythroleukemia cells (MELC) were chosen
since they provide an easily handled model for non-testicular cells.
Our preliminary studies [6] demonstrated the following: i) G is
toxic and is irreversibly cytocidal to MELC after 24 h of exposure
to G (30 μM). ii) G toxicity to MELC depends on the fetal calf
serum (FCS) concentration of the growth medium, e.g., 5 μM G is not
toxic when serum is 10% (v/v) but is toxic when the serum concentration of the medium is reduced to 5%. iii) FCS as well as bovine

257

serum albumin (BSA) potently blocked the steady state uptake of
[14]C-G by MELC and direct and indirect experiments demonstrated high
affinity binding (K_D < 1 μM) of G to BSA and FCS. iv) ^{14}C-G uptake
by MELC is saturable with a K_m of ~8 μM. High affinity binding of
G to human serum albumin has been demonstrated by [7]. Based upon
these data we speculate that contraceptive doses of G are not
acutely toxic in vivo due to the binding of G to plasma proteins,
where protein bound G is not toxic. In the present study we further
characterized ^{14}C-G uptake by MELC. Based upon our results we pro-
pose an unmediated diffusion mechanism for G uptake by non-testicular cells.

EXPERIMENTAL PROCEDURES

MELC strain DS-19 was employed. The origin, culture, counting,
harvesting, and other procedures associated with handling these
cells have been described [8, 9, 10], assay of ^{14}C-G uptake was previously described [10]. G and ^{14}C-G were obtained or prepared, analyzed for purity, and handled as we previously described [10]. All
other reagents were obtained as previously described [10].

RESULTS

We previously demonstrated that BSA potently blocked the apparent steady state level of ^{14}C-G uptake by MELC with an IC_{50} of
~0.03% [10]. In protein-free medium, ^{14}C-G uptake achieves an apparent steady state within one minute (Fig. 1). In the presence
of 0.1% (w/v) BSA, ^{14}C-G uptake reaches apparent steady state between 10 and 20 min of incubation (Fig. 1). The steady state level
of ^{14}C-G uptake in protein-free medium was decreased by reducing
the initial extracellular concentration of ^{14}C-G but apparent steady
state uptake was still achieved within one minute (not shown). Thus,
BSA not only reduces the level of ^{14}C-G uptake, but it also affects
the kinetics of uptake (Fig. 1).

Efflux of ^{14}C-G from MELC was examined as follows. Cells in
protein-free medium were allowed to accumulate ^{14}C-G (6.43 μM) to
apparent steady state (5 min, 24°C), and uptake was determined (this
was considered the zero time point for efflux). Cells were centrifuged, the supernatant medium aspirated, and the cell pellet resuspended in ^{14}C-G free medium at 24°C with or without 2% (w/v) BSA
(Fig. 2). In the absence of BSA there was little loss of ^{14}C-G
from cells (~10% after 1 h, Fig. 2). In the presence of BSA there
was a time-dependent efflux of ^{14}C-G from the cells (Fig. 2). Ki-
netically, this efflux did not occur via a simple one compartment
process (not shown).

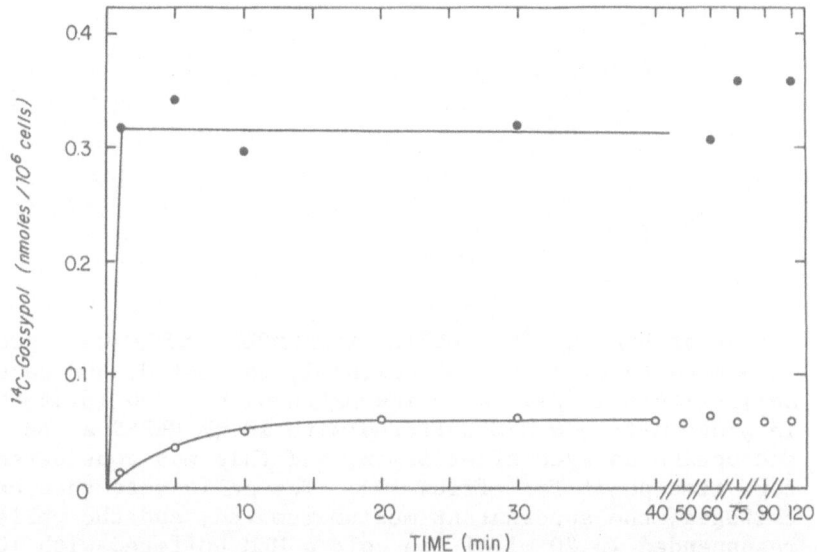

Fig. 1. Effect of BSA on ^{14}C-G uptake by MELC. MELC were grown to a density of 9.2×10^5 cells/ml, harvested, and washed as previously described [10]. Washed cells were resuspended in α MEM buffered with 10 mM HEPES at pH 7.4 with (○) or without (●) 0.1% (w/v) BSA at a final density of 7.9×10^6 cells/ml. Uptake was performed at 24°C and initiated by the addition of cells to the appropriate medium containing ^{14}C-G (6.34 μM).

^{14}C-G uptake was studied to ascertain if the process would behave as expected for a transporter or protein receptor. This reasoning followed from the observation that ^{14}C-G uptake by MELC was a saturable high affinity process [10].

Uptake of ^{14}C-G (6.34 μM₀ at 24°C exhibited a sharp pH optimum between pH 7-7.5 (Fig. 3). Since this is the range of the pka for G, ∿pH 7.2 [11], it might be suggested that the pH optimum for G uptake reflects ionization of G and/or a membrane component.

If a plasma membrane transporter were involved in ^{14}C-G uptake, then a temperature dependence might be expected. When the uptake temperature, in protein-free medium, was reduced from 24° to 4°C, uptake achieved a similar steady state (Fig. 4). Steady state was achieved within one minute at both 4° and 24°C (not shown).

G is probably a substrate for the organic anion transporter of the rabbit kidney [12, S. Hong personal communication]. We previously demonstrated that uptake of the organic anion methotrexate

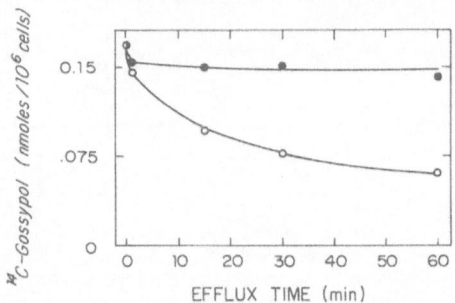

Fig. 2. Effect of BSA on ^{14}C-G efflux from MELC. MELC were grown
         to a density of 1.5×10^6 cells/ml, harvested, and washed.
         Cells (1.4×10^7/ml) were incubated with ^{14}C-G (6.34 µM)
         in protein-free α MEM buffered with 10 mM HEPES at pH 7.4
         and uptake assayed after 5 min, and this was considered the
         zero time point for efflux (◑). The cells were then cen-
         trifuged, the supernatant medium removed, and the pellet
         resuspended in 20 ml of ice cold α MEM buffered with 10
         mM HEPES at pH 7.4, divided into two tubes, centrifuged,
         the supernatant medium aspirated, and efflux initiated by
         addition of 5 ml of α MEM buffered with 10 mM HEPES at pH
         7.4 with (○) or without (●) 2% (w/v) BSA at 24°C. Cell
         associated ^{14}C-G was determined at the indicated times.

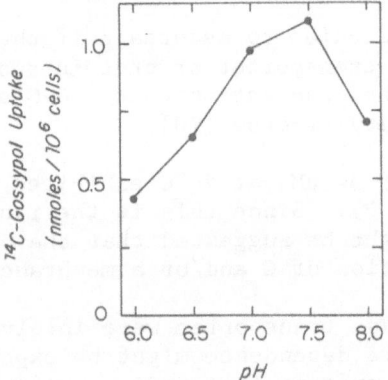

Fig. 3. Effect of pH on ^{14}C-G uptake by MELC. MELC were grown to
         1×10^6/ml, harvested, washed, and resuspended in α MEM
         adjusted to the indicated pH with 10 mM HEPES. Uptake of
         ^{14}C-G (6.34 µM) was assayed after incubation for 10 min
         at 24°C.

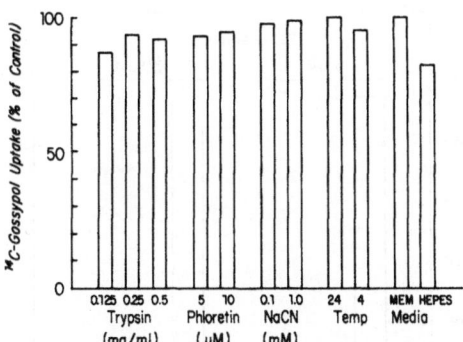

Fig. 4.   Effects of membrane active treatments on ^{14}C-G uptake by
          MELC. Cells were grown to densities of $\sim$10[6] cells/ml,
          harvested, and washed. Cells ($\sim$10[7]/ml) were treated in
          protein-free α MEM, buffered with 10 mM HEPES at pH 7.4,
          for 30 min with the indicated treatments. ^{14}C-G (6.34 μM)
          was then added and uptake assayed after 10 min at 24°C.
          Uptake is expressed as percent of control (no treatment)
          where 100% is equal to $\sim$l nmoles ^{14}C-G per 10[6] cells.

by MELC is affected by the anion composition of the medium [9].
Both anion content and composition were altered for ^{14}C-G uptake by
MELC. The control medium was α MEM buffered with 10 mM HEPES to
pH 7.4. The anions in this medium are primarily inorganic and
permeant, e.g., Cl. The experimental medium was composed of 160 mM
HEPES (an impermeant organic anion) buffered to pH 7.4. Uptake was
assayed in protein-free medium (α MEM) or in 160 mM HEPES (pH 7.4).
There was only $\sim$20% difference in the level of steady state uptake
in these media (Fig. 4). Apparent steady state was achieved within
one minute in both media (not shown). Thus only a small portion,
if any, of ^{14}C-G uptake was dependent upon extracelular anion composition of the medium.

     Plasma membrane transport and receptor proteins are often
trypsin-sensitive. MELC were treated for 30 min at 37°C with 125,
250, or 500 μg/ml of trypsin. Steady state uptake of ^{14}C-G (6.5
μM) was then determined in protein-free medium (Fig. 4). Uptake
was maximally reduced by $\sim$10% (Fig. 4). Thus, most ^{14}C-G uptake
was not through a trypsin sensitive process. A similar result was
obtained when cells were pretreated with the membrane active agent
phloretin at 5 or 10 μM (Fig. 4). When cells were pretreated with
0.1 or 1.0 mM NaCN, there was no appreciable effect on ^{14}C-G uptake
(Fig. 4). These concentrations of NaCN completely inhibited O_2
consumption by MELC (not shown) and presumably ATP synthesis. Thus
[14]C-G uptake does not appear to be coupled with an energy generating
system.

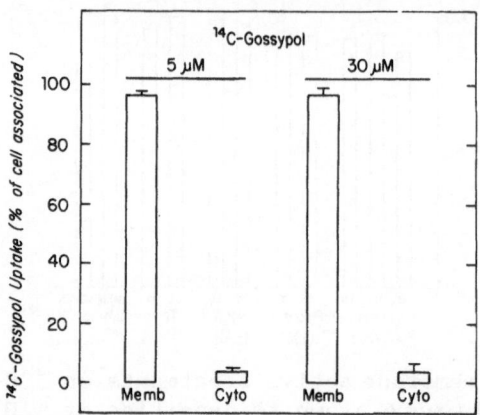

Fig. 5. Crude subcellular localization of ^{14}C-G associated with
          MELC. MELC were grown to density of 1.5×10^6 cells/ml,
          harvested, and washed. Cells ($\sim 8 \times 10^6$ cell/ml) were ex-
          posed to ^{14}C-G, as indicated in α MEM for 10 min. The
          suspension was chilled to 4°C and centrifuged at 500 × g
          for 10 min. The cells were washed once with ice cold
          α MEM. The pellets were lysed by 3 cycles of freezing at
          -70°C and thawing at 37•C and centrifuged at 40,000 × g
          for 1 h. The entire supernatant and the entire pellet were
          dissolved in 10% (w/v) sodium dodecylsulfate by heating at
          100°C for 10 min. These two suspensions were counted for
          radioactivity and percent of cell associated radioactivity
          calculated as the quotient of the radioactivity in the
          pellet or supernatant divided by the sum of the radioac-
          tivity of both.

    We wished to determine how ^{14}C-G distributed between the par-
ticulate and soluble fractions of the cell. MELC were incubated
with ^{14}C-G (5 or 30 μM, a subsaturating and saturating dose, respectively) for 10 min at 24°C. The cells were then chilled to 4°C,
centrifuged, and the pellets washed once with cold buffer. Cells
were then lysed by 3 cycles of freezing and thawing, and centrifuged (40,000 × g, 1 h) and the radioactivity determined in supernatant (cytosol) or pellet (particular) fractions. At both concentrations of ^{14}C-G, $\sim 95\%$ of the recovered radioactivity was in
the particulate fraction (Fig. 5).

DISCUSSION

    The results presented help define the nature of the inter-
action of ^{14}C-G with MELC, i.e., a model for non-testicular
cells. The data in Fig. 1 demonstrate that medium BSA affects the

kinetics of ^{14}C-G uptake as well as the apparent steady state level
of uptake. We previously demonstrated a direct interaction of G
with BSA [10]. One possible explanation for the slowed kinetics of
G uptake is as follows. Both cells and BSA compete for free G.
Under the conditions of this experiment, the cells may represent a
larger sink for G than BSA, i.e., because of the relative concentration of each (see Fig. 1 legend). As free G is depleted, G dis-
sociates from G-BSA complexes, and the cells take up the newly gen-
erated free G. Such dynamics might be of physiological significance
in the circulation since both blood cells and serum albumin [13] are
present at relatively high concentrations.

The data in Fig. 2 demonstrate that BSA also affects the kinetics with which cell-associated G is released from cells. In the
absence of BSA very little G is released (∿10% in 60 min). In the
presence of BSA, approximately 60% of ^{14}C-G is released from cells
after 60 min (Fig. 2). Thus, the ability of cells to retain G is
affected by extracellular BSA. A possible explanation is that BSA
binds G more tightly than cells and shifts the equilibrium from
cell-bound to BSA-bound G. The disposition of cell-bound G that
does not efflux after 60 min (Fig. 2) is currently unknown. A possible explanation is that it has been sequestered in an intracellular target which binds G with a higher affinity than the plasma membrane. An alternate explanation is that more medium BSA is required
for more efflux. Whatever the mechanistic explanations for the data
presented in Figs. 1 and 2, the results indicate that serum albumin
may play a role in G uptake and release by blood as well as other
non-testicular cells.

The following observations led us to consider that ^{14}C-G uptake by MELC might be mediated by a transporter or receptor protein:
i) uptake is a high affinity and saturable process [10]. ii) G
specifically inhibits the anion transporter of human erythrocytes
[6]. iii) G is a substrate for the organic anion transporter of
rabbit kidney [S. Hong, personal communication]. However, the large
body of negative data in Fig. 4 are inconsistent with ^{14}C-G uptake
by MELC via such a transporter or receptor.

Based upon the data shown in Fig. 5, we suggest that ^{14}C-G is
membrane associated. If it is assumed that G were localized to the
plasma membrane, this would translate to ∿1000-fold concentration
of G relative to the initial extracellular G concentration [10].
However, we do not know that G associates with plasma membranes
exclusively. In fact, we have obtained indirect evidence that G
interacts with MELC mitochondrial membranes, i.e., at 1-10 μM G,
O_2 consumption by MELC is stimulated at lower doses and inhibited
at higher doses (unpublished data).

The relative insensitivity of G uptake to various membrane active treatments (Fig. 4) and the presumed membranous localization

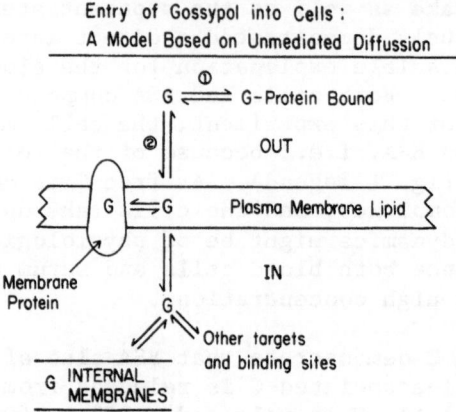

Fig. 6.   Model for G uptake by an unmediated diffusion mechanism.

of G (Fig. 5) form the basis for the following model (Fig. 6). The
role of extracellular protein, e.g., BSA is included in the model
(Fig. 6). We suggest that G enters cells by a partitioning mechanism, i.e., unmediated diffusion. G is hydrophobic and thus may be
very soluble in membranes. It also binds to BSA with high affinity.
We speculate that BSA-bound G is not a substrate for unmediated diffusion into the plasma membrane, rather only free drug is such a
substrate. The level of free drug is determined by the relative
concentrations of extracellular G and extracellular G-binding proteins, i.e., equilibrium 1 (Fig. 6). Free G enters the lipid phase
of the plasma membrane by an unmediated diffusion process, i.e.,
equilibrium 2 (Fig. 6). Once dissolved in the lipid bilayer of the
plasma membrane, G might interact with membrane proteins, internal
membranes, or other intracellular targets (Fig. 6). The capacity
of a cell to accumulate and retain G might therefore be determined
by the membrane composition of a cell. In a particular target cell,
e.g., the testis, there may be a specific binding component with an
affinity for G greater than that of serum proteins or non-target,
hydrophobic, components of the plasma membrane. This would facilitate concentration and retention of G in the target tissue with
subsequent pharmacological action. The data presented here and previously [10] might form the basis of a strategy to search for such
a testicular target. This would involve discrimination of a testicular target that binds G with a higher affinity than serum albumin.

ACKNOWLEDGMENTS

     The authors thank Drs. P. A. Marks and Rifkind of this Insti-
tute for providing MELC, and Kai Yuan Wu for performing the O_2 uptake measurements. The authors wish to thank S. Whaley and P.

Bradshaw for aid in preparation of this manuscript. This work was supported by grants from The Rockefeller Foundation.

REFERENCES

1. National Coordinating Group on Male Antifertility Agents (China): Gossypol - A new antifertility agent for males, Chinese Med. J. (English), 4:217-428 (1978).
2. H. Jackson, Gossypol, in: "Progress Towards a Male Contraceptive," II, Vol. 8 (S. L. Jeffcoate and M. Sandler, eds.), pp. 145-157, John Wiley and Sons, Limited, New York (1982).
3. N. K. Kalla, Gossypol - the male antifertility agent. IRCS-Med. Sci., 10:766-769 (1982).
4. M. B. Abou-Donia, Physiological effects and metabolism of gossypol, Residue Rev., 61:125-160 (1976).
5. L. C. Berardi and L. A. Goldblatt, Gossypol, in: "Toxic Constituents of Plant Food Stuffs" (I. E. Liener, ed.), pp. 211-266, Academic Press, New York (1969).
6. H. C. Haspel, R. E. Corin, and M. Sonenberg, Gossypol, an oral male contraceptive: Effects on human erythrocyte membrane function, Fed. Proc., 41:672 (Abstract No. 2340) (1982).
7. R. E. Royer and D. L. Vander Jagt, Gossypol binds to a high-affinity site on human serum albumin, FEBS Lett., 157:28-30 (1983).
8. P. A. Marks and R. A. Rifkind, Erythroleukemic differentiation, Ann. Rev. Biochem., 47:419-448 (1978).
9. R. E. Corin, H. C. Haspel, and M. Sonenberg, Transport of the folate compoundmethotrexate decreases during differentiation of murine erythroleukemia cells, J. Biol. Chem., 259:206-211 (1984).
10. H. Haspel, Y.-F Ren, K. A. Watanabe, M. Sonenberg, and R. E. Corin, Cytocidal effect of gossypol on cultured murine erythroleukemia cells is prevented by serum protein, J. Pharm. Exp. Therap., 229:218-225 (1984).
11. T. D. Tanksley, in: "The effects of gossypol on some enzyme systems," Ph.D Dissertatation, Texas A and M University, College Station (1968).
12. S. K. Hong, H. C. Haspel, M. Sonenberg, and M. Goldinger, Effects of gossypol on PAH transport in the rabbit kidney slice, Toxicol. Appl. Pharmacol., 71:430-435 (1983).
13. H. A. Sober, Peptides and Proteins, in: "Handbook of Biochemistry, Selected Data for Molecular Biology," 2nd Edition (H. A. Sober, ed.), pp. C36-C39, Chemical Rubber Company, Cleveland (1970).